THE POLITICS OF HEALTH LEGISLATION: AN ECONOMIC PERSPECTIVE

THIRD EDITION

THE POLITICS OF HEALTH LEGISLATION:
AN ECONOMIC PERSPECTIVE

THIRD EDITION

Paul J. Feldstein

Health Administration Press, Chicago

Your board, staff, or clients may also benefit from this book's insight. For more information on quantity discounts, contact the Health Administration Press Marketing Manager at (312) 424-9470.

Library of Congress Cataloging-in-Publication Data

Feldstein, Paul J.
   The politicsof health legislation : an economic perspevtive / Paul J. Feldstein.—3rd ed.
      p. cm.
   Includes bibliographical references and index.
   ISBN-13: 978-1-56793-253-9
   ISBN10: 1-56793-253-3
   1. Medical economics—United States.   2. Medical policy—United States.   I. Title.
   RA410.53.F46 2006
   338.4'336210973—dc22

                                                        2005055090

To two special people,
Rita and Joseph Shore

CONTENTS

ABBREVIATION LIST

AARP	American Association of Retired Persons
ADA	American Dental Association
AARP	American Discrimination Act
AFDC	Aid to Families with Dependent Children
AFL-CIO	American Federation of Labor and Congress of Industrial Organizations
AHA	American Hospital Association
AIDS	acquired immunodeficiency syndrome
AMA	American Medical Association
ANA	American Nurse Association
BBA	Balanced Budget Act
CAB	Civil Aeronautics Board
CAFE	corporate average fuel economy
CBO	Congressional Budget Office
CDC	Centers for Disease Control and Prevention
CFC	chlorofluorocarbon
COLA	cost-of-living adjustment
CON	certificate of need
DOT	Department of Transportation
DRG	diagnosis-related group
EPA	Environmental Protection Agency
ERISA	Employee Retirement Income Security Act
FAA	Federal Aviation Authority
FASB	Financial Accounting Standards Board
FCC	Federal Communications Commission
FDA	U.S. Food and Drug Administration
FTC	Federal Trade Commission
GDP	gross domestic product
HIAA	Health Insurance Association of America
HIPAA	Health Insurance Portability and Accountability Act
HMO	health maintenance organization

HSA	Health Savings Account
ICC	Interstate Commerce Commission
LPN	licensed practical nurse
MCCA	Medicare Catastrophic Coverage Act
MMA	Medicare Prescription Drug, Improvement and Modernization Act [of 2003]
MSA	medical savings account
NFIB	National Federation of Independent Business
NIH	National Institutes of Health
NRA	National Rifle Association
NYSE	New York Stock Exchange
PA	physician assistants
PPO	preferred provider organization
PSRO	Professional Standards Review Organizations
RBRV	Resource-Based Relative Value Scale
RN	registered nurse
S&Ls	savings and loan institutions
SCHIP	State Children's Health Insurance Program
SGR	sustainable growth rate
UAW	United Automobile Workers
USDA	U.S. Department of Agriculture

GLOSSARY

all-payer system: A plan in which all payers—insurers, government, companies, and individuals—pay the same fees for the same medical services.

any willing provider law: Requires all health insurers to be ready and willing to enter into service contracts with any healthcare provider who meets state requirements, practices in the general geographic area, and is willing to meet the insurer's terms and conditions.

antitrust laws: Laws that protect competition by preventing business practices that would result in higher prices or lower-quality services for consumers. The key federal antitrust laws are the Sherman Antitrust Act, the Clayton Act, and the Federal Trade Commission Act.

barriers to entry: Obstacles that would prevent a new participant from entering an industry. Legal barriers include licensing laws, and economic barriers include economies of scale.

budget neutral: When payments to providers under a new system equal the amount spent under the previous system.

cartel: A group of independent entities that organize to limit competition or fix prices.

certificate-of-need (CON) legislation: Requires an entity that wants to construct or modify a health facility, buy major new medical equipment, or offer a new health service to prior approval from a government body. The legislation was meant to eliminate costly, duplicative, or unnecessary healthcare expenditures but also serves as a barrier to entry.

copayment: The predetermined, fixed amount that the individual is required to pay for covered services.

concentrated interest: An issue that has such a large effect on a group that it becomes worthwhile for the group to invest the time, money, and other resources to organize to represent those interests.

diagnosis-related group (DRG): A hospital classification system in which patients are grouped on the basis of diagnoses for purposes of payment to hospitals. Demographic, diagnostic, and treatment characteristics are linked to length of hospital stay and resources consumed

diffuse interest: When the burden of an issue or program is spread over such a large group that the per-person effect is so small that the cost of opposing the issue outweighs the actual cost of the burden.

disproportionate-share hospital: A hospital that serves a large number of uninsured and Medicaid patients.

economic theory of regulation: This theory assumes that political markets are the same as economic markets in that individuals, groups, and firms seek to further their self-interest, and they calculate the benefits and costs to themselves of political action.

fee-for-service payment: A system in which a patient is charged a fee established by the healthcare provider for each service performed.

fee splitting: When a physician refers a patient to a surgeon and receives part of the surgeon's fee in exchange.

free rider: Someone who reaps the benefits of an action without having to pay; when individuals with a common interest organize to achieve favorable economic legislation, all people with that common interest will gain, whether or not they have contributed to the group's efforts.

friend of the court brief: Testimony offered by someone who is not a party in a legal case in order to help the court decide a matter; also called *amicus curiae.*

guaranteed availability: Ensures that an employee is immediately eligible for any insurance benefits offered by an employer without having to meet a waiting period for preexisting conditions.

guaranteed issue: Requires health insurers to provide coverage to those who want to purchase it.

grandfather clause: A provision that exempts a person already engaged in an activity from new regulations that might affect that activity

health maintenance organization (HMO): A managed care plan that offers prepaid comprehensive healthcare coverage for hospital and physician services. The HMOs contract with or directly employ the healthcare providers, using a fixed structure or capitated rates. Participants typically have limited copayments but pay the full costs of services from providers outside the network.

health savings account (HSA): A health insurance program comprising a high-deductible insurance policy and an account into which the employer annually contributes a fixed, tax-free amount of money (tax exempt). Employees can use the money in their healthcare account to pay for medical services. Also called a *medical savings account*.

Medicaid: A health insurance program that provides care for low-income persons who meet a means test. The program is funded by state and federal governments but administered by the states.

Medicare: A federal program that provides medical benefits to the aged. Part A covers hospital services, Part B covers physician and out-patient services, and Part C is a prescription drug benefit.

Medicare Trust Fund: The entity that collects payroll taxes to pay for Medicare Part A.

Medigap: A privately purchased insurance policy that the elderly use to supplement their Medicare coverage. Deductibles and copayments are typically covered.

monopoly: Occurs when there is a single supplier of a product and no close substitutes.

orphan drug: Drugs that drug companies are typically reluctant to develop because they treat rare diseases and only benefit small population groups, thereby making them unprofitable.

out-of-pocket costs: What an individual must pay for medical services after the healthcare plan has paid for the services it covers.

preferred provider organization (PPO): A health plan in which a network of providers offers services to enrolled members at a lower cost than the services of out-of-network providers.

public interest theory of government: Assumes that legislation is enacted to serve the public interest. According to this theory, government's objectives are to improve market efficiency and redistribute income.

redistributive legislation: There are two types of redistributive legislation. The first is based on a charitable motivation, that is, the public's desire to help the less fortunate. The second is universal redistribution, where the motivation of the voting public is primarily to help themselves at the expense of other taxpayers. What differentiates these two types of redistributive programs is whether a means test is involved. Universal programs, such as Medicare, do not have a means test; therefore, everyone is eligible. The proponents of these types of redistributive programs often justify them by saying that unless groups other than the poor are included as beneficiaries there would not be sufficient political support to enact the program. The methods used to finance universal programs, however, are less equitable than the methods used for charitable programs. Usually an excise tax, such as an increase in payroll taxes, is used. These taxes are regressive in that all people must pay the same amount, regardless of income (typically everyone would pay either the same amount or a certain percentage of income up to a maximum level of income).

regressive tax: A system in which everyone pays the same amount, regardless of their income; thus, lower-income people pay a higher proportion of their income for the tax than do higher-income people.

Resource-Based Relative Value Scale (RBRVS): This is the current fee-for-service payment system used under Medicare. Each physician service is assigned a relative value based on the resource cost of performing that service. The relative value is multiplied by a conversion factor to come up with the physician's fee.

single-payer system: A form of national health insurance in which one third-party payer, usually the government, pays the healthcare providers and the entire population has free choice of provider and little out-of-pocket expense.

stagflation: Inflation combined with stagnant consumer demand and relatively high unemployment

stop-loss benefit: This type of coverage limits a beneficiary's out-of-pocket medical expenditure.

vote trading: When legislators offer to exchange their vote on an issue of lesser importance to themselves (their constituents) in order to receive votes from legislators on issues of greater importance (to their constituents)

workfare: A welfare program that requires recipients to perform work in exchange for benefits.

PREFACE

My interest in health politics was first stimulated by economists who extended economic analysis into nontraditional areas, such as regulation and legislation. My 1979 book, *Health Associations and the Demand for Legislation*, focused on one aspect of the economic approach toward viewing health legislation, namely producer regulation. This book continues that analysis.

Producer regulation is only one activity of government. Here I also consider legislation directed toward controlling externalities, such as pollution and medical research, and toward making explicit redistributions among population groups, as occurred with Social Security, Medicare, and the Medicare Modernization Act.

To be useful, an analytical framework for viewing legislative outcomes should be generalizable over a wide range of government activity. That is what I have attempted to do. My purpose, which may seem quite ambitious, has been to use the taxonomy of economics to explain legislative outcomes in the health field. An analytical framework should be explicit in its assumptions as to what motivates the various decision makers. Self-interest, among individuals, groups, and legislators, is assumed to be the underlying motive generating legislative change, thereby giving rise to the hypothesis referred to as the self-interest paradigm, also referred to as the economic theory of legislation.

Economics is exciting because it is a way of thinking. One can use economic analysis to explain various types of events, whether they be historical, current, or political. To the extent that the self-interest paradigm illustrates an economic approach for explaining legislative outcomes and provides insight into previous health legislation, this book will have served its purpose. It is hoped that those interested in health policy find the discussions and analyses useful. To make this book suitable for a diverse audience, no prior knowledge of economics is assumed.

An author is always indebted to others for assistance, critiques, and comments. For previous editions, I particularly want to thank Jack Tobias, the Reference Librarian at the School of Public Health, University of Michigan, for his aid in locating various source materials. Jeremiah German, Stephen Crane, and Kathe Fox made detailed comments on the manuscript for which I am grateful. I was also fortunate to receive extensive and useful comments from anonymous reviewers. Needless to say, not all of those who provided me with comments necessarily agreed with all the analyses presented here. I wish to thank Elzbieta Kozlowski for her excellent research assistance in preparing this new edition.

This third edition updates all of the chapters in terms of material and references. In addition, Chapter 10 (Redistributive Health Legislation Mid-1980s to 2000) examines previous legislation and proposals in terms of competing theories of legislation, including the Health Insurance Portability and Accountability Act, the defeat of President Clinton's healthcare reform proposal, the 1997 Balanced Budget Act, the State Children's Health Insurance Program, and the National Bipartisan Commision on the Future of Medicare. Chapter 11 analyzes President Bush's Medicare prescription drug program and the Medicare Modernization Act enacted in December 2003. These laws and additional legislative proposals provide new material to test the validity of alternative legislative theories. Also new to this edition are chapter objectives and a glossary of key terms. Responses to the end-of-chapter study questions may now be found in the online Instructor's Manual that accompanies this book; for access, email hap1@ache.org.

Paul J. Feldstein
Irvine, California

INTRODUCTION

After completing this chapter, the reader should be able to

- outline the motivation behind the "public interest" and "economic" theories of legislation;
- discuss the accuracy of a theory in relation to its usefulness in understanding legislative outcomes;
- list three different types of legislation, discuss how they differ from one another, and provide an example for each; and
- describe the "public interest" explanation for each of the three types of legislation.

In 1966, the first year of Medicare and Medicaid, total personal expenditures on medical care in the United States were approximately $45 billion. By 2003, almost 40 years later, personal medical expenditures had risen to more than $1.7 trillion.[1] The rise in medical expenditures has exceeded the rate of inflation over that same period and has risen faster than any other sector of the economy. In 1966, 5.7 percent of the gross domestic product (GDP) went to medical care; currently, more than 15.3 percent of GDP is being spent on medical care.

The rapid increase in medical expenditures was caused by several factors: (1) inflation occurred in all sectors of the economy, particularly during the 1970s; (2) the population grew approximately 1 percent per year; (3) the number of aged grew (this group uses about four times as many medical services than the nonaged); and (4) great strides in medicine and improved treatment techniques enabled people to live longer, in less pain, and with fewer debilitating illnesses. As medical facilities expanded, and more technically trained personnel were needed to provide for the greater demands for care, the costs of providing medical services rose similarly.

Economic, demographic, and technological forces have been important in shaping the growth and structure of our health system. Government policies, however, have had an equal, if not greater, effect on the growth in expenditures and the structure of our health system.

self-interest paradigm

The role of government in financing and delivering medical services has sharply increased since 1966. Currently, government expenditures make up about 48 percent of total personal medical expenditures. The role of government, however, is not just limited to financing medical services. State and federal regulations affect all facets of the delivery and financing of medical services. States regulate premiums charged by health insurers, as well as their benefits, the tasks health professionals are permitted to perform, the entry of health providers into various markets, the prices hospitals and physicians charge to Medicare and Medicaid patients, and so on. The role of government in healthcare has become pervasive.

To understand the healthcare system in the United States, how it has changed, and its likely direction, it is necessary to understand how federal and state legislation and regulation have affected the population's use of medical services, the cost of providing those services, the efficiency by which medical services are used and provided, and the large number of uninsured in this country.

The roles of the federal and state governments in health legislation have changed dramatically. Initially, until the mid-1960s, states were more involved in healthcare than was the federal government. States were responsible for public health through, for example, the control of communicable diseases and environmental sanitation. State licensing boards determined the criteria for entry into the different professions, and the practice acts determined which tasks could be performed by which professional groups. Regulation of the health professions continues to be a state function. States also provided for the medically indigent and the mentally ill, generally through institutionalization programs.

Except for the care of disabled and ill seamen and Native Americans on reservations, the role of the federal government in healthcare was relatively small until the early 1900s, when, as a result of great media publicity, Congress enacted the Pure Food and Drug Act. Public sympathy for returning wounded and disabled veterans of World War I led to the federal Veterans Administration hospital system. Throughout the 1920s and 1930s, further federal legislation was limited until a tragedy occurred in the manufacture and sale of drugs, at which time further drug legislation was passed. During World War II, wage and price controls were in effect. However, to forestall a strike for higher wages by ship workers on the West Coast, the federal government ruled that if an employer purchased health insurance for its employees, the employer's contribution would not be counted as part of the employees' income. In this way, employer-paid health insurance became a nontaxable fringe benefit. (Starting in the late 1960s, this "subsidy" for the purchase of health insurance would become an important stimulus for the purchase of private health insurance.)

It was not until after World War II that the federal role in health legislation became more prominent. President Truman's proposal for national health insurance in 1948, which was vigorously opposed by the American Medical Association (AMA), was defeated. However, Truman's proposal for federal construction subsidies for hospitals (widely known as the Hill-Burton Act) was enacted in the late 1940s. During the 1950s and early 1960s there was a great deal of bipartisan support for medical research, which generously funded medical schools. Health manpower legislation, enacted in 1964, provided subsidies for educational institutions and their students. By the 1980s and 1990s, this legislation led to large increases in the supply of physicians and other medical personnel.

It was not until 1965 that the very controversial Medicare program (healthcare for the aged) was enacted. Until Medicare was passed, federal legislation had mainly subsidized the supply of medical services, hospitals, and health manpower. Medicare provided subsidies to pay for medical services for the aged. At the same time, Medicaid (state and federal assistance for the medically indigent) was enacted, without the political controversy that characterized Medicare. The method used to pay hospitals under both of these programs was "cost based." Hospitals had limited, if any, incentives to be concerned with efficiency. Similarly, given their reduced out-of-pocket payments under Medicare and Medicaid, the aged and poor had limited financial incentives to be concerned with their use of medical services. With federal financing of Medicare and federal matching funds to the states for Medicaid, federal expenditures and the federal role in healthcare increased dramatically. Federal expenditures under Medicare and Medicaid rose from $2.5 billion in 1966 to $474 billion in 2004. Initial expectations of the cost of these programs were greatly exceeded.

The role of the federal government continued to expand throughout the 1970s and 1980s. As federal expenditures under these programs began to exceed budgetary projections, the 1970s and 1980s were characterized by regulatory measures that attempted to control the rapidly increasing costs of these programs. Examples of such legislation include (1) the continuation of wage and price controls on the medical sector, until April 1974 (the Economic Stabilization Program was put in place in 1971 to control economy-wide prices and wages and removed in 1972); (2) Medicare utilization review; (3) health planning controls on hospitals' capital investment; (4) a Medicare fee index for physicians; (5) changes in Medicare cost reimbursement for hospitals; and, (6) a new health program that did not require a great deal of money, the Health Maintenance Organization (HMO) Act of 1973.

In the mid-1980s a new Medicare hospital payment system was initiated in which hospitals were paid according to fixed prices per admission

Handwritten margin notes: Hill-Burton Act — strings attached — ① Rolating Mechanism — Facilities that received funding were also required to provide a "reasonable volume" of free care each year for those residents in the facility's area who needed care but could not afford to pay. ③ 20 years of uncompensated care.

(diagnosis-related groups, or DRGs) rather than cost-based reimbursement. Finally, in 1989 a new Medicare physician payment system, which relied on a national fee schedule and limited total Medicare physician payments, was enacted. By controlling what the federal government spent on hospitals and physicians for Medicare patients, the federal government attempted to limit the annual increase in Medicare expenditures.

State Medicaid expenditures also expanded rapidly during the 1970s and 1980s. Unable to use deficit financing and reluctant to raise taxes or reduce state expenditures on politically popular programs, states reduced Medicaid eligibility and limited payments to hospitals and physicians for serving Medicaid patients. As a result, provider participation in Medicaid programs declined. Several states, such as Maryland, New Jersey, and New York, instituted hospital rate-review programs for all purchasers in an attempt to control rising hospital expenditures. At the same time states were reducing their commitment to the Medicaid population, they increased the subsidies provided to medical schools.

While attempts were being made to reduce the rise in federal expenditures, the tax-exempt status of employer-paid health insurance premiums resulted in large annual losses in federal, state, and Social Security tax revenues. (These lost tax revenues were estimated to be in excess of $188 billion in 2004.)[2] The ability of not-for-profit hospitals to finance their capital expenditures through tax-exempt bonds resulted in further lost federal and state taxes.

The 1990s saw continued federal and state reliance on regulatory health policies. The Health Insurance Portability and Accountability Act (HIPAA), enacted in 1996, made it easier for those with health insurance to change jobs and retain their insurance coverage. This Act also resulted in stringent regulations on patient privacy. In response to a backlash against managed care and anecdotal evidence of "drive-through" deliveries, Congress mandated 2-day minimum lengths of stay for normal births. Although there were many debates in Congress on further regulating managed care organizations, including discussions of "patient rights" legislation that would permit HMO patients to self-refer themselves to specialists, allow less restricted access to emergency departments, and establish the right to sue HMOs, such legislation was not enacted..

Regulation at the state level continues to be pervasive. Many states enacted "patient rights" laws guaranteeing a patient's access to specialists, establishing appeal procedures, requiring HMOs to offer a "point of service" option (i.e., allowing patients to visit non-HMO physicians for an extra charge), allowing women in HMOs to go directly to obstetricians and gynecologists without a referral from their primary care physician, requiring the HMO to cover emergency care whenever "a prudent lay person" would consider it necessary, and prohibiting HMOs from using financial incentives to compensate physicians for ordering less care than is medically necessary. Lobbied by medical and dental societies, a number of states enacted "any willing provider" (AWP) laws that permit any physician (or dentist) to participate in an insurer's or HMO's provider network and receive the same payment as negotiated by other physicians. AWP laws reduce price competition among providers; physicians are reluctant to negotiate discounted prices with an HMO if they cannot be assured of an increased volume of patients. Certificate-of-need (CON) legislation, which has been enacted in some states, is also anticompetitive; hospital investment and entry of new healthcare providers, such as home health agencies, are subject to state review. CON has been (and is) an entry barrier to providers who want to enter an existing provider's market.

Health insurers are regulated by the states, and a number of states require health insurers to use various rating (pricing) systems for the individual and small group markets, such as "community" rating (i.e., offering the same premiums for everyone regardless of risk group) and reduced waiting times for coverage of preexisting conditions. Other states require employers to offer their employees health insurance. And each state mandates what benefits (e.g., hair transplants are covered in Minnesota but not in some other states) and which providers (e.g., some states cover naturopaths and others do not) should be included in health insurance sold in their state.

By the late 1990s the federal government's concern over budget deficits had unexpectedly changed. Instead, the government was predicting very large federal budget surpluses into the future. This sudden change in the budget outlook relaxed the fiscal constraints limiting new federal health expenditures. However, despite these large projected budget surpluses, no new large federal program was enacted for the uninsured. Instead, as part of the Balanced Budget Act of 1997, Congress created the State Children's Health Insurance Program (SCHIP), to address the growing problem of children without health insurance. The goal of SCHIP was to expand health insurance to children whose families earn too much money to be eligible for Medicaid, but not enough money to purchase private insurance.

In an attempt to address the long-term solvency of the Medicare Trust Fund, in 1997 Congress also established a Bipartisan Commission on the Future of Medicare. It was believed a bipartisan commission would make it easier to make the difficult political choices to maintain Medicare benefits for the baby boomer generation, who would start retiring in 2011. However, the commission could not achieve a super majority, which was necessary for forwarding its recommendations to Congress.

The disappearance of projected budget surpluses, which many budget analysts had believed were only temporary, did not forestall providing the elderly with new Medicare benefits. During the 2000 election a new prescription drug benefit for the aged became a campaign issue. To eliminate this issue from the 2004 election, and despite large budget deficits, President Bush was successful in having the Medicare Prescription Drug, Improvement and Modernization Act (MMA), which provided a prescription drug benefit for the aged, enacted in December 2003.

To generate support for the MMA from different political constituencies, the Act included many other proposals, the most significant of which was the Health Savings Accounts (HSAs) for the nonelderly. HSAs enabled employers (on behalf of their employees) and individuals to make tax-exempt contributions for high-deductible health insurance plans. These plans would provide employees with an incentive to be cost conscious in their purchase and use of medical services, as the funds in their HSA could be kept and used when they retire.

Rather than being concerned that the Medicare Trust Fund was heading toward bankruptcy, both political parties competed to provide the aged, a politically important voting bloc (particularly in the closely contested state of Florida in the 2000 election) with a new prescription drug benefit. Medicare, which was based on a 1960s-style health insurance system, is characterized by inefficiency and places large cost-sharing burdens on low-income elderly. As the first baby boomers become eligible for Medicare in 2011, Medicare expenditures will increase even faster than previously. Politically, it has proved easier to provide the aged with additional benefits than to reform Medicare for the future.

The rapid rise in medical expenditures and its increasing share of this country's resources represent a massive redistribution of wealth. Two groups have particularly benefited. The first group is the aged, who, as beneficiaries of the federal Medicare program, have received medical services whose value greatly exceeds what they have contributed. The second group is those employed in the medical sector, healthcare suppliers, and health providers, such as hospitals and physicians, whose revenues have risen more than would otherwise have occurred. These two beneficiary groups have provided legislators with the necessary political support for receiving legislative benefits.

These benefits have been financed by the working population, who have had to pay higher health insurance premiums, higher prices for medical services, increased payroll taxes to fund the Medicare Trust Fund (which covers hospital care for the aged), and higher income taxes to pay for other Medicare services (physician, outpatient, and home healthcare) and the Medicaid program (which is funded by general income taxes).

The role of government in financing medical services, as well as through federal and state regulation, is extensive. To understand the reasons for these different types of government intervention and, at times, seemingly contradictory policies, it becomes necessary to have a view of what the government is attempting to achieve. The following is a brief discussion of two competing views of government behavior so as to better understand the type of health legislation and regulation this country has enacted and the likely types of future government policies.

The Public Interest View of Government

Alternative theories of legislative outcomes exist. At different ends of the spectrum are the "public interest" and the "economic" theories.[3] The underlying motivations of the participants and legislators differ in each of these theories, as do each theory's predictions and conclusions. The basic assumption underlying the public interest theory is that *legislation is enacted because well-meaning legislators act according to what they believe is in the public interest.* Although the legislation's (or regulation's) outcome may not always be as satisfactory as desired because of inadequate information or unexpected occurrences, the motivation of legislators is to enhance the public interest.

The traditional or public interest theory assumes that government has two basic objectives: to *improve efficiency* and to *redistribute income in a more equitable manner.*

Efficiency Objective of Government

The first traditional objective of government is to improve the efficiency with which society allocates resources. According to the public interest theory, the reasons for market inefficiency that justify government intervention are twofold: (1) monopolization of a market, such as a merger of all the hospitals in a community into one hospital system; and (2) the existence of externalities, such as air or water pollution that is a by-product of a firm's manufacturing process and that harms members of the community.

A firm has monopoly power when it is able to charge a price that exceeds its cost by more than a normal profit. Monopoly is inefficient because it produces too small a level of service (output). The additional benefit to purchasers (as indicated by its price) from consuming a service is greater than the cost of producing that benefit; therefore, more resources should flow into that industry until the additional benefit of consuming that service equals the additional cost of producing it.

The bases of monopoly power are several: there may be only one firm in a market, such as when there is a natural monopoly, for example, an electric company; competitors may merge to create a single firm with monopoly power; there may be barriers to entry in a market; firms may collude on raising their prices; or, because of a lack of information, consumers are unable to judge price, quality, and service differences among different suppliers. In each of these situations, the prices charged will exceed the costs of producing the product (which includes a normal profit).

The appropriate government remedy for decreasing monopoly power is to prevent anticompetitive mergers, eliminate barriers to entry into a market, prevent price collusion, and improve information among consumers. In other words, the goal is to achieve the conditions of a price-competitive market.

The second situation where the allocation of resources can be improved is when "externalities" exist. Externalities occur when someone undertakes an action and in so doing affects others who are not part of that transaction. The effects on others may be positive or negative. For example, a utility using high-sulfur coal to produce electricity also produces air pollution. As a result of the air pollution, residents in surrounding communities may have a higher incidence of respiratory illness. Resources are misallocated because the cost of producing electricity excludes the costs imposed on others. If the costs of producing electricity also included the costs imposed on others, the price of electricity would be higher and, consequently, demand for electricity would be less, as would the amount of pollution produced. The allocation of resources would be improved if the utility's cost included both types of costs.

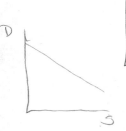

The appropriate role of government in the case of negative externalities is to determine the costs imposed on others and to tax the utility an equivalent (per unit) amount. (This subject is discussed more completely in Chapter 7.)

Redistributive Objective of Government

According to the public interest view of government, the second objective of government, redistribution, results in a transfer of wealth. Whenever a group's benefits from a government program are not equal to the costs of that program, redistribution occurs. If some population group receives benefits in excess of their costs (typically taxes to finance that program), then other population groups must receive benefits that are less than their costs of that program. For example, based on a value judgment of society, those with low incomes should not have to go without medical services. These services should therefore be financed by taxing those with higher incomes. Redistributive programs typically lower the cost of services to a particular group by enabling them to purchase those services at below-market prices. These benefits are then financed by imposing a "cost" on some other group. Those with lower incomes would be expected to receive net benefits (their benefits exceed their costs or taxes) and those with higher incomes should incur net costs (their taxes exceed their benefits) from the legislation.

Crucial to the evaluation of redistributive legislation is determining which population groups are eligible for the benefits and what types of taxes should be imposed to finance those benefits. When eligibility for medical benefits is based on a person's income, and income taxes are used to finance the program's benefits, redistribution will likely occur from high- to low-income groups. The key to evaluating all redistributive programs according to the public interest theory is that the benefits should go predominately to those with low incomes and the costs should be borne by those with higher incomes. The benefits and costs of a redistributive medical program, such as Medicaid, are shown in Table 1.1.

The government uses three *policy instruments* to achieve its efficiency and redistribution objectives: spending money on a program (expenditure policy), tax policy, and regulations.[4] Further, each of these policy instruments can be directed to the demand (purchaser) or supply (provider) side of the market. For example, the government has subsidized (expenditure policy) the purchase of medical services by the aged (demand side) and has also subsidized medical schools to increase the number of physicians (supply side). Tax policy has benefited employees by excluding employer-paid health insurance from taxable income (demand side) and enabled not-for-profit hospitals to pay lower interest costs by enabling them to issue tax-exempt bonds (supply side). State government regulations specify which medical services and practitioners must be included in health insurance sold in that state (demand side), and some states require government approval for building a hospital facility (supply side).

According to the public interest theory, each of the policy instruments, targeted to either the demand or supply side of the healthcare market, should be used to promote economic efficiency (which is defined by the promotion of competitive markets and internalization of externalities) or redistribution (as defined by those with low incomes receiving net benefits).

These policy objectives and instruments, which can be used to classify each type of government health policy, are shown in Table 1.2.

The Economic Theory of Regulation

Dissatisfaction with the public interest theory occurred for several reasons. According to the public interest theory, industries are regulated to prevent monopoly abuses. Thus, the theory would predict that the industries most

TABLE 1.1
Determining
Effects of
Government
Programs

	Low Income	High Income
Benefit	X	
Cost		X

likely to be regulated would be those subject to large economies of scale; a firm would have to be quite large to be efficient, thereby having few, if any, competitors. However, if that is true, why was there such extensive regulation of typically competitive industries (e.g., taxicabs, trucking, and television repairmen)? Further, why were entry barriers established on what were competitive industries? If regulation reduces prices and profitability, firms would not be expected to try and enter the regulated industries. These same issues apply to healthcare. Why do some states erect entry barriers for home health organizations or hospices?

With regard to the redistribution objective in healthcare, why was the hospital portion of Medicare (Part A) financed by a regressive payroll tax rather than an income tax? Why is it that the greatest beneficiaries of tax-exempt employer-paid health insurance are those with the highest incomes?

Dissatisfactions with the public interest theory led to the development of the economic theory of regulation.[5] The basic assumption underlying the economic theory is that political markets are no different from economic markets; individuals, groups, and firms seek to further their self-interest. All the participants are assumed to be rational, that is, they calculate the benefits and costs to themselves of political action. The political market has demanders of legislative benefits and suppliers of legislation, and the price in the political market is political support, which is indicated by campaign contributions, votes, and/or volunteers.

The suppliers of legislative benefits are legislators, and their primary goal is to be reelected. Thus, legislators need to maximize their chances for reelection, which requires political support. Legislators are assumed to be rational and to make cost-benefit calculations when faced with demands for legislation. However, the legislator's cost-benefit calculations are not the costs and benefits to society of enacting particular legislation. Instead, the benefits are the additional political support the legislator would receive from supporting the legislation, and the costs are the lost political support they would incur as a result of their action. When the benefits to the legislators (positive political support) exceed their costs (negative political support), they will support the legislation.

Government Policy Instruments		Government Objectives	
		Redistribution	Improve Efficiency
Expenditures	{ Demand side Supply side		
Taxation	{ Demand side Supply side		
Regulation	{ Demand side Supply side		

TABLE 1.2
Determining Effects of Government Programs

There are two types of demanders of legislation. Population groups seek wealth transfers, such as pension benefits greater than their contributions, subsidized medical benefits, medical education benefits for their children in excess of their tuition, and/or the ability to impose their social beliefs on others. The second group of demanders are firms and industries. Firms undertake investments in private markets to achieve a high rate of return. Why wouldn't the same firms invest in legislation if it also offered a high rate of return? Firms within an industry seek tariffs and entry barriers against potential competitors. Organized groups are willing to pay a price for legislative benefits, political support, which brings together the demanders and suppliers of legislative benefits.

The demanders of legislation calculate the benefits and costs of becoming involved in the legislative process. The costs consist of organizing others, representing their interests before legislators, and providing political support. Demanders involved in the political process are those who have a "concentrated" interest. When legislation has a large effect on an industry's profitability, by either affecting its revenues or its costs, it becomes worthwhile for the industry to organize, to represent its interests before legislators, and to raise political support to achieve the profits that favorable legislation can provide. For this reason, only those with a concentrated interest will demand legislative benefits. For example, assume that there are ten firms in an industry and, if they can have legislation enacted that would limit imports that compete with their products, they would be able to raise their prices and thereby receive $280 million in legislative benefits. These firms have a concentrated interest ($280 million) in trying to enact such legislation. The costs of these legislative benefits are financed by a small increase in the price of their product amounting to $1 per person.

Often, it is not obvious to consumers that legislation enacted to benefit those with a concentrated interest increases their costs. Further, even if consumers were aware of the legislation's effect, it would not be worthwhile (rational) for them to organize and represent their interests so as to forestall a price increase that would decrease their income by $1 a year. The costs of trying to prevent the cost increase would exceed their potential savings. When this occurs, then the costs are said to be "diffuse."

It is easier (less costly) for providers than for consumers to organize, provide political support, and impose a diffuse cost on others. This is why there has been so much producer-type legislation affecting entry into the health professions, which tasks are reserved to certain professions, how (and which) providers are paid under public medical programs, why subsidies for medical education are given to the school and not to the student (otherwise they would have to compete for students), and so on. Most health issues have been relatively technical, such as the training of health professions, certification of their quality, methods of payment, controls on hospital capital investment, and so on. The higher medical prices resulting from regulations that benefit providers have been diffuse and not visible to consumers.

The economic theory of legislation provides an explanation for the aforementioned dissatisfactions with the public interest theory. Firms in competitive markets seek regulation so as to earn higher profits than are available in competitive markets. Prices in regulated markets, such as interstate airline travel, have always been higher than those in unregulated markets, such as intrastate air travel, thereby enabling regulated firms to earn greater profits. These higher prices provided unregulated firms with an incentive to try to enter regulated markets. Government, on behalf of the regulated industry, imposed entry barriers to keep out low-priced competitors. Otherwise, the regulated firms could not earn more than a competitive rate of return. Through legislation firms try to receive the monopoly profits they are unable to achieve through market competition.

When only one group has a concentrated interest in the outcome of legislation and the costs are diffuse, legislators will respond to the political support the group is willing to pay to have favorable legislation enacted. When there are opposing groups, each with a concentrated interest in the outcome, legislators are likely to reach a compromise between the competing demanders of legislative benefits. Rather than balancing the gain in political support from one group against the loss from the other, legislators prefer to receive political support from both groups and impose diffuse costs on those with little political support.

When the beneficiaries are specific population groups, such as the aged, the redistributive effects of the legislation are meant to be very vis-

ible. An example of this is Medicare. By making it clear which population groups will benefit, legislators hope to receive the political support
of the aged and their children, whose potential financial liability is
decreased. The costs of financing such visible redistributive programs,
however, are still designed to be diffuse so as not to generate political
opposition from others. A small diffuse tax imposed on many people,
such as a sales and payroll tax, is the only way large sums of money can
be raised, with little opposition, to finance visible redistributive programs.
These taxes are regressive—the tax represents a greater portion of income
from low-income employees and consumers. Economists have determined
that payroll taxes, even when imposed on the employer, are borne mostly
by the employee. By imposing part of the tax on the employer, however,
it appears that employees are paying a smaller portion of it than they
really are; the tax is less visible. The remainder of the tax is shifted for-
ward to consumers in the form of higher prices for the goods and services they purchase.

Differences in the sources of political support are important for
understanding our two major, visible, redistributive programs. Medicaid is
a means-tested program for the poor funded from general tax revenues.
Because the poor (who have low voting-participation rates) are unable to
provide legislators with political support, support for Medicaid comes from
the middle class, who must agree to higher taxes to provide the poor with
medical benefits. The inadequacy of Medicaid in every state, the conditions necessary for achieving Medicaid eligibility, the low levels of eligibility, and the lack of access to medical providers are related to the generosity
(or lack thereof) of the middle class. The beneficiaries of Medicare, on the
other hand, are the aged themselves, who (together with their children)
provide the political support for the program. As the cost of Medicare has
risen, government has raised Medicare payroll taxes and reduced payments
to providers rather than reducing benefits or beneficiaries from this politically powerful group.

The design of visible redistributive legislation has been greatly influenced by the political support offered by healthcare providers. Physicians
and hospitals have a concentrated interest in the methods by which they
are reimbursed and by which competitors are excluded from participating
in such programs. Physicians have favored payment according to their
"usual, customary, and reasonable" fees, ability to opt out of the government payment system, and exclusion of any payments for competitors.
Hospitals have also received favorable payment systems. (It was only after
rapid increases in hospital and medical expenditures that the government
developed a concentrated interest in changing these self-serving and inefficient payment systems.)

The political necessity of keeping costs diffuse explains why Medicare and producer regulation are financed by regressive taxes, either payroll taxes or higher prices for medical services. Spreading the costs over large populations keeps those costs diffuse. The net effect is that low-income persons pay the costs and higher-income persons, such as physicians or the high-income aged, receive the benefits. Those receiving the benefits and those bearing the costs, according to the economic theory, are not based on income, as shown in Table 1.1, but instead according to which groups are able to offer political support (the beneficiaries) and which groups are unable to do so (they bear the costs). Regressive taxes are typically used to finance producer regulation as well as provide benefits to specific population groups.

Health policies change over time because groups that previously bore a diffuse cost develop a concentrated interest. Until the 1960s, medical societies were the main group with a concentrated interest in the financing and delivery of medical services. Thus, the delivery system was structured to benefit physicians. The physician-to-population ratio remained constant for 15 years (until the mid-1960s) at 141 physicians per 100,000 people, state restrictions were imposed on HMOs to limit their development, advertising was prohibited, and restrictions were placed on other health professionals to limit their ability to compete with physicians. Financing mechanisms also benefited physicians; until the 1980s, capitation payment for HMOs was prohibited under Medicare and Medicaid, and competitors to physicians were excluded from reimbursement under public and private insurance systems.

As the costs of medical care continued to increase rapidly to government and employers, their previously diffuse costs became concentrated. To prevent bankruptcy of the Medicare Trust Fund, the government was faced with the choice of raising Medicare's payroll tax, paying hospitals less for caring for Medicare patients, or reducing benefits to the aged, all of which would have cost the administration political support. Successive administrations developed a concentrated interest in lowering the rate of increase in medical expenditures. (Rather than reducing benefits for the aged, the Medicare tax was increased and Medicare hospital payments were reduced.) Similarly, large employers were concerned that rising medical costs were making them less competitive internationally. The pressures for cost containment increased as the "costs" of an inefficient delivery and payment system grew larger. Rising medical expenditures are no longer a diffuse cost to large purchasers of medical services.

Other professional organizations, such as those representing psychologists, chiropractors, and podiatrists, saw the potentially greater revenues their members could receive if they were better able to compete with physicians. These groups developed a concentrated interest in securing payment for their members under public and private insurance systems and expanding their scope of practice. The rise in opposing concentrated interests weakened the political influence of organized medicine.

Contrasts Between the Public Interest and Economic Theories

The public interest and economic theories of government provide opposing predictions of the redistributive and efficiency effects of government legislation, as shown in Table 1.3. Under the public interest theory, the policy instruments of government are meant to improve market efficiency and to achieve a more equitable distribution of medical services. According to the economic theory, the power of government is used to redistribute wealth to those able to offer political support, while financing that redistribution by imposing costs on those unable to offer political support. Those who are able to offer political support are typically middle- and high-income groups, not those with low incomes.

To test which theory is more accurate, it is necessary to match the actual outcomes of legislation to each theory's predictions. Do the benefits of redistributive programs go to those with low incomes and are they financed by taxes that impose a larger burden on those with higher incomes? Does the government try to improve the allocation of resources by reducing barriers to entry and, in markets where information is limited, encourage the dissemination of information on hospital and physician performance? If, instead, government policies result in greater market inefficiencies and middle- and high-income groups receive net benefits, while those with low incomes bear net costs, then the economic or self-interest paradigm is a more accurate description of the political process.

It might be said that the extraordinary growth in medical expenditures, the resultant inefficiencies, and the poor economic performance could not have been anticipated. If only the policy makers had known, payment systems would have been designed differently. If it were possible to do it over again, a more "rational" system could have been put into place.

These explanations are based on an assumption of ignorance on the part of well-meaning policy makers and legislators. The history of the health field since the late 1940s, however, should not be so easily dismissed or misinterpreted. Health legislation is a continuing process. Those who believe future policies are likely to be more "rational" because well-meaning legislators and policy makers are now better informed are likely to be disappointed once again.

Health legislation and regulation are generally not based on ignorance. Instead, the type of legislation that is enacted (as well as not enacted) is the result of a very rational process. The resulting legislation and regulations are, for the most part, what was intended. If the legislation was "poorly designed," that is, the costs are greater than the presumed benefits or even greater than necessary for achieving its stated purpose, then why not assume that was the real intent of the legislation? This view does not mean to imply that all participants in the policy process have perfect information on the consequences of their actions, but that the process is sufficiently rational to serve as the basis for understanding legislative outcomes.

The economic theory of regulation provides greater understanding of why health policies are enacted and why they have changed over time than alternative theories. The economic theory predicts that government is not concerned with efficiency issues. Redistribution is the main objective of government, but the objective is to redistribute wealth to those who are able to offer political support from those who are unable to do so. Thus, the reason medical licensing boards are inadequately staffed, have never required reexamination for relicensure, and have failed to monitor practicing physicians is that organized medicine has been opposed to any approaches for increasing quality that would adversely affect physicians' incomes. Regressive taxes are used to finance programs such as Medicare, not because legislators are unaware of their regressive nature, but because it is in the economic interest of those who have a concentrated interest.

The structure and financing of medical services is rational; the participants act according to their calculation of costs and benefits. Viewed in its entirety, however, health policy is uncoordinated and seemingly contradictory. Health policies are inequitable and inefficient; low-income persons end up subsidizing those with higher incomes. These results, however, are the consequences of a rational system. The outcomes were the result of policies intended by the legislators.

Criteria for Evaluating Alternative Theories

To be useful, a theory should be able to predict better than alternative theories. A theory does not have to be 100 percent correct to provide a useful framework for understanding health legislation. A theory that explains 70 percent of legislative outcomes in healthcare is preferable to one that can explain only 40 percent. Until a more accurate theory comes along, one that predicts better than random guesses is more useful than no theory at all. Such a theory still provides useful insights.

Theories of Government	Objective of Government	
	Redistribution	Improve Efficiency
Public Interest Theory	Assist those with low incomes	Remove (and prevent) monopoly abuses and protect environment (externalities)
Economic Theory of Regulation	Provide benefits to those able to deliver political support and finance from those having little political support	Efficiency objective unimportant More likely to protect industries so as to provide them with redistributive benefits

TABLE 1.3
Health Policy Objectives Under Different Theories of Government

Another criteria for defining a more useful theory is a theory's generalizability. Constructing a separate theory for each legislative outcome is not as useful as constructing one theory that applies to a wide range of legislation. Unique legislative theories are not theories of legislation. Requiring a separate theory for each piece of legislation is admitting that there are no generalizable principles. If there are generalizable principles, a theory should be applicable for different types of legislation. A theory and its assumptions should provide greater understanding of the legislative process.

Economists have often been criticized because of their simplified assumptions and their disregard for the richness of detail and the complex interactions of personalities, aspects that others believe are necessary for understanding legislation. Many policy analysts emphasize the idiosyncrasies of individual legislators in determining the outcome of legislation. The case-study approach often emphasizes the participants involved. The result is usually a chronological review of what occurred and why as the legislation moved through the various subcommittees and committees, and how it was amended as it made its way to final passage or defeat.

Although case studies can make a valuable contribution to understanding a particular piece of legislation, they do not enable us to generalize across different types of legislation. Case studies may suggest some hypotheses, which can later be tested, but, by their emphasis on detail, generalizable principles are often neglected or downgraded. Further, without some generalizable principles of legislative outcomes to guide the investigator, case studies may neglect appropriate data. When the detail surrounding each piece of legislation achieves overriding importance, then it becomes difficult to develop generalizable principles. Unless one knows what to look for, the underlying motivations of the participants and the organizations they represent might never be questioned.

To construct a generalizable theory, it becomes necessary to simplify the determinants of legislation. Information regarding legislators' personalities and institutional settings may at times have great importance. However, if generalizable principles are to be developed it becomes necessary to cut through much of the detail.

Once generalizable hypotheses have been developed, incorporating institutional detail into the theory may improve its explanatory power. However, the main test of a theory is its ability to predict; to be able to do so, generalizable principles are necessary. Detail may serve to further illuminate what happened. But without a theory, detail merely provides interesting background information.

In constructing a theory of legislative outcome, certain simplifying assumptions regarding human behavior are necessary. For example, legislators are assumed to act "as if" they were solely interested in maximizing their chances for reelection. Knowledgeable students of the legislative process could immediately provide examples of legislators who were more interested in the public interest than in their own prospects for reelection. There are (and undoubtedly have been) legislators who "would rather be right than president." And some legislators are ignorant of the issues. However, if we are interested in predicting the legislature's response to interest-group pressures, it is necessary to have some assumptions regarding legislators' objectives.

If one were to ask legislators what they desired, one could expect impassioned responses dealing with the public interest, this great country, and a place in history. A few legislators might eventually mention "fair trade" for the textile factory in their district or tax breaks for a large employer. Testing our assumption of legislator motivation according to what legislators say or making our assumption sufficiently complex to include multiple motivations is not useful. For predictive purposes, how would multiple, opposing motivations be resolved? Instead, the simple assumption that legislators act "as if" they seek to maximize their reelection chances enables us to predict legislators' responses to differing levels of political support.

The usefulness of these assumptions is not how realistic they are but how well the theory upon which it is based predicts. "The relevant question to ask about the 'assumptions' of a theory is not whether they are descriptively 'realistic,' for they never are, but whether they are sufficiently good approximations for the purpose at hand. And this question can be answered only by seeing whether it yields sufficiently accurate predictions."[6]

The public interest theory offers a set of assumptions regarding the motivations of legislative participants and a set of testable predictions. The self-interest paradigm offers contrasting assumptions and legislative predictions. The purpose of this book, however, is to describe how individuals and groups—acting according to their self-interests, with legislators seeking to maximize their political support—explain legislative outcomes in the health field. Although the process of legislation is complex and the participants are many, the criterion by which this approach should be judged is whether it predicts better than an alternative theory. The richness of detail from any individual legislative outcome could be used to supplement the generalizable principles proposed.

Types of Legislation to Be Examined

The purpose of this book is to demonstrate that legislative and regulatory outcomes in healthcare are consistent with the hypothesis that individuals, groups, and legislators act to serve their own self-interest. A basic assumption underlying this approach is that the legislation that was passed, and the design of that legislation, was as intended by the legislature.

An economic approach to politics is not new. Concerns about the use of government for selfish interest have existed as long as the idea of government itself. Moreover, they have been amply recorded: James Madison and Adam Smith wrote on the subject. More recent formalizations have been provided by such economists as Anthony Downs, James Buchanan and Gordon Tullock, Mancur Olson, Jr., George Stigler, Richard Posner, and Sam Peltzman.[5] No new theoretical contributions are provided in this book. Instead, the economic approach for viewing legislative outcomes is applied to healthcare and used to provide an understanding of the type of health legislation this country has or has not had.

The approach used in this book to explain legislative outcomes—the self-interest paradigm—assumes that individuals act according to self-interest, not necessarily the public interest. Individuals, as legislators or voters, are assumed to act no differently when it comes to politics than they act in private economic markets; they pursue their self-interest. Organized groups that are able to provide greater political support are expected to have greater political influence than groups or voters who are not organized. Organized groups seek to achieve through legislation what they cannot achieve through the marketplace. Such legislative benefits provide producers with greater incomes and organized, politically powerful, population groups with economic gains such as net subsidies or legislation mandating their social preferences.

A theory of legislation, as previously stated, should be applicable to all types of legislation, otherwise it is incomplete and its generalizability is limited. To reduce the large number and different varieties of legislation so that their outcomes can be meaningfully analyzed requires classification. Three legislative typologies have been selected.[7] The basis for these three typologies is the subject addressed by the legislation.

The analytical approach used in this book, namely, the self-interest paradigm, is applied to three types of legislation: *producer regulation*, legislation dealing with *externalities*, and *redistributive legislation*. The most common legislation is regulation that benefits producers.

Producer Regulation

Under the economic theory of regulation, legislation (or regulation) is proposed by trade associations so as to receive legislative benefits for their members. For example, the automobile industry (and the United Automobile Workers [UAW]) lobbied for domestic content legislation. Such legislation, had it been passed, would have raised the cost of imported cars, thereby increasing the demand for domestic cars. Previously, "voluntary" quotas on Japanese cars reduced their availability in this country, with the result that prices and production of U.S. cars increased.[8]

According to the public interest theory, the reasons most often given for producer legislation in medical care are concerns for quality, efficiency, and cost containment; that is, preventing medical prices from rising so rapidly. The validity of these reasons must be examined alongside the effects of policies that purport to achieve these goals.

Health associations' demands for producer regulation are discussed in Chapter 4. The oft-stated rationales for such legislation (quality, efficiency, and cost containment) are compared to the effects producer regulation would have in order to determine their actual versus their stated intent. Chapter 4 examines the different types of health legislation demanded by health associations representing providers, such as physicians, dentists, nurses, hospitals, and health insurance companies.

Since the late 1970s and early 1980s, numerous industries have been deregulated—airlines, railroads, trucking, savings and loan associations (S&Ls), stock brokerage firms, telephone service, and the medical industry. Presumably, the major losers from deregulation have been the regulated industries and their unions who had previously received producer-type regulation. Deregulation led to a revival of the public interest theory. How else could deregulation of protected industries be analyzed? Therefore an opposing theory of legislation—like the self-interest paradigm—should not only be able to explain the regulation of an industry but also why it is deregulated. Chapter 5 discusses the reasons for deregulation of nonhealth-related industries. The deregulation of the medical care industry is discussed in Chapter 6.

Externalities

The second type of legislation relates to market failure or, more specifically, to externalities.[9] Markets may not perform efficiently and government intervention may be justified in several situations. Even if a market is competitive, the firms in that market may, in the process of producing their product, impose costs on persons outside that market. Air and water pollution are two such examples. Congress has enacted legislation directed at water and air pollution.

A public interest theory of legislation would predict that to protect society, Congress would anticipate or respond to the public's demand for protection and achieve this objective in an efficient manner. Medical research provides benefits to all and the public interest theory would suggest that Congress provide an appropriate level of funding for medical research. During the 1950s and 1960s, medical research programs were generously funded by Congress.

It is a task of the self-interest approach, which includes the maximization of political support by legislators, to reconcile the existence of government programs whose ostensible goal is to intervene in situations where externalities exist. This issue is addressed in Chapter 7.

Redistributive Legislation

The purpose of the third type of legislation is redistribution. While all legislation is redistributive in that costs are imposed on some groups and net benefits are received by others, redistributive legislation is meant to be explicit in its effects. Redistributive programs are provided to consumer or population groups, as contrasted to producer legislation which provides benefits to a specific industry. Redistributive legislation confers net benefits on some population groups while financing these benefits by imposing net costs on other population groups. Those burdened with net costs pay taxes that exceed the program benefits they receive.

Redistributive legislation is also politically "visible." That is, the public, particularly the population groups benefiting from the program, must be made aware of the net benefits they are to receive. The political support for redistributive programs is expected to come from the votes of the affected population groups. Examples of redistributive programs are Social Security and, in the health field, Medicare, Medicaid, the Clinton administration's proposal for healthcare reform, and the MMA of 2003, which provided the elderly with prescription drug coverage. Chapter 8 develops the reasons for redistributive legislation, illustrated by numerous examples.

Chapter 9 applies these principles to the largest redistributive program in medical care—Medicare. Chapter 10 analyzes healthcare redistribution proposals and legislation in the 1980 to 2000 period, including the Clinton administration's failed health reform proposal. Chapter 11 analyzes the recently enacted MMA of 2003, and Chapter 12 examines why this country has not had national health insurance.

The stated reason for redistributive legislation is to redistribute income, either in cash or in kind (in the form of services), to those in financial need or to those unable to purchase a service society deems important. One criterion used to establish eligibility for these programs is income levels (e.g., Aid to Families with Dependent Children [AFDC] and Medicaid). Other redistributive programs are "universal," that is, everyone, regardless of financial need or income, is eligible for the program's benefits. For example, everyone is eligible to attend subsidized public colleges and all the aged are eligible for Medicare benefits.

The presumed basis for redistributive programs, at least under the public interest theory of legislation, is society's charitable desire to help its less fortunate members. And, unless everyone was compelled to contribute (through government taxes) to charity, some higher-income individuals could receive a "free ride"—that is, they benefit by knowing that the less fortunate are cared for through the private donations of others. Charity can therefore be considered a "collective" good. Government taxation to provide for charity would, according to this argument, eliminate the "free rider" problem. A self-interest theory of legislation has to explain why redistributive legislation is enacted when the theory's basic assumption is that individuals and groups are expected to act only according to their self-interest. Is the reason for redistributive legislation similar to the reason for producer legislation, namely, to provide politically powerful population groups with an economic benefit?

Thus, government has three traditional roles: to eliminate or control monopoly behavior, to intervene in situations of externalities, and to help those who are less fortunate. Extensive legislation exists on each of these types of legislation at the federal, state, and local levels of government. One could readily conceive of a role for government in each area according to the public interest theory. In the remainder of this book, however, each type of legislation, with applications to the field of medical care, will be examined from the perspective of the self-interest explanation of legislative outcome.

Study Questions

1. What motivations are assumed to underlie the "public interest" and the "economic" theories of legislation (self-interest paradigm)?
2. Must a theory be accurate 100 percent or even 80 percent of the time to be judged useful for understanding legislative outcomes?
3. How do the three types of legislation described in this chapter differ from one another?
4. What are the "public interest" explanations for each of these three types of legislation?
5. What are some healthcare examples of each of these three types of legislation?

Notes

1. U.S. Department of Health and Human Services, Centers for Medicare and Medicaid Services, 2005. [Online information] www.cms.hhs.gov/statistics/nhe.
2. John Sheils and Randall Haught, "The Cost of Tax-Exempt Health Benefits in 2004," *Health Affairs*. February 25, 2004. [Online article] http://content.healthaffairs.org/cgi/reprint/hlthaff.w4.106v1.
3. Throughout this book, the term "economic theory of legislation" is used interchangeably with the terms "economic theory of regulation," "self-interest paradigm," and "interest group theory of government."
4. Nicholas Barr, 1992. "Economic Theory and the Welfare State: A Survey and Interpretation," *Journal of Economic Literature* 30 (1990): 741–803. In his review article, Barr uses a different classification of government interventions: regulation, which can apply to quality, quantity, or price of a product or service; price subsidy, which can be direct or through the tax system; public production, such as when the government is the supplier of the service; and income transfers, which can be tied to specific products, such as food stamps, or general products, as with Social Security. Although public production or provision of medical services occurs in this country, for example, via Veterans Administration hospitals and U.S. Public Health Service facilities, this type of policy intervention occurred many years ago and is unlikely to be considered in the foreseeable future. The lack of use of this policy instrument is also consistent with the economic theory of legislation.
5. Anthony Downs, *An Economic Theory of Democracy* (New York: Harper & Row, 1957); James Buchanan and Gordon Tullock, *The Calculus of Consent* (Ann Arbor: University of Michigan Press,

1962); Mancur Olson, Jr., *The Logic of Collective Action: Public Goods and the Theory of Groups* (New York: Schocken Books, 1971); George J. Stigler, "The Economic Theory of Regulation," *The Bell Journal of Economics* 2, no. 1 (1971): 3–21; Richard A. Posner, "Theories of Economic Regulation," *The Bell Journal of Economics and Management Science* 5, no. 2 (1974): 335–58; Sam Peltzman, *Political Participation and Government Regulation* (Chicago: The University of Chicago Press, 1998); Dennis Mueller, *Public Choice III* (Cambridge, UK: Cambridge University Press, 2003).

For an excellent brief description of the economic theory, also known as "public choice," see Pierre Lemieux, "The Public Choice Revolution," *Regulation* Fall (2004): 22–29.

6. Milton Friedman, *Essays in Positive Economics* (Chicago: The University of Chicago Press, 1953), 15. Friedman provides the following illustrative example: "Consider the problem of predicting the shots made by an expert billiard player. It seems not at all unreasonable that excellent predictions would be yielded by the hypothesis that the billiard player made his shots 'as if' he knew the complicated mathematical formulas that would give the optimum directions of travel, could estimate accurately by eye the angles, etc., describing the location of the balls, could make lightning calculations from the formulas, and could then make the balls travel in the direction indicated by the formulas. Our confidence in this hypothesis is not based on the belief that billiard players, even expert ones, can or do go through the process described; it derives rather from the belief that, unless in some way or other they were capable of reaching essentially the same result, they would not in fact be 'expert' billiard players." (Friedman, 1953, 21)

7. For examples of legislative typologies used by political scientists, see Theodore Lowi, "American Business, Public Policy, Case Studies and Political Theory," *World Politics* 16, no. 4 (1964): 677–715; and Michael Hayes, "The Semi-Sovereign Pressure Groups: A Critique of Current Theory and an Alternative Typology," *Journal of Politics* 40, no. 1 (1978): 134–61.

8. An example of attempted producer benefits in the health field were the efforts by the auto companies and the UAW to have the federal government (as part of the Clinton administration's proposed health plan) pay 80 percent of the medical costs of early retirees. The medical costs of early retirees are paid by the companies and represent an enormous liability for those companies. For example, in 1994, General Motors had an unfunded liability for retiree medical costs estimated at $20 billion; by 2004 this liability, for which General

Motors must set aside reserves each year, had increased to more than $60 billion. If these costs were shifted to the federal government, the company's liability would be reduced and their union employees could receive part of those savings in the form of higher wages. Holman Jenkins, Jr., "Faint, Desperate Hope for Health Care Leadership," *Wall Street Journal*, March 17, 2004: A17.

9. Externalities also occur when individuals contribute to charity, as will be discussed with respect to redistributive programs. Because redistributive legislation is considered separately, this type of externality is excluded from this section. National defense is another example of externalities. Everyone benefits if the country is able to defend itself. Even if citizens do not contribute to the national defense, they cannot be excluded from its benefits; they receive the same protection as those that do contribute. (An important political issue, however, is the appropriate size and composition of defense expenditures.) National defense is not discussed in this section, although the principles can be applied to this subject as well.

AN ECONOMIC VERSION OF THE INTEREST GROUP THEORY OF GOVERNMENT

After completing this chapter, the reader should be able to

- identify the purpose of legislation according to the "economic theory,"
- assess how "concentrated" and "diffuse" interests determine group representation before legislators,
- compare producer and consumer group's successes in the legislative marketplace,
- list legislator objectives and cost/benefit calculations according to the economic theory of legislation,
- explain "vote trading" and how it enables a small group of legislators to receive economic benefits for their constituents,
- compare when "visibility" of legislation is considered desirable and undesirable by its proponents,
- discuss why regulatory agencies more likely represent interests of those they regulate rather than public interest, and
- contrast the public interest view of the government with the economic theory of legislation regarding the effect government policy has on economic efficiency and equity.

The basic premise underlying the economic theory of government is that the motivation used to explain decision making in private markets is no different from the motivation used to explain decision making in public markets, namely, self-interest. Private interests, not public interests, drive legislation. Legislation is a redistributive mechanism. Firms attempt to maximize their profits; consumers and/or population groups seek to maximize their utility, which may involve imposing their social preferences on others or receiving monetary benefits in excess of their contributions; and suppliers of legislation attempt to maximize their political support. Within government, policy makers, bureaucrats, and regulators seek to maximize their own private interests, not any "public interest."

The second basic premise of the economic theory is that the *intended* effects of legislation can be deduced by examining the legislation's *actual* effects. Although lack of information and ignorance may affect legislative outcomes in the short term, over time any information asymmetries can be corrected. Thus, who benefits and who bears the cost of legislation is the most likely indication of what the legislation was intended to accomplish.

The economic theory is a framework for understanding how government does work, rather than how it should work. This chapter presents a more extended version of the economic theory of legislation. First, the demanders of legislative benefits, namely, firms and organized groups are discussed. (An important issue discussed in Chapter 3 is why some groups are more successful than others in being able to achieve their legislative demands.)

Second, the suppliers of legislative benefits, generally considered to be the legislature, the executive branch, regulatory agencies, and the judiciary, are examined. Each of these entities helps to establish the rules of the game under which business firms compete and population groups receive benefits. The main supplier of legislation is the legislature; their output is legislation. The executive branch proposes legislation, but it is up to the legislature to enact it. The legislature can also override executive vetoes. The legislature appropriates funds for regulatory agencies and passes new legislation if it disagrees with judicial rulings. It is important to understand the motivation of these suppliers of legislation and how they respond to the demanders of legislation.

As in any market, there is a price. The price of legislation is political support. Political support—votes, campaign contributions, or volunteer time—is the equilibrating mechanism between the demanders and suppliers of legislative benefits. The amount of political support determines the allocation of benefits among the various demanders.

The Demanders of Legislative Benefits

Imperfections in the Political Market

In a representative democracy, majority rule should determine legislative outcomes. One might expect that for legislation to be enacted it would have to be favored by a majority of the population or by a majority of elected legislators. However, in numerous instances small groups or firms benefit while costs are imposed on the majority. How can government policies that adversely affect the majority be enacted in a system where the majority rules?

Political markets, where benefits and costs to particular groups are distributed by government, differ significantly from economic markets in which consumers express their desires by spending their own money on the goods and services they prefer. They bear the costs of their choices. In political markets, the linkage between the voter and legislation is not obvious— and neither is the link between who receives the program's benefits and who bears its costs. As a result of these imperfections it is possible for organized minorities to gain benefits while imposing the costs on the majority.

The following discussion examines the imperfections that occur in political markets and why groups representing a minority of voters or legislators are able to secure favorable legislation.

First, not all eligible voters vote. There is a cost to voting; the voter must take the time to become informed on the issues and take the time to actually vote. Clearly, it does not pay for voters to invest time on issues that may have a small impact on their well-being. It also does not pay to invest time when their efforts will have little impact, if any, on the outcome.[1] The benefit of voting to the voter is the belief in the importance of the election's outcome and the likelihood that his vote will make a difference in that outcome. On a cost/benefit basis, therefore, many people do not believe it pays to vote.[2]

Second, because it is costly to become fully informed on issues and candidates, voters look for shortcuts to collecting such information. One method of gathering information is to pay more attention to the personalities of the candidates. Another is to rely on ideologies and political parties, which may be similar to brand names, to distinguish between candidates. Alternatively, the voter can rely on a party's political advertising, such as the use of slogans to summarize an issue. Too heavy a reliance on these shortcuts, however, produces voters who are not well-informed.

Given the limited time voters have to become informed on issues and candidates, a voter may concentrate on only those issues of overriding importance. This phenomenon helps explain the rise in political power of single-issue groups, such as "right to life" groups, the National Rifle Association (NRA), acquired immunodeficiency disease (AIDS) advocates, environmental organizations, and gay rights groups. These groups, which have a concentrated interest in a single issue, collect and disseminate relevant information to their members, focusing on their special concerns, thereby economizing on the cost of the voter being informed. By controlling the information flow and summarizing the implications for their members, single-issue groups have greater influence on the voting behavior of their group.

The role of political parties in this regard is of interest. Political parties can be viewed as competing firms, each selling a package of products, a set of government policies, for votes. Firms respond to consumer demands to make a profit. Parties respond so that legislators in their party can be reelected. Party identification is a means of providing, at low cost, information about a candidate to a voter. However, the two-party system in this country may not offer some voters a sufficient diversity of choices. Each political party strives to capture a majority of the voting population by designing their package of policies to appeal to voters in the middle of the issue spectrum. As each party reaches toward the middle, voters farther from the middle believe they have too little choice.

Political parties in the United States do not have as much control over their members as do parties in other countries. Presumably, if a legislator deviates from the party position on important issues, this would affect the party-information role to voters. The party would be expected to protect its "brand name" by making it costly for legislators to deviate. In the United States, however, the brand name of a party connotes different information according to region. More importantly, a legislator is generally not beholden to the party for her election. By raising campaign contributions from nonparty sources and by providing services to their constituents, legislators are able to establish independence from party policies.

Legislators may wish to establish their independence from their party so as not to lose any constituent votes on controversial party issues. Instead, the legislator will attempt to achieve the loyalty of his constituents on issues that are noncontroversial. One such approach is to engage in vote trading that will benefit the district's constituents, for example, pork barrel legislation. Another approach is to offer services to constituents.[3] As the size of government has expanded, together with a myriad of government agencies, constituents often need assistance in resolving problems they have with one or more agencies, for example, eligibility for Veterans Administration benefits. Thus, Congress votes for increases in its staff and resources not to be better able to handle complex national and foreign policies, but instead to be better able to provide services to their constituents. Legislators are able to earn the gratitude and votes of their constituents by this assistance. This activity loosens legislators' needs for strong party ties. As evidence of this, voters do not rely as much on party identification in electing their representatives as they once did.

Another imperfection in the political market is that some legislators face the voters only after a considerable period of time (up to six years in the case of senators); this makes it difficult for voters to register their immediate displeasure on a particular issue. Voters tend to respond to a senator's most recent (past 3 years) performance but not to earlier performance.[4] At election time, in addition to remembering the various issues over the past several years, the voter is faced with making a choice between different sets of issue packages when choosing between senators.

One final distinction between economic and political markets is that legislators do not take into account all the costs of their decisions. Individual legislators are rarely held accountable for the costs of a program or for costs that exceed expectations. Further, the time horizon for members of the House of Representatives is particularly short—it is the next election. These election periods mean that legislation place greater weight on the immediate benefits of a program and a much lower weight on the longer-run costs of that program. Similarly, with regard to the method of financing, legislators prefer borrowing to taxing, which pushes the cost into the future. (Future generations do not vote at the next election.)

These imperfections in the political market suggest that voters are likely to be uninformed on legislative issues, unorganized and so unable to make their voices heard, and unable to provide sufficient support in terms of votes or dollars to have an impact on specific legislation that concerns them. For a group to be effective in the legislative process it is necessary for them to overcome these obstacles.

Because the cost of political participation by individuals is high, compared to expected benefits, voting participation is likely to be low. Further, as most legislative issues are not controversial and not very visible to the public, individuals have a low demand for legislation. Instead, legislation is demanded by those who are organized, act in their own interest, and are willing to provide political support to receive legislative benefits.

Organized Interest Groups

In competitive markets, persistent or long-run excess profits cannot exist. Firms earn a normal rate of return, sufficient to allow them to stay in business. However, all firms would like to make higher profits. If the market in which a firm competes expands and the firm makes excess profits, additional firms will be attracted to that industry. As new firms enter and production expands, the excess profits once enjoyed by the firm decline until they are back to normal. The only way firms in a competitive industry can earn excess, or above normal, profits is to prevent other firms from entering their industry. As there is no legal way to do this, the current firms in that industry are likely to try and change the legal requirements governing that industry, such as raising competitors' costs or restricting their entry.[5]

Similarly, a particular population group organized for some common purpose might be the demanders of legislation. The motivation is the same. This population group might be categorized by age, sex, income, race, or a single issue. If such a group can receive particular legislative benefits, for example, a subsidy or a tax advantage, then that group will be better off than it would have been otherwise. A single-issue group may also benefit by imposing its preferences on the rest of the population, such as permitting prayer in the schools.

For a group to be successful in the legislative arena, it is necessary that the costs of organizing, representing its interests, and providing political support be less than the value of its expected legislative benefits. Groups that most often meet these criteria are organizations of producers. Producers are said to have a "concentrated" interest in regulation. Any legislation affecting their industry can have a major impact on each firm's profits (by affecting the firm's costs, prices, or entry of competitors). The unions in those industries also have a concentrated interest through the regulation's effect on the number of employees and their wages. Often the interests of the employees and the firms in an industry coincide, as in the case of legislation affecting substitutes, such as quotas or tariffs on imported goods.

Groups with a concentrated interest have an incentive to organize and represent their interests before the legislature. The revenue effects of protective legislation are potentially so large as to make it worthwhile to organize, raise funds to hire lobbyists, become informed on regulations affecting their interests, and actively promote their interests.[6] The members of such groups are also likely to be more informed as to the positions taken by their legislators (or those to whom they provide political support) at election time. For these reasons, Downs concluded, "Democratic governments tend to favor producers more than consumers in their actions."[7]

Trade associations, professional associations, labor unions, agricultural cooperatives, and corporations are groups that have organized for some other purpose; thus, these groups have a cost advantage when it comes to organizing for political benefits. These organizations have already incurred the organizational costs necessary for representing their political interests; they have an advantage compared to others who have not yet incurred such organizational costs. Lobbying and offering political support becomes a by-product of the organization's other functions.

The gains producer groups receive from legislation impose small costs on a broad population base. Thus, legislation favoring any producer group has a relatively small effect on an individual. And individuals are, for the most part, unaware of the effect. For example, legislation providing large benefits to firms (and employees) in an industry will lead to a small increase in costs to consumers; for example, restricting lower-cost imports leads to price increases of domestic equivalents. Consumers purchase many goods and services. If the price of one service is increased because of restrictive legislation, the effect on the consumer's income is relatively small—too small for consumers to organize themselves, to be informed on all such legislation, and to represent their interests before the legislature. The cost of being involved greatly exceeds the savings from preventing the legislation. Clearly, it does not pay for consumers to incur the costs to forestall such a small burden. Consumers are therefore said to have a "diffuse" interest in the enactment of restrictive legislation; the increased prices they have to pay have a small effect on their overall budget.

Industries with many firms are more likely to seek anticompetitive restrictions than are industries comprising few firms. When few firms are in an industry, it is easier (less costly) for these firms to collude on prices and marketing arrangements and to detect which firms are cheating on the agreement. Industries with a large number of firms, such as physicians, find it more difficult (costly) to reach an agreement among all producers. Similarly, it is difficult to detect cheaters; firms also try and "free ride" on the efforts of others.[8] For industries with a large number of producers, legislation is a less costly method of monopolizing the industry than attempting to do so without the use of government.[9]

Those who participate in the legislative process and in regulatory hearings do so based on a rational calculation of the costs and benefits to themselves. It does not pay for consumers to participate. Thus, the process is dominated by those who have a lot to gain (or to lose). Those with a concentrated interest find it both worthwhile and necessary to participate. Those with diffuse interests—consumers—are unlikely to participate.

This does not mean to imply that concentrated interests always get the legislation they desire. But it does suggest that concentrated interests always have an incentive to represent their interests and provide political support to legislators when the potential gains are significant compared to their costs. When there are opposing groups, each with a concentrated interest, then the cost to a group of achieving its objective is increased.

Legislation and regulation change when new groups with a concentrated interest arise. For example, if the regulatory costs imposed turn out to be particularly high to some groups, or if a change in technology changes the industry's cost for producing the service, other groups may develop that have a concentrated interest in that industry's regulations.[10] *When a group's costs change from being diffuse to concentrated, then it will be in the group's interest, in terms of benefits and costs, to represent those interests and provide political support.*

Health policies in the United States have changed, not because of legislators' efforts to improve efficiency or equity, but because those who previously had a diffuse interest (e.g., incurred a diffuse cost) developed a concentrated interest in the outcome and therefore provided political support for changes in policy. For example, only after health insurance premiums and Medicare expenditures rose rapidly did business and government develop a concentrated interest in holding down hospital and physician expenditures.

The Suppliers of Legislative Benefits

The Legislature

People, in general, are interested in the welfare of others. They are concerned about what is good for the country, and they are also concerned for themselves. For the most part, given the time they spend on their jobs, people are predominantly concerned with their own affairs; they are attempting to further their own careers or self-interests. The motivations of those employed in the public sector are the same as those employed in the private sector. Although they are concerned with what is good for the country, they also act in their own self-interest. While acting according to their own self-interest they may also be acting in the public interest. If they are, however, it is incidental. For example, businesses introducing a higher-quality product or firms introducing technology that reduces costs and thereby increases market share do so because they expect to profit from these actions, not because they will benefit the public. The same is true for legislators and bureaucrats. Their actions are undertaken to benefit themselves; only as a by-product may they also benefit the public.

Acting according to one's own self-interest is the basic assumption underlying an economic approach explaining legislative outcomes. One should expect this to be the case regardless of whether the individuals are in the public or private sectors. This does not mean that every individual always acts in this way, but it is a useful assumption for predicting outcomes in both economic and political markets.

As mentioned previously, it is assumed that legislators are primarily interested in maximizing their chances for reelection. Regardless of what a legislator's motivations may be, unless they are reelected they will not be able to achieve them. Accordingly the late Illinois Senator Everett Dirksen's first law of politics was reputed to be "get elected," and his second law of politics was "get reelected." And reelection requires political support.[11]

In deciding which legislation to support and which to oppose, legislators base their decisions on which legislative positions provide the greatest amount of political support.[12] Like other rational participants in the political process, legislators also make implicit cost/benefit calculations. The benefits to legislators from providing legislation to an organized group is the political support received from that group; in other words, the cost to the legislators of providing those legislative benefits is not the dollar cost of the legislation, as they do not bear it, but instead it is the loss in potential political support from their actions. As long as legislators receive net positive benefits from providing legislation, they are expected to do so.

The previous discussion of interest groups described why the demand for legislation is often made by organized groups representing minority interests. The method by which Congress (and other bodies, such as state legislatures) is structured also makes it possible for minority interests to prevail in the legislative arena while imposing the financing burden on the majority.

Because the legislature as a whole cannot deal with all the issues that come before it, some legislative functions are delegated to committees. To improve the efficiency of the legislative process, committees with jurisdiction over different policy areas were established. The committee structure enables the legislature to divide up work, develop expertise in complex areas, and provide for a more efficient size for group discussion. However, this organizational efficiency is not without cost. The legislature provides each of the relevant committees with near monopoly power over its area of jurisdiction. Approval by the relevant subcommittee and consequently the parent committee is necessary for legislation to be initiated and funds appropriated.

The committee system also provides the link between the interest groups that are seeking benefits and the legislature, which provides the benefits. To maximize their contributions, legislators have developed reputations on certain issues and created a system of specialized, standing committees that facilitate repeated interactions and long-term relationships between groups providing political support and the members of relevant committees. Interest groups have an incentive to reward legislators who have developed clear reputations with large contributions, sufficiently large so as to make it worthwhile for the legislators to develop reputations and reduce uncertainty.

The committee system in the U.S. Congress has three distinctive features: (1) the committees are standing, not temporary (this promotes repeated interactions and long-term relationships between interest groups and the members of the relevant committees); (2) legislators retain their committee membership for as long as they are reelected (i.e., committee assignments are stable); and (3) the committees have specialized jurisdictions and legislators may join a limited number of committees (the restrictions prevent legislators from opportunistically joining committees that are dealing with hotly contested issues and, thereby, competing with existing members for special-interest contributions).[13]

Membership on committees is generally based on self-selection. Legislators seek those committees that are important for their reelection. Those with strong special-interest constituencies have a strong incentive to be a member of the committees that deal with that special-interest legislation. Thus, legislators whose constituents are farmers seek membership on the agricultural committees, and legislators from urban areas select committees whose jurisdiction deals with urban affairs. Interest groups desiring legislative benefits seek out legislators on the relevant committees and subcommittees that deal with their problems. In this manner legislators are able to provide legislative benefits in return for political support.

An important method by which minority interests are successful in receiving legislative benefits is through the process of vote trading.[14] Vote trading occurs when legislators offer to exchange their vote on an issue of lesser importance to themselves (their constituents) in order to receive votes from legislators on issues of greater importance (to their constituents). For example, assume that there are only three legislators. Only legislator A favors a subsidy to construct a hospital in Illinois. And only legislator B favors a subsidy for constructing a hospital in Pennsylvania. Legislator C opposes both measures. By agreeing to vote for each other's subsidy, both legislators A and B receive their subsidies, each of which would otherwise be opposed by a majority of the legislators. If it were not for vote trading, it would be difficult for legislators with narrow constituent interests to get sufficient votes from other legislators to achieve a majority vote for their special interests.

As the workload of the legislature increases, legislators find it necessary to delegate some of their rule-making authority. The mechanism by which this is done is to create administrative agencies. These regulatory agencies are also able to provide political benefits. Each regulatory agency reports to a particular legislative subcommittee. The interest groups affected by the regulatory agency are the same groups that provide political support to the legislators who have oversight responsibility for the regulatory agency. The regulatory agency therefore has to act in a manner consistent with the legislator's desires; otherwise the legislator would not receive political support from the groups affected by the agency's decisions. For this reason, regulatory agencies will not act independently of their oversight committee.

Given the limited time available to the legislator and the need to allocate that time so as to maximize the chances of reelection, it is not in a legislator's interest to be overly concerned with the oversight function. Only if there are complaints from constituents or from those providing political support does the legislator verify that the agency is acting according to the legislator's wishes. There is little need for the legislator to be concerned with the agency's performance if there are no complaints.

Legislators attempt to maximize political support, given the structure of the legislature and its rules, in the following manner.

One interest group.

The simplest case occurs when only one organized interest group has a concentrated interest in a particular piece of legislation and the costs are diffuse. The legislator will favor that legislation if the political support provided by that group exceeds the cost, both in terms of loss in political support and the legislator's opportunity cost of producing that legislation.

The cost of producing legislation is the legislator's time. The legislator's limited time has to be apportioned among a great many bills introduced during each session of the legislature. For each bill considered, members of legislative committees must hold hearings, draft and amend bills, negotiate among themselves, and rally popular support through media interviews and meetings with constituents.[15] Time spent on any one bill means there is less time to spend on others. That is the real cost of legislation. Legislators could receive political support by enacting other legislation, or they could provide constituent services, which are also a source of political support. The method by which the legislature is organized also affects the time and ease of passing (or changing) legislation. The committee structure of the legislature, whether there are one or two houses, the rules under which each house operates, whether filibusters are permitted, the type of voting procedures in each house, and so on, all affect the time, hence cost, of producing legislation.

Competing interest groups on producer-type legislation.

Legislators face a difficult decision when there are competing interest groups, each willing to provide political support to have its way on regulation. If the legislator accepts political support from one group, she foregoes receiving political support from the other group. (The excluded groups may even decide to back a challenger to the legislator.) The legislator is likely to receive a greater total amount of political support in this situation if she can provide some benefits to each group. A compromise is likely to be reached that provides some benefits to each opposing interest. An example of this type of compromise was airline regulation.

The airlines were important beneficiaries of regulation, as were the airline unions, whose members received above-market wages because of the entry restrictions in the airline industry. As other organized interest groups, such as representatives of small communities, began to participate in the regulatory process, the profitability of the airlines declined. Small communities (represented by their legislators) were subsidized by requiring airlines to serve these communities. The airlines were in part rewarded by being awarded routes in more profitable markets. The regulators also established a method of pricing, typical of regulated industries, that set price proportional to distance rather than to cost. Because the actual costs of travel per mile were lower for long distances, setting prices proportional to distance subsidized short trips. The more profitable markets, those with high prices compared to costs, subsidized small communities as well as those making shorter trips. Such systems of cross-subsidies are typical of situations where there are opposing interest groups in the regulatory process.

Visible legislation.

Producer-type regulation, such as import quotas, tariffs, and entry restrictions, is anticompetitive and is generally not a visible issue to the public. The segments of the population who bear the costs of these producer benefits have a diffuse interest in the outcome of this type of regulation.

However, some types of special-interest legislation are more visible in their effects. Legislative benefits to particular population groups, such as subsidized pensions for the aged (Social Security), subsidized healthcare (Medicare), and subsidized education for middle-class children (public universities) have more obvious beneficiaries. In these cases, legislators seek political support from the benefited population groups. Similar to producer regulation, the cost of these benefits is diffuse and spread over other population groups.

When organized opposition to a visible type of legislation does not exist, then legislators go overboard in their support; they do not face budgetary constraints. They gain the political support of members of groups backing the legislation and lose no support, because organized opposition is absent. Program expenditures are greater than even the beneficiaries expected. An example of this legislation was medical research throughout the 1940s and 1950s. Expenditures for medical research, as approved by Congress, provided more money than the research agencies requested and more than could be usefully spent. (See Chapter 7.)

Another example of a popular, visible type of legislation was the competition between the two political parties to receive the aged's political support by increasing Social Security benefits before each election. Finally, both parties agreed to a formula for increasing Social Security benefits without unduly jeopardizing the Social Security system.

Opposing interest groups on visible legislation.

When legislation benefiting specific population groups is opposed by other organized population groups, legislators face a difficult choice. The legislator, when confronted with these opposing groups, will lose political support from one group if forced to choose. The best strategy to follow in a situation of controversial, visible legislation—if compromise is not possible—is to not vote on the issue. When it becomes imperative to solve a crisis, as occurred in 1983 when the Social Security system's financial solvency was threatened, the political leadership from both political parties form a bipartisan commission to resolve the issue. The bipartisan commission protects legislators from being attacked for their vote by legislators from the opposing party. Another way to avoid a loss of political support is to enact symbolic legislation. Legislation is enacted, thereby satisfying one group; however, the legislation contains limited, if any, enforcement mechanisms, thereby ensuring that the legislation will not achieve its stated goals. Early environmental legislation has often been symbolic. (See Chapter 7.) Symbolic legislation relies on the public's lack of knowledge of the specifics of visible legislation. Fortunately for Congress, most legislation is not of the visible, controversial variety.

Producer groups.

Legislation benefiting particular population groups also occurs when a producer group, acting in its own interest, supports legislation favoring a consumer group, such as the Food Stamp Program, nutrition programs, environmental programs, and Medicare. In some such cases, the legislation to aid a population group actually originated from a producer group. As a means of increasing the consumption of farm products, for example, agricultural committees promoted school lunch and milk programs. (See Chapter 8.)

When an organized population group is successful at obtaining legislation, legislators design the program in such a way as to also benefit the industry suppliers. Medicare provided care to the elderly but was also structured to satisfy the legislative demands of medical and hospital providers (who initially opposed the legislation). In the case of environmental legislation, many firms actually favored the regulations that would have imposed costs on new entrants to that industry. By granting grandfather clauses, these firms received a competitive cost advantage over new firms. Even though legislation may impose costs on an industry, it does not impose those costs evenly on all suppliers.

Legislators require political support to be reelected. At times the political support is provided by a single organized group. At other times legislators refrain from making any choices for fear of losing political support from one of several opposing groups. However, whenever there is a possibility for legislators to extract political support from more than one group, such as from a population group and a producer group, they will find a way to do so.[16]

The Executive Branch

The executive branch (the administration) is both a demander and a supplier of political benefits. It proposes policies to Congress, and Congress decides whether to enact them. To receive congressional support for its policies, the executive branch, acting as a supplier of political benefits, can provide political support to legislators by judicial and governmental appointments, by locating projects in their districts, and by providing the support of a popular president at election time. The executive branch also appoints agency managers and judges (with the consent of Congress) and has an important influence on the shape of the overall government budget and on departmental expenditures.

The motivation of the executive branch is assumed to be similar to that of the legislative branch, namely, reelection. However, there is an important distinction between the two. The executive branch, because of its stated functions, faces certain constraints on its efforts to maximize political support that are not found in the legislative branch. For example, the executive branch is held responsible for this country's foreign affairs, which constrains its support for politically popular legislation to restrict foreign imports such as textiles. Another important constraint on the executive branch is its concern over the performance of the economy. The president is held responsible for inflation and recession. A prosperous economy with rising incomes, low inflation, and low unemployment is believed to provide electoral benefits to the party in control of the executive branch. Neither large deficits nor the taxes to erase those deficits are politically popular. Further, both may have an adverse effect on the economy. The executive branch therefore has a concentrated interest in constraining expenditures so that they do not result in deficits or necessitate tax increases. (Individual legislators are not usually held accountable by their constituents for increases in government deficits.)

The executive branch's concern over spending and its distribution has had important consequences for health policy, at times bringing it into conflict with Congress. An example of this occurred when President Ford vetoed a renewal of the Nurse Training Act. Health programs have always been politically popular and Congress, more mindful of the immediate political benefits than the subsequent budgetary costs of the Nurse Training Act, easily overrode President Ford's veto.

One method used by various administrations to circumvent its concern over the budgetary impacts of politically popular legislation is to shift the costs of such programs to others. Presidents Nixon, Carter, and Clinton proposed employer-mandated national health insurance programs. In each case, the administration sought to receive political support for proposing a new, highly visible benefit to the voting (working) population. Business would have been required to pay for the government-mandated benefits to their employees. The cost of financing an employer-mandated program is no different from one financed by the government. However, by requiring business to pay for the benefits the government did not have to propose an explicit tax on employees. Requiring business to provide the benefits would make it appear that business firms were financing the program.

However, these costs would eventually have been shifted to their employees who would have ended up paying for the mandated benefits through reduced wages.

Had these national health insurance proposals been presented in the above manner, their political appeal would have been greatly diminished. Those employees without health insurance who would have been covered by the mandated program would have had to pay the full costs. Unless they were receiving some net subsidy, why would the employees have favored such a program when they had previously chosen not to have health insurance?

Another advantage of shifting the financing cost to business and off the government budget would occur if expenditures under such a program exceeded expectations, as has occurred under Medicare; the additional financing burden would fall on businesses and their employees through an increase in the payroll tax (and the wage base) rather than on the government.

As government expenditures under the Medicare program began to exceed their budget projections, successive administrations have been faced with politically difficult choices. One approach was to fund rising Medicare expenditures through further increases in the Medicare portion of the Social Security tax. An alternative approach was to ask the aged beneficiaries to pay a greater portion of the program's cost. A third choice was to pay physicians and hospitals less. An administration would not expect to receive political benefits from any of these actions. However, the political burden of finding a solution to this dilemma has typically fallen more heavily on the executive branch than on the individual members of Congress, because the executive branch is held more responsible for budgetary consequences. (Successive administrations have determined that increasing the Medicare portion of the Social Security tax and the wage base to which it applies, as well as paying hospitals less, would cost them less political support than decreasing benefits to the aged or increasing their costs.)

Executive branch behavior with regard to the health field can be explained by its desire to maximize political support while being constrained by the budgetary implications of its actions. Successive administrations have continued to propose politically popular health programs, such as funding for medical research, health professional education, and new health benefits for the aged under Medicare. Such legislation is both highly visible and valued by the public, according to public opinion polls. At the same time, successive administrations have tried to reduce the rise in expenditures of existing health programs, such as Medicare, by paying providers less and thereby forestalling the need to call for tax increases to fund those programs or impose costs on politically powerful beneficiaries (i.e., the aged). The aged have been important beneficiaries of visible redistributive legislation, as most recently indicated by the new Medicare prescription drug benefit.

Agency Bureaucracies

A regulatory agency's performance depends on the goals and objectives of those in charge of the organization. Their motivations are assumed to be job security and higher salaries, both of which result from being the managers of a growing agency. Promotions and job prestige are more likely to occur when an agency's budget is expanding.[17]

To achieve these goals, agency managers engage in several types of behavior that maximize the agency's political support. In fact, if the agency loses the support of its legislative sponsors, the job security of its managers and the very existence of the agency itself may be threatened.[18]

A regulatory agency, therefore, is dependent on the policies and desires of its legislative sponsors. A regulatory agency is unlikely to act in a manner consistent with that of the public interest *unless* the agency's oversight committee so intends. In initiating legislation, a legislative committee has a certain purpose or set of purposes and would want the agency to behave in a fashion consistent with its intentions. The congressional committee holds oversight hearings to evaluate the agency's performance, is able to veto the president's appointments to policy-making positions within the agency, and recommends the size and scope of the agency's budget to the Congress. Through the use of these methods, the oversight committee is able to ensure that the agency is behaving as the legislators intended, rather than doing what others may perceive to be the public interest. A lack of congressional oversight hearings does not mean Congress is neglecting its duties. Instead, it is more indicative that the congressional committee is satisfied with the agency's performance.

Agency behavior can best be understood by examining legislative behavior. Both the agency and legislators attempt to maximize their political support. The groups that provide political support to the agency are the same as those that provide political support to those legislators serving on the committee with jurisdiction over the agency. The only difference is that the agency also tries to provide the members of the legislative committee with political support. The agency provides services to constituents in the legislator's district and attempts to generate support by stimulating the demand for its services.[19]

There are a number of examples in the health field where regulation has not achieved its stated objectives. One can only infer from this that the *stated* objectives were different from the *intended* objectives. For example, for years there has been concern over the quality of care provided by nursing homes. State regulatory agencies have long had at their disposal various mechanisms to ensure that nursing homes provide a certain standard of care. The state agency is permitted to make unannounced visits and deny reimbursement to the home. Additional legal remedies are often not needed to ensure quality. However, state regulatory agencies rarely use their power to make unannounced visits or shift patients to another nursing home. State nursing home associations have a concentrated interest in how existing regulations are applied. Neither the state regulatory agency nor the legislators who have oversight responsibility are likely to change their behavior as long as the major source of their political support comes from the association whose members are regulated.

When Medicare was enacted, healthcare providers were paid according to their existing, preferred payment systems. Payment was on a fee-for-service basis; that is, a fee was charged each time the patient received service from a provider. However, alternative delivery systems, such as prepaid organizations (HMOs), charge an annual fee per patient regardless of the number of times a patient sees a physician or enters the hospital. These prepaid organizations have a different incentive than fee-for-service providers, whose incentive is to provide more services. HMO incentives are to provide fewer services, thereby reducing their costs, and to offer additional benefits to attract enrollees. Fee-for-service providers (and their insurers) compete with HMOs. At the time Medicare was enacted, the American Medical Association (AMA) and the American Hospital Association (AHA) were the two most important health associations. At that time, these organizations, particularly the AMA, provided a great deal of political support to Congress. Therefore, it is no surprise that the agency administering the Medicare system did not permit prepaid organizations to be paid according to an annual capitation fee; they were paid the same as fee-for-service providers. This policy, in effect, eliminated any financial incentive for prepaid organizations to recruit Medicare patients. (In 1985 this policy was changed to allow HMOs to be paid an annual capitation fee.)

An agency must avoid adverse publicity to retain political support.[20] Criticism of the agency makes it appear that the legislative sponsors of the agency have not been performing their oversight function. An agency therefore will attempt to prevent "service" failures in the industry it regulates. One such example is the way the U.S. Food and Drug Administration (FDA) treats the drug industry. If a new drug causes medical problems or death to a small number of those taking it, the regulatory agency, that is, the FDA, would receive adverse publicity for approving the drug. Unfortunately, it is not possible to anticipate all the side effects of new drugs, particularly when they are taken in conjunction with other drugs. It is only after a drug has been introduced that these problems come to light. To minimize the possibilities of adverse publicity, however, the FDA has raised the testing requirements for drug approval. Increasing test requirements increases the costs of new drugs and reduces their potential profitability; consequently, fewer drugs are made available. As a result of FDA policy, many people have been denied the benefits of new drugs while the drugs await approval. It has been estimated that the "cost" of fewer new drugs and the drug lag, in terms of forgone benefits to consumers, has been far greater than the cost of permitting new drugs to enter the market early.[21]

Thus, there is a trade-off between possible deaths due to too rapid introduction of a new drug and deaths that could have been prevented had that drug been on the market sooner. The first type of death is "visible"; they are actual people with families and their pictures may appear in the papers. The second type is "statistical"; deaths that could have been prevented. For an agency concerned about adverse publicity, it is more important to prevent visible deaths. By placing too great an emphasis on preventing visible deaths, however, the agency gives too little emphasis to statistical deaths, which are many times greater. The FDA's weighting scheme may be quite different from that of society and those who would prefer to purchase the drug.

However, increased testing, which increases the time and cost of developing new drugs and, consequently, reduces the rate of new drug innovation, does not necessarily harm all firms in the drug industry. Firms are able to charge higher prices for their existing drugs, and these drugs retain their market share for a longer period of time because the entry of new drugs has been limited.

In addition to maximizing its political support, a regulatory agency attempts to achieve and maintain a monopoly position over the provision of its services.[22] If Congress were to establish a competitor agency, the managerial goals of the initial agency would be threatened. The agency may see part of its appropriations go to its competitor, and the performance of the agencies could then be compared.[23] Thus, any attempt to decrease the monopoly power of an agency is likely to bring forth strong defensive actions. The following two examples illustrate how a health agency responded when its monopoly position was threatened.

After World War II, Congress wanted to increase funds for medical research. A representative of the U.S. Public Health Service, the federal agency responsible for medical research, testified that the agency could not profitably spend the additional funds. This spokesman was quickly retired by the agency. His replacement welcomed all the additional funds Congress decided the agency needed. The U.S. Public Health Service was fearful that if it did not go along with congressional interests, Congress would set up another government agency to carry out its desires. Rather than have these funds go to a competitive agency, the existing agency accommodated congressional interests. (The role of Congress in medical research is discussed more completely in Chapter 7.)

In the 1970s, conquering cancer was perceived as having large public support. To demonstrate their concern, several legislators favored establishing a separate, highly visible cancer center that would be independent from the National Institutes of Health (NIH), which at that time was the main government agency for medical research. The threat of a competitive agency that would draw funds away led to the NIH's vigorous defense of its research efforts and a downgrading of the idea of a separate cancer establishment. NIH was able to generate support from medical schools and other medical research institutes they supported. (These constituencies were afraid that they might receive less funding from a competitive agency.)

To achieve their goals, agency managers require increased budget appropriations. The managers of an expanding agency are thereby able to justify increased staff, increased responsibilities for themselves, and, consequently, higher salaries. When an agency bargains with its oversight committee over its annual budget, the outcome usually favors the agency. This is true for several reasons.

In bargaining with the legislature, the bureaucratic agency has more information available on the cost of providing its services. Because there are no competitors, the legislature cannot simply compare the agency's cost of providing the service with that of another organization. Further, the agency has more at stake over its budget than does the legislature. Thus, the agency will devote more time and effort toward justifying its need for a larger budget. The legislative subcommittee with jurisdiction over the agency has limited time to devote to the agency's budget. Legislators are involved in many other activities and whether or not the agency's budget is somewhat larger than necessary will have no adverse effect on their chances for reelection.

The agency is also fairly well-informed as to the value the legislature places on its services, that is, the legislature's demand for the agency's output. The agency is responsive to the organized interests affected by the agency. These same interest groups lobby the legislature for the benefits provided by the regulatory agency, and the legislature will seek to accommodate them. The agency will try to benefit legislators by, for example, locating agency facilities in the legislators' districts.

Government agencies were an important source of financial support to groups that had a similar political sympathy, according to one study of interest group financial support.[24] By providing funds to groups for training, staff assistance, or other purposes, the agency also builds support from these groups to lobby Congress to continue and expand these programs. This symbiotic relationship enables the agency to increase its demand by organizing constituents that would have had a difficult time organizing themselves.

Because of the agency's control over information and its ability to marshal constituency support, it has a strong position with the legislative subcommittee in negotiating its appropriation.[25]

Agency growth, however, has not been particularly noticeable in the health field, despite the fact that health expenditures, both public and private, have been increasing rapidly. An important reason for this is that when Medicare was enacted, hospital and physician organizations insisted on being paid by nongovernment agencies. In most cases, these "intermediaries" between the Medicare patient and the health provider were hospital-controlled Blue Cross associations and physician-controlled Blue Shield plans.

In summary, the hypothetical goals of agency managers are job security and higher salaries, both of which result from promotions and the increased prestige of being managers of an agency with a large budget. To achieve these goals the agency must first have the confidence and political support of those legislators with oversight responsibilities for their agency. To do so means that the agency attempts to minimize any adverse publicity, to provide services for those legislators, and to generate favorable support from those having an interest in the agency's functions. To ensure that increases for their agency's functions go to their agency and not to competitors, managers are expected to oppose new agencies with similar functions and to favor eliminating competition ("duplication") among agencies.

One implication of an agency's need for political support is that the agency ends up protecting an industry that it is ostensibly meant to regulate in the public interest. However, in doing so the agency is merely following the legislators' desires, as the regulated industry also provides political support to those regulators.

The Antitrust Laws

The antitrust laws are generally assumed to be an activity in which the government acts in the public interest. Antitrust law was developed in three statutes enacted around the beginning of the 1900s, the Sherman Antitrust Act (1890), the Clayton Antitrust Act (1914), and the Federal Trade Commission (FTC) Act (1914). These laws were designed to prevent monopolization and promote price competition. In price-competitive industries, prices of goods and services are lower and output is greater than if those same industries were monopolized. Profits are also lower in price-competitive industries. Consumers are better off—that is, they pay lower prices and have greater choice—when the market in which they buy their goods and services is price competitive. Given that the antitrust laws place the benefit of consumers over the interests of producers, are the antitrust laws evidence of the public interest theory?

To be consistent and generalizable, the economic theory should be able to explain the enactment of the antitrust laws using a self-interest group perspective.[26]

The United States underwent an industrial transformation in the late 1800s: railroads connected major cities; new industries, such as mining, steel, and oil developed; and banks formed to provide the funds to finance these industrial developments. These new industries monopolized the sale of their services, either through mergers or informal collusion. After the Sherman Antitrust Act was enacted to deal with these monopoly abuses, mergers continued, so the Clayton Antitrust Act (as well as the FTC Act) was enacted to strengthen the Sherman Antitrust Act, which was perceived as being ineffective in stopping the monopoly abuses at that time.

Proponents of the public interest theory claim the enactment of the antitrust laws was the result of populist sentiment against monopoly abuses.

According to the economic theory of regulation, the main groups having a concentrated interest in the antitrust laws at that time, and consequently those with an incentive to try and influence the legislative process, were farmers, large manufacturing companies with dominant market shares, and small manufacturing companies with limited market penetration. Large manufacturing companies opposed enactment of the antitrust laws because they would have been adversely affected by antitrust restrictions on their ability to merge with competitors. They would be accused of monopolizing the market. Similarly, their practice of interlocking directorates, which enabled collusion between competitors, would be banned.

Favoring enactment of the antitrust laws were small businesses who believed predatory price competition by large firms disadvantaged them. Small businesses thought they would benefit by making such actions illegal. For small businesses, the purpose of the laws was not to promote competition but to prevent larger, more efficient firms from driving small firms out of business. According to its proponents, the purpose of the laws was to limit the economic power of large firms, not to achieve greater economic efficiency. Some states had actually enacted antitrust laws before 1890 and small businesses favored them.

Agriculture was a major part of the economy around the turn of the century, and agricultural interests strongly affected how senators voted. Farmers, similar to any producer, benefit when their products are sold to competitive purchasers, rather than to monopolist buyers. By making monopolies illegal, the antitrust laws prevented monopoly purchasers of their products.

Agriculture, however, was partially exempted from the antitrust laws, thereby enabling agricultural organizations to form cooperatives, which permitted them to monopolize and charge higher prices for their products. (The Capper-Volstead Act of 1922 exempted agricultural cooperatives from the antitrust laws. States with a large percentage of their populations on farms supported the exemption.)[27]

The Judicial System

According to the economic or self-interest theory of government, the legislature supplies legislation in return for political support. An independent judiciary, however, can nullify special-interest legislation. If a judicial system is able to invalidate the legislature's actions, interest groups would not be willing to pay as high a price for the legislation. What role, therefore, does an independent judiciary play in an interest group theory of legislation?

The federal judicial system was designed to be protected from current political pressures. The authors of the Constitution intended that there would be three branches of government and that the judicial system be independent. Federal judges, under Article III of the U.S. Constitution, are appointed rather than elected, their appointments are for life, and Congress is forbidden to reduce their salaries.

The other two political branches of government can influence court decisions through several methods. The executive branch exerts its influence through its appointment of judges; however, this process may take many years before it affects desired legislation. The executive branch can also fail to enforce decisions that it opposes. Congress can fail to appropriate sufficient funds for salary increases and for judicial staff, create additional federal jurisdictions that vitiate existing courts, and pass new laws, with the concurrence of the administration. Except for the latter, these approaches, however, must be viewed as long-run attempts to control the decisions of federal judges.

Rather than being viewed as an obstacle to the provision of special-interest legislation, however, an independent judiciary is viewed as an important part of the interest group theory of government.[28]

If one Congress "sells" special-interest legislation, it cannot ensure that a future Congress will not overturn it. A new Congress with a different composition and other interest groups will not have to abide by the decisions of a previous Congress. Thus, if a subsequent Congress amends or nullifies special-interest legislation, the value of that legislation will be worth less than if the legislation had some long-term durability. A special-interest group would not be willing to "pay" as much for legislation that lasts only a short period or if there is uncertainty as to how long the legislation would last. Legislators would like to receive as high a price (political support) as possible for their services, so it is in their self-interest to increase the durability of special-interest legislation.

Legislative durability is achieved in two ways. First, the difficulty of enacting and reversing legislation adds stability to enacted legislation. Before it may be passed, proposed legislation must go to a committee, committee hearings have to be held, a majority vote of the committee members must approve the proposed legislation, and the bill must be approved by a majority of the legislature. The legislation must then go through the same process in the other house of congress. In other words, proposed legislation must be approved by a majority in two legislative bodies. Along the way, opponents could filibuster the bill, and at the end of the process the legislation could be vetoed by the executive branch. These procedures reduce the amount of legislation produced and consequently raise the cost to a subsequent Congress of overturning previously enacted special-interest legislation. Given the limited time available to legislators, the time spent overturning previous legislation could be spent on new legislation that generates political support.

Also providing durability to contracts entered into by a particular Congress is an independent judiciary that is willing to interpret the law according to congressional intent. A legislature is able to extend the life of its legislation, thereby increasing its value, as long as the judiciary accepts congressional deals as given. If the courts interpret the law according to the discussions by Congress and the intent of the act at that time, then a Congress is able to provide a special-interest group with a long-term contract.

If a judiciary were more susceptible to the intent of a current Congress, that is, if it were not independent, then court decisions would rely more heavily on current political pressures than previous congressional intent. Thus, it is in the economic interest of Congress to have an independent judiciary that will interpret the law as the enacting Congress intended.

Examples of "dependent" judiciaries were the regulatory agencies established by Congress, such as the Interstate Commerce Commission (ICC) and the Civil Aeronautics Board (CAB). Each Congress determined the budget of these agencies, and the members of the regulatory agencies served specific terms. Because regulatory agencies are more dependent on the current Congress, an interest group would not be willing to pay as much for legislation establishing a regulatory agency as it would for more secure legislation. Regulatory agencies, however, may be more suitable for legislative benefits that depend on local variations in services and rate setting. In this way a special-interest group can bypass dealing with separate state legislatures. Federal regulatory agencies may also be a way for Congress to bypass the independent judiciary if previous legislation would conflict with the new special-interest legislation. An example of this latter case was the regulation of prices and entry used in the railroad and airline industries, which was in conflict with the Sherman Antitrust Act. The fact-finding function of enforcement proceedings is assigned to the regulatory agency rather than to the courts.

This view of the judicial system as a mechanism that provides long-term contracts to politically powerful interest groups has several implications. The perception that the courts are above politics enhances the value of previous political contracts. Rather than being a constraint on special-interest legislation, ". . . they enforce the 'deals' made by effective interest groups with earlier legislatures."[29]

The self-interest theory of the federal court system (and its interpretation of the Constitution) does not imply that all legislation and judicial decisions are necessarily against the public interest. It is merely that the independent judiciary and the Constitution are viewed as a means of providing durable protection to politically powerful special interests. First Amendment rights are viewed "as a form of protective legislation extracted by an interest group consisting of publishers, journalists, pamphleteers, and others who derive pecuniary and nonpecuniary income from publication and advocacy of various sorts."[30,31]

The independent judiciary is important for understanding the change that has occurred in the regulatory environment governing the medical sector. Antitrust laws protect both consumers and potential producers from monopoly power. Some protectionist legislation, enacted at the behest of powerful health interest groups at a state level, have had the effect of providing these health interest groups with monopoly power; restrictions were placed on price competition and on the formation of alternative delivery systems for providing medical services. The independent federal judiciary has been called on to resolve conflicts between federal law (the Sherman Antitrust Act) and state protectionist legislation. These decisions by the judiciary, particularly by the Supreme Court in 1982 (discussed in Chapter 6), have had a profound effect on the structure of the medical care system in this country.

Concluding Comments

Economic markets reflect the desires of those willing to purchase specific products. Producers respond to purchasers' demands. There is a close matching of costs and benefits in economic markets; those receiving the benefits of their purchases pay the full costs of the goods and services received. In political markets, however, the legislative benefits provided to a group exceed their associated financial costs. Those groups receiving legislative benefits are able to achieve them by imposing part or all of the cost on others.

The ability of certain groups to successfully use the legislative process to redistribute wealth away from others to themselves results from imperfections in the political marketplace. Voters are generally uninformed on specific legislative issues. Many voters do not even vote, and when they do, they vote on sets of packages rather than expressing their preferences on each issue of importance to themselves.

These differences between political and economic markets make it worthwhile for organized groups to provide political support and be more successful in political markets than in economic markets. Groups with a concentrated interest, generally producers, are more likely than consumers to be successful in the legislative arena. The costs of organizing themselves, representing their interests, and providing political support to legislators are lower to groups with a concentrated interest than the value of their expected legislative benefits. The costs of providing legislative benefits are imposed on those with a diffuse interest. It is less costly for consumers to pay slightly higher prices for particular goods or services (generally "invisible" costs used to finance producer benefits) than to incur the greater burden of organizing themselves and representing their interests to forestall these higher producer prices. Health policies change when diffuse costs increase so that those who bear it develop a concentrated interest in decreasing those costs.

The motivation of the suppliers of legislative benefits makes it possible for organized groups to receive benefits at the expense of politically unorganized groups. Those who run for political office, as well as those who work for the government, are no different from anyone else. They are concerned with their self-interest. To maximize their chances for reelection, legislators require political support. As such, legislators are more likely to respond to the demands of those offering political support.

The approach legislatures use to organize themselves also enhances the ability of organized groups to secure favorable legislative benefits. Congress relies on committees and subcommittees to sort out the various demands for legislation. Legislators on subcommittees having jurisdiction over particular special-interest groups, therefore, have an undue influence over legislation affecting those groups. Thus, legislators receiving political support from particular organized constituencies are often the same legislators proposing legislative benefits to those same groups. Vote trading also enables legislators representing minority interests to enact legislation on behalf of their constituents' interests.

In addition to legislators, the other participants affecting legislation and regulation are the executive branch, regulatory agencies, and the federal judiciary. The executive branch also seeks to maximize its chances for reelection; unlike legislators, however, it faces certain constraints in its attempt to maximize political support. The executive branch is held responsible for the budgetary implications of its actions and the conduct of foreign policy. Regulatory agencies are not independent organizations. The managers of such agencies require the backing of their legislative sponsors if the agency is to receive annual increases in its appropriations. Thus, the actions of regulatory agencies are expected to reflect the desires of those legislators having jurisdiction over their agency rather than the manager's perceptions of the public interest. Finally, the federal judiciary is viewed, according to the economic version of an interest group theory of government, as providing durability to legislation enacted by Congress.

To be generalizable, a theory has to be stripped of much detail. The hypotheses must be abstractions from reality. The resulting theory may then appear to be too simplistic. However, the true test of a theory is how well it predicts, not whether it includes all the appropriate institutional detail of the legislative process. Further, to be useful for understanding legislative outcomes and for predicting likely changes in the future, a theory does not have to be 100 percent accurate; a theory merely has to predict better than an alternative theory. When evaluating the economic theory of legislation, this criterion for judging the usefulness of a theory should be kept in mind.

In subsequent chapters, the self-interest approach to legislation will be used to explain why specific health legislation was enacted. Although the public interest is always promoted as the *stated* goal of legislation, whether the public interest is improved is incidental to the actual intent of the legislation. As discussed in the Chapter 3, however, it first becomes necessary to explain why certain health associations were more successful than others in achieving their legislative goals.

Study Questions

1. What is the presumed purpose of all legislation according to the economic theory of legislation?
2. How do the concepts of "concentrated" and "diffuse" interests determine whether a group represents its interests before legislators?
3. Why are producer groups more likely than consumer groups to be successful in the legislative marketplace?
4. What objectives are legislators presumed to have and what types of

cost/benefit calculations are they presumed to undertake, according to the economic theory of legislation?

5. Explain how "vote trading" enables legislators representing minority economic interests to receive legislative benefits for those interest groups.

6. When is the "visibility" of legislation considered desirable by its proponents and when is it considered undesirable?

7. Why are regulatory agencies more likely to represent the interests of those whom they regulate rather than the public's interest?

8. Contrast the public interest view of government to the economic theory of legislation in terms of the likely effect of government policy on economic efficiency and the equity of redistribution policies.

Notes

1. Much has been written on voting behavior. A classic book on this subject is Anthony Downs, *An Economic Theory of Democracy* (New York: Harper & Row, 1957).

2. Voter turnout was found to be proportionately smaller the larger the population in an area (indicating that a voter in a more populous area has less likelihood of affecting the vote outcome) and the more one-sided the election. When presidential and senatorial elections were held at the same time as local elections (meaning the election tended to have greater importance), the voter turnout was greater. Yoram Barzel and Elliott Silberberg, "Is the Act of Voting Rational?" *Public Choice* 16, (Fall 1973): 51–58.

3. Morris P. Fiorina, *Congress: Keystone of the Washington Establishment* (New Haven, CT: Yale University Press, 1977).

4. Sam Peltzman, "How Efficient Is the Voting Market?" *Journal of Law and Economics* 33 (1990): 27–63.

5. There are many other methods besides limits on entry whereby legislation can affect a firm's profits. For example, firms or participants in an industry (e.g., farmers and hospitals) can be granted a subsidy. Again, the motivation underlying each type of legislation is the same: firms desire to become more profitable than if left to the outcome of a competitive market. For a more complete discussion of these methods, see Chapter 4.

6. Several factors affect a group's demand for legislation. (The first may be considered a movement along a demand curve for legislation, whereas the others are equivalent to shifts in the demand for legislation.)

    (a.) In any economic market as the price of a good increases, the quantity demanded of that good drops. The same is true in political markets. The higher the political support required (the price), the lower the quantity demanded of legislation. It is assumed that the demanders are aware of the value of legislative benefits. Therefore, they would be willing to pay, in terms of political support, a price that does not exceed the value of their legislative benefits.

(b.) The value of legislation to a group and what it is willing to pay for those benefits is affected by the durability of the legislation. The more permanent the legislation, the greater its value.

(c.) When the demand for a producer's product increases, the value of legislation, and hence the producer's demand, also increases. That is, the value of legislation to a group is greater the larger the market in which that legislation is applicable. For example, as the amount of dollars consumers spend on health services has grown, so has the value of legislation that limits the number of health professionals who can practice in that market.

(d.) When opponents are also willing to provide political support, then the group demanding legislative benefits will have to pay a higher price in terms of political support. Thus, whether or not there is opposition to a group's demand for legislation will affect the price a group has to pay for legislative benefits, as well as the amount of legislation they receive.

7. Downs, *An Economic Theory of Democracy*, 297.

8. Gary Becker, "A Theory of Competition Among Pressure Groups for Political Influence," *Quarterly Journal of Economics* 98 (1983): 371–400.

9. A public relations campaign by an industry seeking protection against foreign imports attempts to exert political pressure by claiming "fairness" in reducing imports that compete with their products. In this manner the industry hopes to sway legislators not dependent on their votes. Robert Baldwin, "The Political Economy of Trade Policy," *Journal of Economic Perspectives* 3, no. 4 (1989): 119–135.

   Regulation and monopolization of an industry become more profitable when the overall demand for the industry service is "inelastic." That is, when supply is restricted an increase in the price of the product would result in an increase in total industry revenues.

10. When imperfect information exists, there is opportunity for "political entrepreneurism." A political entrepreneur, who is usually a politician, helps to improve the performance of the political marketplace, particularly with respect to "visible" redistribution. For example, in the special Fall 1991 Senate race for an open seat in Pennsylvania, a relative unknown, Harris Wofford, ran against the

Republican nominee, Richard Thornburg, who had been the U.S. Attorney General and was strongly favored to win the election. Wofford's main campaign issue, which Thornburg ignored, was healthcare reform. Wofford was successful in making healthcare reform a salient issue in the minds of the voters; thus, he changed the outcome of the election. By demonstrating healthcare reform as a winning issue in a state race, he captured the attention of the Democrats, who then made it one of their campaign issues in the 1992 presidential election. For a discussion of political entrepreneurship, see Roger Noll, "Economic Perspectives on the Politics of Regulation," in *Handbook of Industrial Organization*, vol. 2, eds. R. Schmalensee and R.D. Willig. (New York: Elsevier Science Publishers, 1989), 1253–1282.

Similarly, political candidates often compete over defining the issue agenda future elections will be fought over. Their goal is to make electorally prominent the issues on which their policy positions are popular and undermine the importance of issues on which their views are unpopular. Amihai Glazer and Susanne Lohmann, "Setting the Agenda: Electoral Competition, Commitment of Policy, and Issue Salience," *Public Choice* 99 (1999): 377–394.

11. The above discussion assumes legislators are not monopolists; that is, they face competition in their bid for reelection, not only in the general election but also with a possible challenge in the primary. This concern over challengers causes the legislator to respond to political support. Some legislators, however, are either unopposed or win by such large margins that they do not have to respond to the political support offered by an interest group. The interest group has no alternative but to deal with the particular legislator. In these situations the legislator has greater flexibility to act on issues.

12. Although political support is often thought of as being votes, volunteer time, or money, political support may also be an interest group's ability to disrupt legislative programs. For example, during the negotiations leading to the passage of Medicare, legislators were concerned that if physicians and hospitals were not paid according to their payment preferences, they would not participate. Legislating benefits for the elderly but not being able to ensure that they would be delivered would have had the effect of nullifying the program. Congress could then have lost the political support they thought they were going to receive by passing the program in the first place.

13. Randall S. Kroszner and Thomas Stratmann, "Interest Group Competition and the Organization of Congress. Theory and

Evidence from Financial Services Political Action Committees,"
American Economic Review 88 (1998): 1163–87.

14. Some persons draw a distinction between logrolling and vote trading. Logrolling is used when the groups involved consist of a majority; in vote trading, the participants are a minority.

15. Isaac Ehrlich and Richard A. Posner, "An Economic Analysis of
Legal Rulemaking," *Journal of Legal Studies* 3 (1974): 257–86. See
also, Mark Crain, "Cost and Output in the Legislative Firm,"
Journal of Legal Studies 8 (1979): 607–21.

16. Milton Friedman explains the 1986 tax reform legislation that eliminated many of the loopholes providing advantages to special-interest
groups in the following way: "From Congress's point of view, tax legislation has an . . . important function: It is a way to raise campaign
funds. . . . That is why members of Congress put such a high value on
being assigned to the Ways and Means or Finance committees. . . .
The Senate Finance Committee discovered that this process had come
to a dead end . . . the tax space was overcrowded with loopholes.
There was no room to add anymore without destroying the tax base
altogether. . . . Senator Packwood's approach was an ingenious solution to the potential collapse of tax reform as a source of campaign
funds. . . . [It] wipes the slate clean, thereby providing space for the
tax reform cycle to start over again. . . . If my interpretation is correct, the improvement will turn out to be temporary. . . . As members
of Congress try to raise campaign funds, old loopholes will be reintro-
duced and new ones invented. . . . The process will be strictly bipartisan—as it always has been. The only partisan element will be the
rhetoric used to defend the changes."

    In a letter to the editor on this subject, Ralph Nader said that
his recent experiences convinced him that Friedman was completely
correct in his analysis of Congress's interest in tax reform. Milton
Friedman, "Tax Reform Lets Politicians Look For New Donors,"
Wall Street Journal, sec. A, July 7, 1986.

17. The following references concern the behavior of regulatory agen-
cies: Aaron Wildavsky, *The Politics of the Budgetary Process* (Boston:
Little, Brown, 1964); Gordon Tullock, *The Politics of Bureaucracy*
(Washington, DC: Public Affairs Press, 1965); Anthony Downs,
Inside Bureaucracy (Boston: Little, Brown, 1967); William A.
Niskanen, *Bureaucracy and Representative Government* (Chicago:
Aldine Atherton Publishing Company, 1971); William A. Niskanen,
"Bureaucrats and Politicians," *Journal of Law and Economics* 18
(1975): 617–44; Albert Breton and Ronald Wintrobe, "The
Equilibrium Size of a Budget-Maximizing Bureau," *Journal of*

Political Economy 83 (1975): 195–207; M.D. McCubbins, R.G. Noll, and B. Weingast, "Administrative Procedures as Instruments of Political Control," *Journal of Law, Economics and Organization* 3 (1987): 243–277.

18. An example of what occurs when an agency's policies (the FTC) diverge from those of its sponsors (the Congress) is discussed in Barry R. Weingast and Mark J. Moran, "Bureaucratic Discretion or Congressional Control? Regulatory Policymaking by the Federal Trade Commission," *Journal of Political Economy* 91(1983): 765–800.

19. In their work on the economic theory of regulation, Stigler and Peltzman do not distinguish between agency and legislative behavior. This is presumably because they expect the actions of both groups to be similar, that is, the agency is a creation of and controlled by the legislature. Their concern, therefore, is just with the legislature. George J. Stigler, "The Economic Theory of Regulation," *The Bell Journal of Economics* 2, no. 1 (1971) and Sam Peltzman, *Political Participation and Government Regulation* (Chicago: The University of Chicago Press, 1998).

20. Media coverage influences the general public's opinions and Environmental Protection Agency (EPA) decision makers respond to the public's concerns. Coverage of pesticides in the *Washington Post* has influenced the EPA's special review decisions; evidence indicates that the effect of media coverage is nonlinear. The media's influence is very powerful when coverage levels are high. J. Andrew Yates, and Richard L. Stroup, "Media Coverage and EPA Pesticide Decisions," *Public Choice* 102 (2000): 297–312.

21. Drug legislation is also covered in more detail, together with appropriate references, in Chapter 7.

22. Bureaucracies are generally monopolist suppliers. The U.S. Postal Service, the Department of Defense, municipal garbage collectors, and the local health department, for example, are all monopolist sellers of their services. In fact, various government study groups (commissions) often recommend that duplication of government agencies should be eliminated. Thus, if there are overlapping jurisdictions, reorganizations eliminate them, thereby ensuring that the agency has a monopoly.

   In economic markets, a monopolist charges a higher price than if competition existed. The result of monopoly behavior is that prices are higher, profits are greater, and output of that service is reduced. Bureaucracies, however, are not organized for profit. The agency cannot keep the difference between their total revenues and their total costs. Therefore, they receive no benefit from increasing the profits of their agency. Further, bureaucratic agencies do not sell their services on a per-unit basis, as does a private firm. Instead, an agency that has monopoly power is likely to be less efficient in carrying out its objectives and would generally receive a greater appropriation from the legislature to cover the costs of its activities than if it had to compete with another agency.

23. From the perspective of economic efficiency it would be worthwhile to decrease the monopoly power of an agency. One way this has been achieved is by contracting out the agency's function to the lowest bidder. An example of this approach is in municipal services, for example, garbage collection. The cost savings have been dramatic. Another method has been to ask existing government agencies to bid against one another on performing a government function. This approach was used during the Vietnam War when the Coast Guard received a contract over the Navy for performing certain naval combat functions in Vietnam's rivers.

    Permitting agencies to offer bids on functions performed by other agencies would force those other agencies to hold down their costs. It would be embarrassing to an agency manager if at appropriation hearings another agency offered to perform certain functions for half the appropriation.

    Finally, agency efficiency would increase if agencies with a national jurisdiction were subdivided into separate regional entities. In this way, cost and productivity comparisons could be made between the various regional agencies.

    The above suggestions, which have been made many times by others, assume that legislators are concerned with agency efficiency. If instead the legislators are more concerned with maximizing political support, and the existing agency structure helps them achieve this goal, then it is unlikely that legislators would favor such radical changes.

24. Jack L. Walker, "The Origins and Maintenance of Interest Groups in America," *The American Political Science Review* 77 (1983): 390–406.

25. Perhaps the most well-known observations on agency size are attributed to C. Northcote Parkinson. Parkinson's two axioms were "An official wants to multiply subordinates, not rivals," and "Officials make work for each other." Parkinson finds empirical support for his "laws," the most notable being the British navy from 1914 through 1928. Although the number of ships decreased by 67 percent and the number of officers and men actually on ships decreased by 31

percent, the number of admiralty officials increased by 78 percent. This led one observer to comment that Britain had ". . . a magnificent navy on land." Bureaucratic expansion occurs regardless of whether the workload decreases. Similarly, as increasing numbers of British colonies declared their independence, the British Colonial Office continued to expand. As the number of farmers in the United States declined, the U.S. Department of Agriculture's budget and personnel increased. C. Northcote Parkinson, *Parkinson's Law* (Boston: Houghton Mifflin Co., 1957), 35.

26. For a discussion on the origins of the antitrust laws, see George J. Stigler, "The Origin of the Sherman Act," *Journal of Legal Studies* 14 (1985): 1–11; William F Shugart and Robert D. Tollison, "The Positive Economics of Antitrust Policy: A Survey Article," *International Review of Law and Economics* 5 (1985): 39–57; and Carlos D. Ramirez and Christian Eigen Zucchi, "Understanding the Clayton Act of 1914: An Analysis of the Interest Group Hypothesis," *Public Choice* 106 (2001): 157–81.

27. Stigler, "The Origin of the Sherman Act."

28. The discussion in this section is based on the article by William M. Landes and Richard A. Posner, "The Independent Judiciary in an Interest-Group Perspective," *Journal of Law and Economics* 18 (1975): 875–901.

29. Ibid., 894.

30. Ibid., 893.

31. Controversy occurs when the independent judiciary acts in a truly independent fashion. When the courts provide the politically powerless, namely criminals, with rights not provided to them explicitly by the Constitution, as was done by the Warren Court, there is debate about whether the courts have gone too far. An interest group view of government that interprets legislation and even the Constitution as protection for the powerful would not expect that the framers of the Constitution wanted to confer such rights on powerless, unrepresented groups. Whether (and how) the poor and powerless should be protected by society is a value judgment and is separate from the analytical issue of what the framers of the Constitution had as their intent.

THE RELATIVE SUCCESS OF HEALTH ASSOCIATIONS

After completing this chapter, the reader should be able to

- explain the necessity for an organization to overcome the "free rider" problem in order to achieve its legislative objectives,
- identify health association approaches to overcoming the "free rider" problem,
- discuss association characteristics that lead to legislative agenda achievement,
- describe how the federal government's "budget-neutral" Medicare financing methods affect the AMA and the AHA's ability to represent their constituents' interests, and
- analyze whether the American Dental Association or the American Nurses Association are positioned to represent their members' legislative interests more successfully.

Some health associations, such as the AMA, have been much more successful in the legislative arena than others, such as the American Nurses Association (ANA). The most direct measure of this success is the relative incomes of their members. Throughout the post–World War II period physicians have earned "excess" rates of return; these rates of return were greater than what would have been necessary to produce the same supply of physicians. Nurses, during different time periods, have either earned lower or similar rates of return to those earned in professions with comparable training. Nurses have not earned excess rates of return.[1]

Although an association's success is affected by a number of factors, such as whether other concentrated groups oppose their legislative proposals, there are several characteristics of an association and of its members that affect its ability to achieve favorable legislation. These attributes are useful predictors for judging the success of an association. The following is a brief discussion of the determinants of an association's success in the legislative marketplace.

Similarity of Members' Interests

When the members of a group have similar interests, the costs of organizing the group are less than if the members disagree on what they want. When members' interests differ, negotiation among those with divergent views must occur before they can arrive at a mutually agreeable position. Large differences in members' positions or in their perceived interests may cause defections from the group. These defecting members may then claim that they speak for the industry or profession. Legislators will not be certain who speaks for the members' interests when there are multiple spokespersons and each subgroup provides political support and presents different proposals. Differences in interests among group members will also lessen the likelihood that members will contribute to a group whose legislative proposals differ from their own.

Consumers have different interests. They have different occupations, live in different regions, and have different values. Thus, it is very difficult, in other words, costly, to organize consumers around one particular economic issue. Further, any economic policy may have a relatively small effect on consumers' incomes. (The effect of that policy on consumers is said to be "diffuse.") Consumers may not purchase particular products very frequently and, when they do, the effect of a given policy on the prices they pay may be relatively small. When consumers favor a specific visible issue, it is easier to organize and represent that specific issue. For example, opposition to gun control and abortion are two issues a number of people feel strongly about. Therefore, it is much easier to organize consumers on these issues than on others. However, given the heterogeneity of consumers and their interests, it is generally difficult to organize consumers into political groups.

Producers in a particular industry, on the other hand, generally have homogeneous interests; they want to increase their incomes. The revenues of firms in an industry come from similar sources, and producers are aware of the way in which policies that affect their costs or the demands for their product or service can also affect their incomes. Because producers' interests are similar, it is less costly for them to organize and represent their interests. For this reason we observe so many more organizations representing producers than consumers.

A potential problem for producer associations occurs when certain subgroups seek to receive a competitive advantage over other producers in that association. When this occurs, the producer association must continue to represent the common interests of all producers—otherwise the association will fractionate into separate groups, each seeking to gain advantage. Should this occur, no one group will then be interested in representing the common interests of all producers.

Dental Associations

Dental associations have a relatively homogeneous membership. Dentists are predominantly in fee-for-service practice, most often as solo practitioners. (About 80 percent are in solo practice, 13 percent belong to a partnership, and a small number of salaried dentists work in hospitals and offices of physicians.)[2] General dentists represent the vast majority of all dentists. About 80 percent are general dentists versus members of different specialty groups. Dentists who become specialists are required to limit their practice to their specialty. Specialists in dentistry, therefore, are limited to a smaller portion of the total market for dental care and cannot compete with general dentists. Dentistry has handled the specialty "problem" by not permitting specialists and general dentists to become competitors. General dentists were able to impose these conditions on specialists, and the dental associations were then able to continue to represent the common interests of all.

American Nurses Association

Nurses have not had similar interests. There are about 2.7 million registered nurses (RNs) in the United States. Approximately two-thirds of RNs work in hospitals; the remainder work in other settings, such as public health agencies, physicians' offices, and academia. Even those nurses employed in hospitals may be specialized, such as nurse anesthetists and critical care nurses. In nonhospital settings, nurses' roles also vary, from a general nurse in a physician's office to a privately employed nurse-midwife. Nurses, therefore, have specialty nursing associations that more closely represent their professional roles,and there is greater similarity of interests among nurses within these associations than within the ANA. Consequently, only 5.6 percent of nurses are members of the ANA (the ANA has 150,000 individual registered nurse members.)[3]

The number of nurses within a specialty is sufficiently large, in the tens of thousands, to support a national specialty association at a reasonable cost. Nurses in specialty roles and general-duty nurses are not in competition with each other. There are no barriers in the path of general-duty nurses who desire to take additional training and move into specialty roles.

In addition to a lack of similar economic and professional interests, many nurses have not looked at nursing as a long-term career. Many nurses have viewed nursing as an occupation until they became married. After marriage, many nurses left the profession to raise a family. Once their children had grown, some returned to nursing but others did not. Many nurses did not view themselves as the primary wage earner in the family. Instead, they viewed their income as supplementing their spouse's income. The economic benefits of joining a national nursing association were, therefore, questionable.

The political effectiveness of the ANA has been further weakened by the types of legislative issues they have favored. Rather than representing the common economic interests of nurses, nursing associations have lobbied for broader (nonnursing) social issues. It is unlikely that nurses (or other professions) will be willing to provide financial support to the ANA (or their professional association) for achieving broad societal changes. Instead of concentrating their political support on issues that affected their members' economic interests, nursing associations backed legislation on the nuclear freeze and women's rights, in addition to those that affected their members' economic interests. In more recent years, the focus of nursing associations has become more targeted to nursing issues.

American Medical Association

The AMA, considered to be the most successful health association, has, until relatively recently, been able to deal with a membership whose interests are not always homogeneous. As early as 1883, the AMA was concerned about the growth of specialization and the formation of separate societies to represent those physicians.[4] As the number of specialties began to rise, it became more and more difficult for the AMA to represent physicians whose field of practice and method of practice were changing.

The growth of physician specialty societies threatened the role of the AMA as the representative of organized medicine. Specialists wanted to restrict certain tasks to those physicians who were specially trained to perform them. At the same time, specialists, if they were not busy, wanted to be able to perform generalist tasks.[5] From a generalist's perspective, if specialists were successful in limiting the services generalists were permitted to perform, there would be less demand, hence income, for generalists. Conflicts between specialists and generalists become a problem when there is insufficient demand facing each practitioner and when specialty services begin to cover a significant portion of all physician services. To prevent themselves from being limited to a smaller market, generalists wanted to be able to continue performing all tasks.

Board certification was a compromise between specialists and generalists. Generalists were still permitted to perform all medical services, but board certification helped to distinguish between physicians who were specially qualified, in terms of education, training, and examination, to perform the same tasks.[6]

The AMA was able to overcome the potentially divisive issue of specialty societies by understanding and representing the common economic interests of all physicians; namely, the maintenance of fee-for-service practice without government interference. They were able, until the late 1960s, to maintain tight control over the supply of physicians. By being able to understand the common economic interests of all physicians they were able to mobilize all physicians, as in their legislative defeat of President Truman's proposal for national health insurance and the modifications included in the original Medicare Act to benefit physicians and preclude competition by HMOs and preferred provider organizations (PPOs).

The characteristics of physicians have changed with a consequent change in their economic interests. There are a greater number of female physicians; more physicians belong to medical groups, which in turn are becoming larger; and more physicians receive a significant portion of their patients, hence income, from large healthcare organizations, such as HMOs and PPOs, as well as managed care insurers.[7]

As its membership has declined, from more than 70 percent of all physicians in 1962 to about 35 percent, or 250,000 physicians, in 2004, the AMA has had to search for common interests among the increasingly diverse physician population. (About 80,000 of its members are medical students and residents who pay deeply discounted annual dues.) To attract younger physicians, the AMA has been more vocal on such issues as tobacco subsidies, boxing, seat belts, patient safety, and disease prevention. These broader issues helped create a new image for the AMA, but the organization has not neglected the economic interests of all physicians. For example, the AMA opposes payment reductions in the Medicare program, a program it once strenuously opposed, as Medicare is a major source of income for many physicians.

The growth in the number of physicians and the federal government's actions to reduce Medicare expenditures have placed great strains on the AMA. The supply of physicians has risen from 142/100,000 population in the early 1960s to 300/100,000. (There are about 870,000 physicians currently.) To maintain their incomes as the number of patients per physician declines, the different physician specialties are engaged in competition with each other. Specialists would like to restrict the tasks that nonspecialists can perform, and family practitioners would like to be able to continue to perform a broad range of services. Each organization is supported by large numbers of physicians.

In 1992 the federal government initiated a new physician payment system for Medicare patients. The Resource-Based Relative Value Scale

(RBRVS) has several parts, but the aspect that caused each specialty to come into conflict with every other specialty was the rearrangement of the physician fee structure under Medicare. Fees for cognitive services were increased while fees for performing procedures were decreased. This rearrangement of physician fees was intended to be "budget neutral," that is, the total amount spent by the government on physician Medicare services was supposed to be unchanged. Thus, the only way in which one physician specialty could receive higher fees was to cause a decrease in fees for other specialties. Changes in a specialty's fees had a direct effect on the incomes of physicians in that specialty.

To protect their member's interests, each physician specialty had to engage in the political process. As the separate specialty societies competed (politically) among themselves to ensure that their members received a "fair" share of government expenditures, the AMA found it difficult to take sides lest it antagonize one or more of the physician specialty societies. The main role of the AMA was to ask for "more" and try to represent the common interests of all physicians.

"Budget neutrality" brought to the forefront the divergent economic interests of different physician specialties and, in doing so, has strengthened the role of the specialty societies. The specialty societies now have an important lobbying function, to represent their members' interests regarding changes in Medicare physician fees. The rise in each specialty's political power made it more difficult for the AMA to speak for all physicians on all issues. The AMA had to negotiate with the separate physician specialty societies that maintain their own Washington lobbyists.

Given the increasing divergence of economic interests among physicians, the AMA finds it more difficult to find a common set of economic goals for which it can claim to be the physician's representative. The viability of the AMA depends on its ability to have sufficient dues revenues to perform its functions and find a common set of economic interests. Some such issues are higher Medicare physician payments (the annual percentage increase in RBRVS fees), limits on malpractice awards, and changes to the antitrust laws to allow independent physicians to collectively bargain with large health insurers.

American Hospital Association

The AHA has been the major trade association for hospitals. Its constituency, however, has been very diverse. Its membership consists of large and small hospitals, hospitals located in urban and rural areas, hospitals that are major teaching institutions, not-for-profit hospitals, and for-profit hospitals. Each state also has its own state hospital association. In the past, particularly from the late 1940s through the 1970s, the AHA was generally able to represent the common interests of all hospitals. The AHA was successful in having legislation enacted that increased revenues and decreased costs to all hospitals. For example, the AHA successfully lobbied for hospital construction subsidies (the Hill-Burton Act in 1948), for federal subsidies to increase the supply of nurses (the Nurse Training Act in 1964), and for generous federal payment to hospitals under Medicare. It was relatively easy to represent the common interests of all hospitals at a time of expanding federal budgets. There was no need for either the government or the AHA to choose which hospitals would benefit.

The success of the AHA's lobbying efforts under Medicare, however, resulted in rapidly rising hospital expenditures, duplication of expensive services, and inefficiency in the provision of hospital services.

Successive administrations, both Republican and Democratic, attempted to reduce Medicare hospital expenditures and, as a result, developed an adversarial relationship toward hospitals. As hospitals had to compete, legislatively, for a more limited share of federal expenditures, it became more difficult for the AHA to represent its members' common interests. If small and rural hospitals were to receive increased funding, it would be at the expense of urban hospitals. Under a system of "budget neutrality," where the total amount of money spent by Medicare on hospitals was fixed, increased funding for one type of hospital had to come from funding for another group of hospitals. As federal efforts to reduce hospital expenditures intensified, each group formed its own association as it tried to protect its own interests while trying to shift the burden to other hospitals.

Faced with limited Medicare funding, a diverse membership, and additional trade associations, the AHA has attempted to work with its separate constituencies on lobbying activities of general interest to hospitals. A recent example was including a moratorium on the development of new specialty hospitals in the 2003 MMA. (Hospitals were concerned that these new competitors, which were partly owned by physicians, were taking profitable orthopedic and cardiovascular patients away from the general hospitals.) To remain as the spokesperson for all hospitals, the AHA has changed its organizational structure to be more responsive to its constituencies. The AHA now relies on the use of ad hoc committees to develop policy. The AHA's regional advisory boards have been transformed into regional policy boards for purposes of debating policy options, and the Board of Trustees, rather than the House of Delegates, is designated as the final policy-approval authority.[8]

The AHA has also been able to work with competitive organizations, such as the Federation of American Hospitals (the association representing for-profit hospitals), when there are general hospital issues common to the membership of both organizations.

The AHA has a unique advantage over other health associations when representing general hospital issues.[9] Hospitals, after all, are located in every congressional district. By notifying its local and state hospital associations when pressure needs to be placed on legislators, the AHA is able to energize influential hospital board members, local businesses dependent on their hospital, and communities and labor organizations whose business and jobs are affected by the fortunes of their hospital that they should lobby their congressperson. These concentrated interests at the grassroots level are very persuasive to legislators from both political parties.

The "Free Rider" Problem

Until the mid-1960s, it was generally believed that the common interests of individuals or firms would lead necessarily to an organization to represent those interests. However, this reasoning was faulty; it neglected an important aspect of organizational development, the problem of "free riders."[10]

When individuals with a common interest organize to achieve favorable economic legislation for themselves, all individuals with that common interest gain, whether or not they participate in the organization. For example, if some dairy farmers form an organization and contribute to having representation for increasing milk price supports, then, if the legislation is enacted, all dairy producers benefit—even those who have not contributed to the association. Establishing high price supports for milk is a "collective" good—no dairy producer can be excluded from benefiting from the policy. Because a producer cannot be excluded from the resulting legislation, there is no incentive for the individual producer to contribute to the group's efforts. The individual producer who does not contribute can get a free ride, thereby obtaining the legislative benefits without sharing in the costs of producing those benefits.

Unless a group can overcome this free rider problem, it may be unable to raise sufficient funds from those likely to benefit to lobby for their desired policy. Overcoming the free rider problem is an important determinant of the legislative success of a group.

Labor organizations are a prominent example of an organization overcoming the free rider problem. A labor union negotiates wages for all employees in a plant. It would clearly be in the economic interest of each employee not to join the union and thereby save himself the union dues. However, if each employee acted according to her individual interests, it is unlikely that an effective union would be formed to serve the common interests. For this reason, unions seek a "closed shop." In other words, once a union has been certified in a plant, all employees are required to join. If not, some employees would receive a free ride on the union's collective bargaining activities. The union would be unable to raise sufficient dues to undertake its collective bargaining activities. Congress and the states have granted unions special exemptions from the antitrust laws to overcome the free rider problem.

Producers in an industry, however, cannot coerce one another to contribute to the industry's trade association. Instead, trade associations attempt to overcome the free rider problem in one of several ways. One method is to tie membership in the national trade association to membership in a local association in which the firm or individual is economically motivated to join. (ADA uses this method as will be discussed later.) The local association then remits part of the firm's dues to the national organization. Another approach is for the association to require any person desiring certification to become a member of the association; assuming certification leads to a higher income, the individual then has an economic incentive to join. However, in 1978 the Supreme Court declared this approach illegal in the case of the National Society of Professional Engineers.

The most common approach for overcoming the free rider problem is for the trade association to sell "private" services to its member firms and withhold these services from nonmembers (or sell them at a much higher price). The "profits" from selling these private services are then used to support the lobbying activities of the industry. The lobbying efforts of an association are a byproduct of the services the organization sells to its membership.[11] If the association has a monopoly position over the sale of those private services, it is more likely that the individual will purchase the services from the association and that the association will be able to charge a high price. Unless the association can find unique services to sell, however, competitive sellers of such services will be able to provide them at a price lower than that offered by the association.

American Medical Association

In the past, a physician desiring hospital privileges was required to be a member of the county medical society. Unless a physician had hospital privileges, he could not provide a complete medical treatment to the patient. If a patient had to be hospitalized, a physician without hospital privileges had to refer the patient to a physician with such privileges. This placed the referring physician at a competitive disadvantage. Membership in the county medical society was particularly important for specialists, such as surgeons, whose place of practice was the hospital. Membership in the county society also offered physicians greater protection against medical malpractice. Not only was it easier for a physician to purchase such coverage but other physicians would be more likely to testify on their behalf. Thus, the county medical society was in a powerful position. If the county society chose to deny membership to a physician, the physician would not be able to prac-tice in the community.[12]

Until 1949 the AMA used to be a federation of state and county medical societies. So if physicians joined the county medical society, they were automatically members of the national organization, the AMA. Part of each physician's dues were then remitted to the AMA. The AMA was thus able to overcome the free rider problem through this agreement with their constituent societies. In 1950 the AMA, presumably in an attempt to increase its revenues, created a separate dues-paying membership. (This was the period of intense AMA opposition to national health insurance proposals.) Physicians could join just the county and state medical soci-eties and would not have to join (and thus not remit part of their dues) to the AMA. Many state medical societies, however, continued to include the AMA's dues as part of their own dues structure. (These state societies were referred to as being "unified.") AMA dues were relatively low during this time (in 1958 annual dues were $25). Physicians perceived that the bene-fits of membership exceeded the relatively small cost. AMA membership was quite large, representing approximately 74 percent of all physicians. The free rider problem was not extensive.

As the dues increased, however, the number of unified medical soci-eties declined. In recent years, only two state medical societies were uni-fied. Because the the county medical society offers physicians more limited benefits, state and county medical societies are fearful of losing members if they continue to be unified and include the AMA's annual dues with their own. As the cost of the annual AMA membership rose (as of 2005, to $420 a year) compared to perceived benefits, AMA membership declined to 30 percent of all physicians. Many physicians decided to take a free ride on the AMA's legislative efforts.

To raise sufficient funds to continue its lobbying efforts, the AMA has tried to sell private services to physicians, thereby making it worthwhile for them to join. Savings on participation in retirement plans, such as Keogh investment plans; educational programs; and journal subscriptions are impor-tant inducements for membership. The AMA also offers a broad range of insurance services and personal services, including credit cards, savings on medical supplies, technology discounts from IBM and Dell, and loan con-solidation. In addition, the AMA provides incentives to state medical soci-eties, including offering the state additional delegates in the AMA's House of Delegates, if they become unified state medical societies.[13]

In 2002, the AMA's House of Delegates, concerned over the AMA's declining membership, the decrease in dues revenue, and annual deficits, voted to transform the AMA once again into an umbrella organization for national specialty societies and eliminate individual memberships.[14] The new umbrella organization would be responsible for general advocacy and ethics issues affecting all physicians and would rely on a certain percentage of annual membership fees from all national specialty societies. This approach for financing the AMA's advocacy efforts, however, has met with opposition from several specialty societies. Specialty societies are concerned that they will have to raise member dues to fund the AMA and that they will then lose membership as physicians might not want to be forced to pay the higher dues and/or be forced into joining the AMA. For example, the American Academy of Pediatrics has 55,000 dues-paying members but fewer than 7,000 belong to the AMA.

As an umbrella organization, the AMA could claim to represent the interests of 90 to 95 percent of all practicing physicians; a far larger percentage than they represented previously, even though the physicians would not be paying their dues directly to the AMA. This greater constituency would carry more weight when the AMA discusses legislative issues with policy makers and politicians.

Therefore, to overcome the free rider problem, the AMA has reverted to an organizational structure it rejected almost 60 years ago. It remains to be seen whether the new financing formula will be acceptable to a majority of the AMA's diverse and often contentious members, a federation that includes about 165 specialty societies and state associations.

American Dental Association

The ADA has been among the more effective health associations in overcoming the free rider problem. Membership in the ADA is tied to membership in the local dental society.[15] Part of the dues is remitted to the national organization. A dentist, however, does not need a hospital to practice. Thus, other inducements are necessary to have dentists join their local society. Malpractice insurance, which is sold by the state dental association, is the main benefit. Another service some state dental associations provide is the use of credit cards in patient payment and collection. The ADA also provides some private services in return for part of the dentist's dues: life and disability insurance, retirement plans, and educational programs. Currently, about 70 percent of dentists are members of the ADA and their local societies.

The dues that can be charged for "private" services to induce dentists to join their local societies are less than if membership were required to earn a living, as was previously the case for physicians. For example, a Florida dental society found that nonmembers cited the high annual dues as the main reason for not joining.[16]

American Nurses Association

The ANA is a federation of 54 state nursing associations. A registered nurse who is a member of a state nursing association is automatically a member of the national nursing association. This organizational structure was adopted in 1982. In some states nurses can join the ANA directly and receive benefits from the national association but not benefits from their state association. Although the ANA claims to represent the nation's 2.6 million RNs, as of 2004 only about 6 percent, or fewer than 160,000, RNs were members of the ANA. This low membership percentage has been fairly constant over time.[17]

There are several reasons why such a small portion of all trained nurses are members of nursing associations. Previously, the number of employed nurses as a percentage of the total number of nurses (the participation rate) was approximately 50 percent. Starting in the late 1960s, the participation rate increased, in part because of increased nurses' wages, to where it is now—approximately 80 percent. Those nurses who are not working are generally not seeking employment. Further, many employed nurses are not all working full-time (about 28 percent of employed nurses work part-time). Nurse employment, as mentioned above, tends to vary according to the life cycle of the nurse. After graduation, the nurse participation rate is high. After marriage and the birth of children the participation rate falls, and then it increases as the children become older. In addition, nurses have generally not been the primary earner in a family. Thus, many nurses have not viewed membership in nursing associations as important to their careers or their ability to find a job. Nurses typically sought jobs in locations where their spouse was employed. To many nurses the costs of ANA membership exceeded any economic advantages.

In addition to all of the aforementioned reasons, it has been very difficult for the ANA to overcome the free rider problem. To increase membership, the ANA and state nursing associations are involved in several activities. They are attempting to become the collective bargaining unit for representing hospital-employed nurses. (In 1999 the ANA House of Delegates formed, within the ANA, the United American Nurses, whose purpose is to provide collective bargaining services to nurses.) Once a hospital signs a collective bargaining contract with a nursing association, all RNs in that hospital, as well as future employed nurses, become members of the state and, consequently, the national association. This is the strategy used successfully by unions. The ANA, however, faces intense competition from other unions for representing nurses. These other unions, particularly the Service Employees International Union and the California Nurses Association, have been targeting nurses in other unions to switch to their unions. These intra-nurse organizations have weakened the ANA's role as the representative of nurses.[18]

State nursing associations are also offering various "private" services, such as professional liability insurance, life and health insurance, loans, retirement plans, and discounts on purchases of automobiles, to induce nurses to join. As indicated by its low membership statistics, the ANA has a long way to go before it can state before any legislative body that it represents all nurses. (Before the ANA can represent the interests of nurses, it must first determine what those common interests are, i.e., whether the issues are related to women's concerns generally, broad health issues, or more narrow issues representing the economic self-interest of RNs.)

American Hospital Association

There are about 5,800 AHA-registered hospitals in the United States. Of these, close to 5,000 hospitals, or more than 80 percent, belong to the AHA. Membership dues vary according to the type and size of the organization (hospitals, healthcare systems, postacute patient care facilities, and hospital-affiliated educational programs). The AHA also has 37,000 individual members. Hospitals can also join their state associations without having to join the AHA.[19]

When hospitals were reimbursed according to their costs, the size of their membership dues was not a concern. As hospital occupancies fell and the hospital market became more price competitive, hospitals have been attempting to reduce their costs. In the years ahead, more hospitals will likely attempt to receive a free ride from the AHA's legislative activities. Similar to the other associations discussed here, the AHA offers a number of private services, such as educational programs and data-reporting services, to make it economically beneficial for hospitals to remain as members.

Costs of Organizing a Group

The greater the costs of organizing a group, the less likely that the group will be formed. Greater similarity of interests among its potential members and ease in overcoming the free rider problem, as in the case of unions, lower the costs of organizing a group and increase the likelihood that an association will be formed.

Another important organizational cost relates to a group's size. The larger the group, the more difficult it will be to organize its members. Although unions are very large today, the first unions to organize were small craft unions, such as printers, workers in the building trades, and shoemakers. Employees in large factories, such as automobile production workers, organized later because of the greater costs to organize.[20] These union locals are then joined together in a national organization, which in turn provides collective benefits to each local. (A trade-off exists with regard to the optimum group size. The larger the interest group, the greater will be its organizational costs; however, the larger the group, the more likely are politicians to be receptive to its demands.)

This pattern of growth was very similar for the AMA. Physicians were more likely to join the county society for the benefits the local society could provide. The AMA was then a federation of local societies, as were unions.

In addition, the fewer the number of members in a group, the easier is it for the group to monitor the performance of its members. Peer pressure can be placed on each firm or professional to contribute to the group. Each firm will perceive that it has a large stake in the outcome because the benefits will be distributed over a smaller number of firms.

Size of the Potential Benefits

As the potential benefits from legislation increase, the rewards to the firms from organizing are greater. If the potential benefits are relatively small, then each firm is unlikely to contribute (invest) a great deal of money to receive small benefits. However, as the potential benefits increase, so should the firm's willingness to invest.

One major reason changes in the payment and delivery of medical services occurred is that the potential benefits of instituting changes became very large to two groups: the federal government and business. (Government and business developed a "concentrated interest" in cost containment.) As expenditures for medical care kept rising rapidly, the federal government and business had to keep funding these increases. Businesses found it increasingly difficult to pass on these cost increases in the form of higher prices. The federal government was concerned about having to continually raise the Medicare payroll tax (and the wage base to which it applied) to pay for hospital benefits under Medicare. The potential savings from more stringent cost-containment policies made such efforts worthwhile to both groups.

Conversely, in those cases where the benefits from regulation have declined, the regulated firms and their associations were not willing to spend a great deal to maintain those legislated benefits. An example of this occurred in the railroad and airlines industry. The respective regulatory agencies had set high (relative to their cost) prices for both rail and air travel. However, profits from these high (relative to cost) prices were eroded by entry of new firms (trucks), and by nonprice competition from existing firms (the airlines). These regulated firms eventually concluded that the benefits of regulation were no longer sufficient to spend the necessary funds to maintain their regulated status. (The reasons for deregulation are discussed more fully in Chapter 5.)

Uncertainty

If the effects of legislative change are uncertain, that is, if it is not clear who will benefit and who will lose or what the size of those expected benefits or losses will be, then a group is less likely to organize to achieve favorable legislation or forestall unfavorable legislation. Advocates of the status quo are more often represented than proponents for change because both the size of the benefits and the number of recipients are more uncertain than the number of those benefiting from the change.

Those benefiting from the status quo are more knowledgeable regarding any change in their status. There is often more information available to the existing firms than to potential beneficiaries or losers. When legislation is proposed that will impose costs on existing firms (e.g., mandating pollution-control devices on electric utilities), these same firms will be more knowledgeable about the costs of that legislation than will the beneficiaries of the legislation's positive effects. Thus, the existing firms are more likely to organize and represent their interests.

Greater certainty about the effects of legislation and about which groups receive the benefits or bear the burden increases the likelihood that those groups will organize to represent their interests. Research that provides information as to the consequences of legislation, and the subsequent publicizing of that information, should increase certainty as to the legislation's effects. This should increase the number of groups organizing to represent their interests.

The following examples illustrate the importance of uncertainty in determining legislative outcomes.

An example of producer groups that have been legislatively successful are the auto industry and the auto union, who were able to impose "voluntary" import quotas on Japanese autos in the early 1980s. The auto industry has few firms and one union, the United Automobile Workers (UAW). Auto plants are also located in many states, which increases the number of senators who would favor such protectionist legislation. The benefits of such a restriction to both the industry and its union are known with fairly high certainty. The costs are diffuse; they are borne by auto purchasers. Although the higher auto prices that result from this protection are obvious to some auto buyers, they are not obvious to many others.

Further, the proponents of voluntary quotas attempt to create uncertainty about the cost of this protection by claiming that if auto workers were laid off, the public would have to pay increased taxes to care for unemployed workers. Thus, the costs to the public of restrictive trade policies are diffuse and uncertain. (To limit the effect of such protectionism on their sales, Japanese auto firms have built plants in the United States.)

Previously, medical societies were successful in having state legislation enacted that made it difficult for persons to start prepaid (HMO) health plans. (These plans could not advertise, they had to be nonprofit, they could not exclude any physician from participating, and physicians had to make up a majority of the board.) Organized medicine viewed such organizations as competitors to solo, fee-for-service physicians and wanted to eliminate such competition. Few of these organizations were available before the mid-1970s; thus, the public was unaware of the advantages of participating in this form of medical delivery system. The public also had a diffuse interest with regard to medical expenditures. The potential beneficiaries of prepaid plans therefore did not organize to represent their interests. Physician organizations, because they had a concentrated interest in how medical services were paid for and delivered, understood the potential consequences to their members if prepaid health plans were established.

Another example where current producers are more knowledgeable about the effects of proposed legislation is the issue of PPOs. A PPO is an organization of providers who have agreed to sell their services at a lower price than the prevailing market price. To receive the price reductions, patients can only go to those providers who participate in the PPO. PPOs may be started by insurance companies or by providers themselves. If PPOs did not exist, then patients would not be locked in to a particular set of providers (e.g., hospitals, physicians, and dentists). Although all dentists are able to join a PPO, they would have to accept lower fees to do so. PPOs are therefore a means of stimulating price competition among providers.

The ADA and state dental societies have attempted to prohibit the development of dental PPOs by making them illegal. Aware of the negative effect on their members' incomes if dental PPOs are established, dental societies in various states have lobbied their legislatures to have them prohibited. The beneficiaries of dental care PPOs, namely the patients and purchasers of dental services, generally do not know what PPOs are, let alone know their beneficial effects. This lack of information and uncertainty over the size of the benefits has kept the public out of the controversy and left it up to the dental societies and the insurance companies to determine the outcome of state legislation regarding dental PPOs.

Similar in its effects to having PPOs being declared illegal, are any willing provider laws (promoted by medical and dental associations). These anticompetitive laws enacted by states allow any provider to participate in a PPO. Any willing provider laws discourage providers from discounting their fees to insurers as they cannot be assured of receiving a greater volume of patients.

The development of new healthcare delivery systems has been inhibited because of lack of information and uncertainty. Existing providers have a better understanding of the adverse effects on their incomes of new delivery systems, such as HMOs and PPOs, while the beneficiaries—the public—are unaware. Potential new firms are not represented in the legislative arena. Existing physicians, and the medical societies that represent them, are already organized and are aware of the effects of innovation on their incomes. This is why changes in the status quo in medicine have taken so long.

Concluding Comments

It is to be expected that groups with a special interest will lobby for their members' interests before Congress. However, to understand why certain special-interest groups are more successful than others in achieving their legislative demands requires an analysis of the organization of an interest group itself. If a group is to be formed, health professionals and firms must find it in their interest to join. If they can be coerced into joining, no one can receive a free ride. If coercion is not possible, then sufficient economic incentives must be provided to make it economically worthwhile to join. Otherwise the organization will not be able to raise sufficient funds to lobby for the group's legislative interests.

In the past, membership in the county medical society was a necessity if a physician wanted to practice in a hospital and earn an income. At that time it was important for the national organization (the AMA) to convince the local organizations to belong to the national organization. The membership structure of the ADA required dentists who joined the local society to be members in the national organization, too. Local associations have been more important to the careers and income goals of health professionals than national associations. Important to the success of the national organization is its ability to tie membership in the local society to the national association.

To induce health professionals to join their local society requires that the perceived benefits of membership exceed the professional's costs (dues). The medical society offered the strongest of incentives, a physician's ability to practice. Other societies (and medical societies currently) attempt to sell private services to their members, including journal subscriptions, educational programs, retirement plans, and malpractice insurance. To the extent that these can be offered at a lower price than the individual can otherwise purchase them, the individual has an incentive to join. However, the amount of dues that can be raised in this way to support lobbying efforts at the national level depends on the value to the practitioner of these economic incentives.[21]

American Nurses Association

The nursing associations have had the most difficulty in organizing their members. The interests of their members are not as similar nor as singular as those of other professions. Nurses have fewer incentives to join their local society, there are a greater number of members to organize, and their members are less aware of the potential legislative benefits of membership. Nursing associations have been ambivalent in acting as a unionizing agent for nurses. However, as other unions have tried to organize nurses, nursing associations have begun to assist in unionizing for fear of losing members. Unless nurse associations can replicate the unions in overcoming the free rider problem, it is unlikely that the reasons for low membership in state and national nursing associations can be easily overcome.

American Dental Association

The ADA has many of the necessary ingredients for a successful health association. Its members are relatively homogeneous, and they are required to join the national organization as a condition of joining the local dental society. However, the amount of dues the local society can charge is limited by the nature of the economic benefits they can provide. The ADA has been relatively successful in the legislative arena. Also, state dental societies have been able to reduce the potential for price competition among dentists by limiting dentists' productivity increases; the tasks that can be performed by nondentists, such as dental auxiliaries, have been limited by state law so that productivity increases do not exceed increases in demand for services. Further, potential substitutes such as denturists (dental technicians that sell dentures directly to the public) are legal in only seven states, and this only since 1977. (In two of the seven states, denturists either have a limited scope of practice or they need to work with a dentist.)[22] Dentists have been relatively successful in reducing—to a great degree, legislatively—their competition.

Although the ADA has many attributes of a successful association, it is concerned over its ability to be the sole representative and voice of the dental profession. Strains within the dental profession have emerged. For example, various groups within dentistry, such as dental examiners, dental schools, and dental researchers, believe themselves to be underrepresented in ADA's House of Delegates. There is also a growing divergence among dentists in their economic interests; for example, solo-practice dentists are opposed to corporate dental clinics. These concerns led to the formation of a special study group to examine fragmentation of the association and the profession.[23]

The changing economic situation facing dentistry, starting in the early 1980s, has also been an important reason for the profession's concern. There was a large increase in the number of new dentists by the mid-1980s because of the past expansion of dental schools. As a result of government funding of dental schools and the applicability of the antitrust laws to all the health professions in the early 1980s, competition among dentists increased. Consequently, there was an increase in the number of corporate dental clinics, advertising, and dental PPOs as well as a greater emphasis on cost containment by business and insurance companies. In 1980 there were 60 dental schools, and first-year enrollees were 6,132. However, by the late 1980s the dental profession was successful in reducing entry into the profession. By 2005 the number of dental schools was reduced to 56 with a corresponding decrease in the number of first-year students, to 4,300.[24] As the supply of dentists increases at a slower rate, eventually some of the competitive pressures facing dentists will begin to moderate.

American Hospital Association

The AHA faces difficult times in its role of hospital advocate. The federal government is attempting to limit increases in Medicare hospital expenditures; there is increased competition among hospitals; many hospitals have consolidated into large systems, physicians are shifting more inpatient services into an outpatient setting where they may have a financial interest; and the growing divergence in economic interests between different types of hospitals—small and rural hospitals, teaching hospitals, large hospital systems, and for-profit hospitals—makes it more difficult for the AHA to lobby for legislation beneficial to all its constituencies. Increased legislative benefits for one group of hospitals in a Medicare budget-neutral environment is likely to come only at the expense of other hospitals.

However, the ability of the AHA, working through its state associations, to energize board members and constituents of local hospitals, located in each congressional district, has made the AHA a formidable interest group.

American Medical Association

Although still politically influential, the AMA is unlikely to recover the legislative influence it once had. This decline in influence is due to four reasons. First, its membership has become more heterogeneous with differing economic interests: there are wide age differences among physicians, more women and minorities have entered the profession, and more physicians are working as part of large managed care organizations rather than as fee-for-service practitioners. With the rapid expansion in the supply of physicians, physicians are engaged in greater market competition. Physicians disagree on the use of report cards and "pay for performance" for evaluating physicians. And favoring one type of payment and delivery system (solo practice and fee-for-service) over others (group practice and capitation), brings the AMA into conflict with physicians who work in these other settings.

Second, the new Medicare physician-payment system forced each medical specialty into conflict with every other specialty. The "budget neutrality" of the legislation split the medical profession into specialty groups with opposing concentrated interests. Increased fees for one physician group can only come at the expense of others. Each specialty was forced to represent its interests in the legislative marketplace.

Third, the sharp decline in the AMA's membership and dues has decreased the funds available for lobbying and limited its ability to claim before Congress that it represents the interests of all physicians.

Fourth, the rise of competing groups with a concentrated interest has affected the AMA's legislative success.[25] Podiatrists and chiropractors have formed their own lobbying organizations, as the potential benefits from organizing have increased.[26] Other professionals, such as physician assistants (PAs) and nurse practitioners, are also seeking to have greater leeway in the types of tasks they are permitted to perform and to be reimbursed independently of the physician for their services under public programs. Being included in public programs, such as Medicare and Medicaid, offers greatly increased incomes to members of these other professions. Changing legislation to enable members of these other associations to perform a greater number of tasks offers large potential rewards to these practitioners.

Other interest groups have also formed to represent their members' interests. Business groups, such as the Business Roundtable, realize that large savings can be achieved from increased legislative involvement. Businesses are opposed to legislation that would increase their employees' health costs (such as the AMA-backed patient's bill of rights and allowing physicians to collectively negotiate with insurers), while favoring legislation (such as managed care) that offers the potential for reducing the rise in their employees' health insurance premiums. Similarly, the large potential savings to the federal government from reducing expenditures on public medical programs provides the federal government with an incentive to represent, legislatively, its own interests more strongly.

An increase in the number of organized groups with divergent economic interests raises the cost and thereby diminishes the likelihood that any one group will be successful in achieving all of its legislative aims. The rise of opposing interest groups diminishes the AMA's political influence.

Study Questions

1. Why is it necessary for an organization to overcome the "free rider" problem if it is to be successful in achieving its legislative objectives?
2. What are some of the approaches health associations use to overcome the "free rider" problem?
3. Discuss the characteristics that an association should have if it is to be successful in achieving its legislative agenda.
4. How has the federal government's "budget-neutral" financing methods under Medicare (RBRVS for physicians and DRGs for hospitals) affected the AMA's and the AHA's ability to represent their constituents' interests?
5. Of the ADA and the ANA, which organization is more likely to be successful in representing the legislative interests of its members?

Notes

1. Data on internal rates of return to a physician's education from the 1930s through the 1980s are summarized in Paul J. Feldstein, *Health Care Economics*, 6th ed. (Clifton Park, NY: Thomson Delmar Learning, 2005), 340–42. Data on nurses' incomes compared to those of comparable professions are presented on pages 397–399.
2. Bureau of Labor Statistics, U.S. Department of Labor, "Dentists," *Occupational Outlook Handbook, 2004–05 Edition*, http://www.bls.gov/oco/ocos072.htm.
3. American Nursing Association, "Who We Are: Frequently Asked Questions: Membership," http://www.nursingworld.org/about/faq.htm; U.S. Department of Health and Human Services, Bureau of Health Professions, Division of Nursing, *The Registered Nurse Population: March 2000: Findings from the National Sample Survey of Registered Nurses*, http://bhpr.hrsa.gov/healthworkforce/reports/rnsurvey/rnss1.htm.
4. James G. Burrow, *AMA: Voice of American Medicine* (Baltimore, MD: The Johns Hopkins Press, 1963), 7–8.
5. If limits were placed on the tasks physicians could perform, then different educational and licensure requirements would be appropriate. There has never been a career ladder in medicine. All physicians take

the same basic four years of college, then four years of medical school, and then a residency requirement. It does not matter that the training of a family practitioner can be accomplished in fewer years or with a different curriculum than for a neurosurgeon. Thus, a physician can be an anesthesiologist with no additional training, with additional training, or with board certification. They can all perform the same procedures and charge the same price. A career ladder would make it easier to become a physician; nurses could become physicians with some additional training. It would have been more difficult for the AMA to limit the supply of physicians if advancement had been based on tests and additional training.

6. Malpractice should be an effective limitation on the tasks performed by a physician. However, the malpractice system has not always performed up to expectations in this regard.

7. American Medical Association, *Physician Characteristics and Distribution in the U.S.* (Chicago: American Medical Association, 2005).

8. American Hospital Association, "About the AHA," http://www.aha.org/aha/about/about.html.

9. Michael Heaney, "At the Root of its Success: AHA's Lobbying Muscle Comes from Strong Network of Local Advocates," *Modern Healthcare*, July 19, 2004, 23.

10. For a discussion of the free rider problem, as well as its application to unions, see Mancur Olson, *The Logic of Collective Action* (Cambridge, MA: Harvard University Press, 1965).

11. Ibid., 133. Also, in a study of a large number of interest groups, Walker found that the proliferation of nonprofit interest groups in the past 20 years, that is, groups whose constituents were not members of the same occupation, was a result of financial support from outside sources, rather than from the sale of private services to its members. These groups were generally the least homogeneous in membership. Examples of these "citizen" groups are civil rights groups, peace organizations, and groups representing the handicapped. The funding required to start and maintain these groups came from government agencies through grants and contracts, for example, to increase public understanding or train professionals. The government agencies attempted to further their own political objectives through this funding to outside groups (p. 402). Other sources of funds for such groups came from patrons of political action, for example, the UAW and aging organizations. Without such outside support these groups would not have been able to overcome the free rider problem and generate sufficient funds to

organize. Jack L. Walker, "The Origins and Maintenance of Interest Groups in America," *The American Political Science Review* 77 (1983): 390–406.

12. The Mundt resolution, which was declared unconstitutional in the mid-1960s, required the entire medical staff of a hospital to be members of the county medical society in order for the hospital to be approved for intern and residency training. Physicians wanted their hospitals to have interns and residents, as they increase physician productivity. Membership in the county medical society was also a prerequisite if a physician wanted to take examinations for various specialty boards. For a more complete discussion of the control mechanisms used by organized medicine over the behavior of individual physicians, see Reuben Kessel, "Price Discrimination in Medicine," *Journal of Law and Economics* 1 (1958): 20–53.

13. For more information on the AMA and its membership services, see the AMA web site: http://www.ama-assn.org.

14. Michael Romano, "AMA Approves Plans to Become Umbrella Group," *Modern Healthcare*, June 24, 2002, 8–9.

15. For more information on the ADA, see the ADA web site: http://www.ADA.org. Membership in the ADA is a three-tiered system. "The system by bylaw, that a dentist must pay dues to the component society, constituent society, and ADA in order to join the local dental society."

    In April 1972, four dentists sued the ADA on grounds that the three-tiered membership system violated the antitrust laws. The dentists lost and the ADA's membership system was retained.

16. *The ADA News*, October 24, 1983, 2. At the time the annual dues were $400.

17. For more information on RNs, see the following web site: http://www.nursingworld.org.

18. Melanie Evans, "Laboring for Nurse Unions," *Modern Healthcare*, May 23, 2005.

19. For more information on the AHA, see the AHA web site: http://www.aha.org/aha/about/index.html.

20. Olson, *The Logic of Collective Action*, 66.

21. The less price-elastic the demand for these private services, the higher the price at which they can be sold.

22. The seven states are Maine (1977), Arizona (1978), Colorado (1979), Oregon (1980), Idaho (1982), Montana (1984), and Washington (1994). For more information, see: http://www.international-denturist.org/index.html.

23. "Final Report of the Special Committee on Fragmentation of the

Association and the Profession," mimeograph (Chicago: American Dental Association, April 14, 1986).

For information on current ADA policies, see: http://www.ada.org/prof/resources/positions/doc_policies.pdf.

24. Data for 2005 are from ADA web site: http://www.ada.org/ada/prod/survey/faq.asp#schools.

25. According to Becker, the political effectiveness of a group is determined not just by its absolute efficiency, that is, "its absolute skill at controlling free riding—but by its efficiency relative to the efficiency of other groups." Gary S. Becker, "A Theory of Competition Among Pressure Groups For Political Influence," *Quarterly Journal of Economics* 98 (1983): 371–400.

26. In addition to a change in the magnitude of benefits (or costs), other reasons an unorganized constituency may become legislatively involved are the ability to overcome the free rider problem and a reduction in both the costs of information and the costs of organizing.

THE DEMAND FOR LEGISLATION BY HEALTH ASSOCIATIONS

After completing this chapter, the reader should be able to

- provide examples of "demand-increasing" legislation favored by health associations,
- describe methods associations have used to discourage price competition,
- explain how the price competition for patients was eliminated with the initial benefit structure hospitals designed for Blue Cross,
- compare heath professionals as a complement or a substitute depending on who receive fees for service,
- identify medical association approaches for decreasing competition from substitute providers,
- assess the political positions of hospital and nurse associations in regard to an increase of foreign-trained nurses to alleviate nursing shortages,

Health interest groups demand legislation that is in their members' interests. It is necessary, however, to go beyond that statement. Health associations, such as the AMA, have claimed that they are educational organizations, not trade associations representing the narrow economic interests of their members.[1] Further, such associations claim that the legislation they favor is in the public's interest; they are concerned with quality rather than economic interests. Thus, it is important to be specific about the types of legislation on which health associations take a position. For example, do health associations such as the AMA favor measures that increase quality, regardless of the effect on their members' incomes, or do they favor only those quality measures that increase their members' incomes?

It is necessary to use a framework for examining health legislation. The framework lets us understand which types of legislation are in the economic interests of health associations' members. It indicates the types of legislation health associations favor or oppose, because it is not always obvious how certain types of legislation promote the economic interests of association members. The AMA has had a great deal of political influence at both the state and federal level. Understanding which legislation is preferred and which is opposed by the AMA explains much of the type of health legislation this country has or has not had, particularly in the period up to the 1980s. This model also helps to predict the types of legislation health associations will favor or oppose in the years ahead.

First, it is necessary to describe what is meant by the economic interests of health association members. After all, some health associations, such as the AHA and the Association of American Medical Colleges, represent nonprofit organizations. Once the economic interests of health association members are defined, it becomes possible to demonstrate how particular legislation works to enhance members' interests. The validity of the proposed framework can be tested by how well it predicts the political positions of the various health associations. Without a definition of interests and a legislative framework, it would not be obvious how specific legislation promotes the economic interests of the members of a health association. The final section of this chapter discusses the implications of the political behavior of health associations on the financing, quality, and organization of the healthcare delivery system.

The Motivation of Health Associations

Health associations demand legislation that serves the interests of their members. Without a definition of those interests, however, it would not be obvious how specific legislation promotes the members' perception of these interests.

Health professionals and health organizations, such as hospitals, have many goals. Even within the same profession, individuals place different weights on what they perceive to be their self-interest. The tendency, therefore, is to make the definition of self-interest complex. However, if the definition is complex and encompasses this diversity, or if different motivations are specified for each piece of legislation, then it is not possible to develop a good predictive model. Although it may seem more realistic to develop a complex goal statement, it is easier to evaluate the effects of legislation using a simple one. Besides, *unless the membership easily understands the goal that its association is pursuing, the members may be distressed over the activities in which the association is engaged.* The true test of whether the simply defined goal accurately measures member self-interest is how well it predicts the association's legislative behavior.

The legislative goal of associations with individuals as members—whether physicians, dentists, nurses, or optometrists—is assumed to be maximizing the incomes of its current members. Health professionals are no different from other individuals; they will say that they have many goals, and that income is only one of them, but income is the only goal that all the members have in common. (Goals such as increased autonomy and control over their practice are highly correlated with increased incomes. Thus, income is a more general goal.)

Nonprofit institutions—including hospitals, some Blue Cross plans, medical and dental schools—cannot retain profits. Medical and dental schools are assumed to be interested in maximizing the prestige of their institution. Prestige for a medical school is defined as having students who wish to become professors and researchers themselves, a faculty that is primarily interested in research, and a low student-to-faculty ratio. Little prestige accrues to a medical school that trains students to enter family practice or to practice in underserved areas.

Until the mid-1980s, when hospitals were reimbursed according to their costs, hospitals were also interested in maximizing their prestige, which is indicated by its size and the number of facilities and services it offers. Administrators of large, prestigious hospitals were held in esteem by their peers and earned higher incomes. Each hospital attempted to become a medical center. The availability of a full range of services also made it easier for the hospital to attract physicians to its staff.

Beginning in the early 1980s, however, hospital objectives began to change. The payment system for hospital care went from cost-based reimbursement to fixed prices; hospitals engaged in price competition to increase their volume of patients from insurers and HMOs; and low-cost substitutes for hospitals, such as outpatient surgery centers, began to reduce hospital utilization, as did utilization review programs under managed care.[2] As these changes occurred, hospitals became more concerned with survival than with emulating major teaching institutions. Even teaching hospitals began to act as though their futures were in doubt. Hospitals began to minimize their costs, dropped money-losing services and patients, and gave greater consideration to the profitability of their investments. To succeed in a more competitive environment, hospitals attempted to minimize their costs and to act as though they were trying to maximize their profits.

Blue Cross and Blue Shield plans were originally started by hospitals and physicians, respectively. Hospitals provided the initial capital to Blue Cross plans and controlled the organization. The same was true for medical societies and Blue Shield plans. It was not until the 1970s that these nonprofit organizations separated from the providers that controlled them. Until that time, therefore, the objectives of Blue Cross and Blue Shield plans were to serve their providers' interests.

During the period when Blue Cross and Blue Shield were controlled by their respective providers, their methods of provider payment and their benefit structure were in accordance with the economic interests of hospitals and physicians. These policies also coincided with the interests of the organizations' managers. Nonprofit organizations wanted to grow. A larger organization provides management with greater responsibility, and that justifies higher incomes. Like any nonprofit bureaucracy, these organizations also had some form of satisfying behavior as a goal; namely, extra personnel, larger facilities, and higher wages than if these organizations were in a very competitive industry.

As the healthcare sector became more competitive in the early 1980s, competition between Blue Cross and Blue Shield plans and commercial insurance companies increased. To survive in this new marketplace, Blue Cross and Blue Shield plans began to merge. Starting in the early 1990s, Blue Cross plans, such as California Blue Cross, began converting themselves into for-profit organizations. The behavior of both nonprofit and for-profit Blue Cross plans became similar to for-profit insurance companies. By attempting to minimize costs, increase market share, and respond to employer demands on benefit design, Blue Cross and Blue Shield acted as though they were attempting to maximize profits. An adversarial relationship began to replace the previously cooperative association with hospitals and physicians.[3] In analyzing the legislative behavior of Blue Cross and Blue Shield plans, it is important to keep in mind the periods when their objectives differed.

Although differences existed in the objectives of health associations representing health professionals, hospitals, medical and dental schools, and Blue Cross and Blue Shield plans, the members of these associations all tried to make as much money as possible. They would then retain it for themselves, as did health professionals, or spend it to achieve prestige goals, as medical schools did and hospitals previously did. The incomes of employees of prestigious institutions are likely to exceed those of less prestigious institutions. Thus, the objective underlying the demand for legislation is the same for each health association. *Each association attempts to achieve for its members through legislation what cannot be achieved through a competitive market, namely, a monopoly position.* Increased monopoly power and the ability to price as a monopolist seller of services was, and is, the best way for an association to achieve its goal.

Framework for Analyzing Legislative Behavior

There are five types of legislation that health associations demand on behalf of their members: demand-increasing legislation, legislation to secure the highest method of reimbursement, legislation to reduce the price and/or increase the quantity of complements, legislation to decrease the availability of and/or increase the price of substitutes, and legislation to limit increases in supply. As government policy shifted from increasing to decreasing health expenditures (given the concern over the Medicare Trust Fund deficit and rising Medicare Part B expenditures) the emphasis devoted to each of these types of legislation by health interest groups has changed over time.

This model has several caveats. The above model should predict an association's political position on legislation according to the earlier definition of its members' interests. However, it may occasionally be observed that an association takes a political position different than what is expected. Before concluding that the above framework is inaccurate, the following must be determined.

Is the association's preferred position no longer politically possible? No health professional association favors reexamination for licensure. Some of its members may not be able to pass the exam. If the examination is made so simple that all members can pass, then nonmembers would claim they should be allowed to enter the profession because they could pass the examination. If there is a great deal of pressure from the media, for example, for reexamination, the profession may propose a less costly alternative—continuing education. The association would not normally propose continuing education, as it imposes some costs on its members, but to forestall an even more costly policy the association comes out in favor of it. Thus, the association's policy on continuing education, although not its preferred position, is consistent with the model's predictions.

Another example where it may appear that an association's political position diverges from its members' interests occurs when the cost of taking a position exceeds its potential benefits. The AHA's position on the applicability of minimum wage laws to hospital employees is an example. Minimum wage laws increase the cost of labor to hospitals. For many years the AHA was successful in exempting hospitals from such legislation. As hospital wages began to increase, most hospital employees earned in excess of the minimum wage. Thus, the law's applicability to hospitals would have had a small effect. When removal of the hospital exemption was once again proposed, the AHA decided not to oppose it. Not only would the effect have been small, but the AHA determined that the legislation would have passed over its objections. The AHA decided that it would be a needless loss of political capital to oppose it.

Except for these caveats mentioned, health associations are expected to act in accordance with their members' economic interests. The five types of legislation each association either favors or opposes are based on the above economic framework.

Demand-Increasing Legislation

An association favors demand-increasing legislation because an increase in demand, with a given supply, will result in an increase in price, an increase in total revenue, and consequently, an increase in incomes or net revenues.

The most obvious way to increase the demand for the services of an association's members is to have the government subsidize the purchase of insurance for the provider's services. Health providers, however, do not want the government to insure everyone. Instead, the providers' demand for insurance subsidies was always proposed in relation to specific population groups in society, such as people with low incomes. The reason for selective government subsidies is twofold. First, people with higher incomes presumably have private insurance coverage or can afford to purchase a provider's services. The greatest increase in demand would result from extending coverage to those unable to pay. Second, extending government subsidies to those currently able to pay for the services would greatly increase the cost of the program to the government. A greater commitment of government expenditures would result in the government's developing a concentrated interest in controlling the provider's prices, utilization, and expenditures. Thus, when health associations favor demand subsidies, they are always in relation to specific population groups or services rather than to the population at large.

The American Medical Association.

Examples of the above approach include the AMA's positions on national health insurance, Medicare, and Blue Shield. The AMA successfully defeated President Truman's national health insurance proposal in 1948 because subsidies would have been provided to all, regardless of income level. The AMA's opposition to Medicare was similarly based on the fact that all the aged, regardless of income, were to be subsidized (see Chapter 9). Instead, the AMA favored a system of tax credits for purchasing health insurance, which would decline as a person's income rose.

During the 1990s, as concern with the federal deficit increased and federal funds to subsidize those with low incomes were less available, the AMA favored an employer mandate, whereby employers are required to purchase health insurance on behalf of their employees. An employer mandate would increase the demand for physician services by requiring the working uninsured to have private coverage. It would also move low-income employees and their families off Medicaid onto private insurance, which also reimburses providers at a higher rate.

In the 1930s and 1940s when medical societies developed (and controlled) Blue Shield, it only provided coverage for physician services (not for physician substitutes) and paid the physician's bill in full only if the patient's income was below a certain level (originally $7,500 a year). A low-income person purchasing Blue Shield would increase her use of physician services and not be concerned with which physician had a lower price. (The demand for physician services was increased, and physicians did not have to compete on price for that business.) If the subscriber's income exceeded $7,500, the physician was permitted to charge the patient an additional amount above the Blue Shield payment (referred to as "balance billing"). Higher-income patients could afford to pay more.

The American Dental Association.

The ADA's major demand-increasing effort has been to expand private insurance coverage for dental services. Insurance is generally purchased for events that are very expensive, such as hospital care and in-hospital physician services, and that have a low probability of occurring. Dental expenditures, which are relatively small, expected, and not catastrophic, are therefore not insurable in the same sense as hospital or surgical services; in fact, dental prepayment is not really insurance but a form of forced savings.

If special incentives to purchase dental insurance did not exist, most people would just pay for dental care when they needed it. The use of dental services is also highly related to income.[4] Thus, a major reason for the growth in dental insurance has been the favorable tax treatment of employer-paid health insurance premiums. Such contributions are not considered part of the employee's income; the employee does not have to pay federal, state, or Social Security taxes on employer-paid health benefits.

During the 1970s, when the demand for dental insurance grew rapidly, the top income-tax bracket was 70 percent. In addition, the person would have to pay Social Security and state income taxes on additional earned income. For middle- and high-income people, the after-tax value of a $1,000 raise would be reduced by these three taxes, leaving the individual with perhaps half of that amount to spend on out-of-pocket medical payments, dental care, vision benefits, and so on. If instead the employer used the $1,000 to purchase more comprehensive health insurance for the employee, the employee could receive $1,000 worth of health benefits.

The exclusion of employer-paid health benefits from the employee's taxable income results in a large revenue loss to the federal and state governments. The lost federal income tax revenue and Social Security tax revenue (excluding state taxes) from this tax exclusion in 2004 was estimated to be about $190 billion dollars.[5] The beneficiaries of this tax exclusion are clearly those in the upper-income groups. Eliminating or "capping" the amount of employer-paid health benefits that are excluded from taxable income has been advocated in some healthcare reform proposals as a means of raising revenues to finance health benefits for those with low incomes. Economists have also favored eliminating or reducing this tax-subsidy for the purchase of health insurance because it would make employees more cost conscious in their choice of health plans; selecting a more expensive health plan would have to be paid with after-tax dollars.

The ADA's major legislative strategy has been to defeat any such tax cap. If a tax cap were passed, employees would want less comprehensive health benefits because they would have to pay for additional benefits with after-tax dollars. The ADA believes, and rightly so, that if the tax discount for purchasing dental insurance were eliminated, the incentive for employees to purchase such insurance would decline. With less dental insurance, consumers would have to pay the full price of dental care. The demand for dental care would decline and consumers would be more inclined to "shop" among dentists for the lowest price.

Additional approaches ADA has used to increase the demand for dental care involve lobbying to include dental benefits in federal employees' health benefits; permitting dependents of military personnel to have free choice of civilian dentists, even though military dental clinics are available; including dental benefits as part of Medicare Part B; lobbying for increased funding of dental benefits as part of state Medicaid programs; and promoting the inclusion of dental care as part of the benefits of HMOs.[6]

The American Nurses Association.

The ANA has favored three types of demand-increasing legislation. The first are proposals that increase the demand for medical services. An example is the ANA's support for national health insurance. Increases in demand for medical services would increase the demand for institutions in which registered nurses are employed, thereby increasing the demand for registered nurses. However, because health insurance coverage for hospital care is more extensive than for any other delivery settings (and two-thirds of registered nurses work in hospitals), nurse associations have also favored other demand-increasing proposals.

For example, the ANA has favored requiring minimum nurse staffing ratios in hospitals as well as mandating a minimum number of registered nurses on the staffs of nursing homes and home health agencies for certification purposes. In 1999, the California state nurse's association was successful in having the state enact minimum nurse-to-patient staffing ratios that were higher than current hospital staffing ratios. Nurse associations in a number of other states have similarly promoted nurse-to-patient ratios in hospitals and other healthcare facilities.

Second, nurse associations have opposed hospital attempts to substitute lower-paid nurse aides to perform more of the tasks currently performed by registered nurses, which would decrease the demand for registered nurses.[7]

A third type of demand proposal nurse associations favor is one that widens the nurse's role, that is, increases the number of tasks nurses are legally able to perform. The registered nurses' value to the institution increases as they are permitted to perform more, and higher valued, tasks. The demand for their services will increase, and consequently, their incomes will increase. In attempting to increase their tasks, nurses have come in conflict with the AMA, however. The AMA fears that relaxing state laws that limit the scope of what nurses with advanced training can do would decrease the demand for physicians.[8]

As nurses work to increase their roles, they wage a struggle in the legislative marketplace to prevent other health professionals, such as licensed practical nurses from performing tasks previously reserved to registered nurses. The ANA is also in competition with physician's assistants over which profession will be able to perform tasks previously reserved to physicians.

The health professional association that is successful in enabling its members to increase their role, while preventing other health professionals from encroaching on their own tasks, will be able to increase the demand, hence the incomes, of its members. Examples of the legislative conflict over state practice acts are the optometrists' attempts to increase their role at the expense of ophthalmologists—as well as the struggles of psychologists versus psychiatrists, obstetricians versus nurse-midwives, and podiatrists versus orthopedic surgeons.

The American Hospital Association.

The initial approach hospitals used to increase the demand for their services was the establishment and control of Blue Cross. When hospitals started Blue Cross, Blue Cross only paid the costs of hospital care. Even if it was less expensive to perform diagnostics in an outpatient setting, for a patient with Blue Cross coverage it was less expensive to have it performed in the hospital. Patients with Blue Cross did not have to pay any additional hospital costs. High-cost hospitals were not at a price disadvantage with low-cost hospitals, thereby precluding price competition for Blue Cross patients. Further, every Blue Cross plan required the participation of at least 75 percent of the hospitals in its area. This requirement precluded Blue Cross from contracting with only a lower-cost panel of hospitals.

As the price of hospital care became free to Blue Cross subscribers, hospital use increased. Hospitals were reimbursed generously by Blue Cross for their services.

Legislatively, the AHA favored government subsidies to stimulate the demand for hospital services by the aged and the poor. Medicare, which provided generous hospital coverage for the aged, increased the demand for hospitals by a high-user group with generally low incomes. Hospitals have been in the forefront of lobbying efforts to receive federal subsidies for "uncompensated care"; that is, the provision of hospital care to the poor, for which they are not reimbursed. In the 1990s' debate over national health insurance, the AHA favored an employer mandate, which would increase the demand for private health insurance by those who are uninsured and by those whose hospital bills are being paid by Medicaid.

The Association of American Medical Colleges.

The Association of American Medical Colleges has favored legislation, at both state and federal levels, that provides such schools with unrestricted operating subsidies. Such subsidies would increase the demand for medical and dental schools by enabling them to set tuition levels greatly below the actual costs of education. With artificially low tuition levels and limits on the number of students they would accept, there would be an excess demand for their spaces. As long as there is an excess demand for a medical education—and the schools do not willingly expand their spaces to satisfy this demand—then the schools can determine the type of educational curriculum that comes closest to meeting their (and the AMA's or ADA's) preferences.

Without excess demand for a medical education, the schools would have to respond, that is, compete for applicants as would any other supplier, by providing the type of service demanders were willing to pay for. These schools currently have a monopoly over the provision of medical and dental education. By charging tuition levels that are so low as to encourage excess demand for such an education, the schools are able to select the type of students they prefer. The schools are thereby able to establish the training times and educational requirements for entering the profession. These policies are also in the economic interest of physicians and dentists as they lead to a smaller supply of physicians and, consequently, higher incomes.

Another method health providers use to increase the demand for their services, primarily at the state level, is to mandate that all health insurance sold in that state include coverage for certain services or providers. Examples include mandating insurance coverage for hair transplants and obesity treatments or covering providers such as acupuncturists and chiropractors. Although these types of services and/or providers may be beneficial, the effect of state mandates is to increase the cost of health insurance, leading to an increase in the number of uninsured persons. Unless these services and providers were required by state legislatures, many individuals would not choose to spend their money on these benefits. About 1,500 state mandates have been enacted in the 50 states.

Legislation to Secure the Highest Method of Reimbursement

Regardless of whether an association member's goal is income, prestige, or growth, the method by which the provider is reimbursed is crucial to attaining that goal. High prices, resulting in large net revenues, increase incomes and enable institutions to achieve their objectives through the expenditure of those revenues. The method of reimbursement, or the method providers use to charge for their services, has been crucial to understanding provider economic behavior.

Eliminating price competition.

Health associations have used two basic approaches to achieve the highest possible reimbursement for their members. The first has been to try to eliminate price competition among their members. The ability to engage in price competition is more important to new practitioners or firms desiring to enter a market. For example, new competitors must be able to let potential patients know (through advertising) they are available, and new surgeons must be able to provide primary care physicians with an incentive (fee splitting) to switch their surgical referrals away from established surgeons.

To prevent price competition from occurring, health associations have termed the elements of price competition, such as advertising and fee splitting, "unethical behavior" and have prohibited such behavior in their state practice acts.[9] The medical and dental professions have used strong sanctions against practitioners who engaged in unethical behavior. A physician could have his license suspended and be assessed financial penalties. Previously, medical societies were able to deny hospital privileges to physicians who advertised or engaged in price competition.[10] Without hospital privileges a physician could not offer her patients a comprehensive set of medical services. As physicians new to an area had the greatest incentive to engage in such "unethical" behavior, they were given probationary membership in the local medical society. They were thereby placed on notice that they could lose their hospital privileges if they engaged in such behavior. (Since the application of the antitrust laws to healthcare in 1982, such anticompetitive behavior by medical societies is no longer permitted.)

A number of studies have shown that restrictions on advertising raise the price of optometric services from 20 to 50 percent.[11] (Most of the studies on advertising in the health field have been conducted on prescription drugs and optometric services.) The American Optometric Association has claimed (without offering evidence) that higher prices reflect higher-quality services. In 1980, the FTC attempted to resolve the issue of quality and advertising. The FTC took seven people with similar visual conditions and trained them at two optometric schools with regard to the optometric exam. When these seven subjects went to specified optometrists, they recorded the price charged, the amount of time spent by the optometrist, and specific information on the tests and procedures performed. The subjects went to cities where advertising was prohibited as well as to cities where it was permitted. In cities that permitted advertising, they visited optometrists who advertised and those who did not.[12]

The researchers concluded that removing advertising restrictions would cause prices to decline by more than 20 percent. Further, nonadvertising optometrists *in markets where advertising occurs* provide service of superior quality to those of optometrists in nonadvertising markets. Optometrists who do not advertise (in markets where other optometrists advertise) compete by lowering their price—but not by as much as optometrists who advertise—and by spending more time with their patients. Thus, optometric services are lower in price and, on average, higher in quality where advertising is permitted than where it is prohibited.

Price competition and advertising are not necessarily related to providing low-quality services. Defining such practices as unethical could only be interpreted as a means of preventing price competition.

As a result of the FTC's successful suit against the AMA (upheld by the U.S. Supreme Court in 1982), state medical and other professional societies can no longer penalize their members if they advertise or engage in other anticompetitive activities. All professionals are now permitted to advertise. After the Supreme Court ruling, however, the AMA, ADA, and other professional groups that are regulated at the state level made a final attempt at forestalling competition by trying to have Congress grant them an exemption from the FTC's jurisdiction. They were unsuccessful. Anticompetitive behavior in healthcare is now subject to the antitrust laws.

A more recent example of the AMA's attempt to eliminate price competition among physicians has been the AMA's lobbying of Congress for an exemption from the antitrust laws to allow competing physicians to collectively negotiate prices for their services with insurers. (Currently, such price fixing is illegal but does not apply to employees, union members, or merged corporations that no longer operate as competitors.) Allowing physicians, who are competitors, to agree on prices and withold their services if their demands are not met is similar to physicians organizing a cartel. The purpose of a cartel would be to raise physician fees. For example, all the anesthesiologists in a market could get together and decide on the prices they wanted to charge. In 2000, the AMA was successful in having the House (but not the Senate) vote to allow physicians to bargain collectively against managed care organizations (the Campbell bill).

Price discrimination.

The second approach health providers use to secure the highest possible payment for their services is to engage in price discrimination, which means charging different patients or payers different prices for the same service. These different prices do not result from differences in costs, but from the patient's or payer's ability to pay. Charging according to ability to pay results in greater revenues than a pricing system that charges everyone the same price.

Organized medicine's desire to maintain a system whereby physicians can price-discriminate influenced the financing and delivery of medical services for many years. Once medical insurance was introduced, organized medicine attempted to retain the physician's ability to price-discriminate. For example, when medical societies started Blue Shield plans, the physician's fee was paid in full for those subscribers whose incomes were below a certain level. Physicians were permitted to charge higher-income patients an amount in addition to the Blue Shield payment. The Blue Shield income limits were eventually eliminated as the large majority of subscriber's incomes exceeded the income limit and had other insurance options. Blue Shield insurance was not worth as much to high-income people if they had to pay a large amount, in addition to the annual premium, each time they went to the physician. As Blue Shield organizations dropped their income limits so as to be able to compete and enroll more high-income subscribers, some medical societies dropped their sponsorship of the Blue Shield plans.

Once income limits were removed, physicians could still maintain some ability to price-discriminate by deciding when they wanted to participate in Blue Shield and when they wanted to charge the patient directly. In the latter case, the patient would then receive payment from Blue Shield for an amount less than the physician's charge. For persons with higher incomes, physicians would charge the patient directly, which would provide them with a higher payment than if the physician participated in Blue Shield.

The physician-payment system under Medicare was based on the same principle. Physicians could decide to participate in Medicare on a case-by-case basis. If they thought they could make more money by charging the patient directly, they would do so. When they accepted the Medicare fee, the patient was responsible for a 20 percent copayment. When the physician chose not to participate, the patient had to pay the physician's fee, which was greater than the Medicare fee, and the patient was responsible for the difference in the fees as well as the copayment. By having the option of participating when they wanted to, physicians were assured of payment from low-income persons, while still being able to charge a higher price to higher-income patients. The method of pricing and flexibility of physician participation under Blue Shield and Medicare was crucial to their acceptance of these plans.[13]

Organized medicine's desire to maintain physicians' ability to price-discriminate limited the growth of prepaid health plans. HMOs charge patients the same premium regardless of income level. When fee-for-service physicians charge higher-income patients a higher fee, then a plan that charges all persons the same premium is a form of price competition; it limits the physician's ability to price-discriminate.

In his classic article, "Price Discrimination in Medicine," Reuben Kessel describes how county and state medical societies attempted to forestall the development of prepaid group plans.[14] When physicians moved into an area with the intention of joining a prepaid plan, local medical societies prevented them from receiving hospital privileges. Unless the plan had its own hospital, which was unlikely, this effectively eliminated competition. Several successful antitrust suits were brought against medical societies for this behavior.[15] (Such suits are costly, however, and take years to resolve.) Medical societies were subsequently successful in having restrictive legislation enacted at a state level that effectively limited the growth of these plans. For example, one such restrictive statute permitted only the medical profession to control and operate such plans. In 1976, Blue Shield of Spokane, Washington, agreed to discontinue its practice of discriminating against physicians who offered their services through an HMO. Blue Shield ended its boycott only after the FTC ordered it to do so on the grounds that it was anticompetitive.

In the mid-1980s, the federal government offered to pay HMOs an annual capitated price for each Medicare enrollee (referred to as Medicare risk contracts). Any HMOs enrolling Medicare beneficiaries were reimbursed 95 percent of the average area per capita cost of the combined amounts of Parts A and B of Medicare. The HMOs can keep the difference between the amount the government pays them and the costs of providing care for their aged enrollees. This approach increased the choices available to the Medicare patient. To attract Medicare patients from the fee-for-service system, HMOs offered additional benefits. The AMA opposed this approach and attempted to delay its implementation.

Increasing payment under public programs.

As government Medicare and Medicaid payments to healthcare providers have risen, such payments represent a significant portion of a provider's revenues. An important role of any health association today is to lobby for increased government payment for their member's services. Physician and hospital Medicare payments, for example, are annually updated, and the extent of that update not only affects the profitability of physicians and hospitals when serving Medicare patients, but also the federal government's expenditures under Medicare Parts A and B. The government has an incentive to limit Medicare hospital and physician payments, as Part B expenditures are funded from general revenues and contribute to the federal deficit and Part A expenditures affect the solvency of the Medicare Trust Fund.

In the past several years, the formula used to update Medicare physician fees led to projected *decreases* in physician fees. For example, Medicare physician fees were projected to decline by 4.5 percent in 2004, resulting in a loss of $3 billion in Medicare physician payments.

The AMA successfully lobbied Congress to have this fee reduction reversed and instead have Medicare physician fees increase by 1.5 percent. The increasing role of government in provider payment has required each association to devote significant resources for lobbying to ensure that its members receive the highest reimbursement possible under these public programs.

The American Dental Association.

Dental societies have acted similarly with respect to advertising and price competition. Until the successful FTC suit against the AMA in the early 1980s, dental societies included bans on advertising in their state practice acts. Since the FTC suit, a number of cases have been brought against dental societies for their failure to eliminate anticompetitive behavior. Various dental societies have prohibited advertisements on quality, prohibited practice by a dentist under a trade name (which would adversely affect corporate dental chains), and placed restrictions on prepaid dental plans.[16]

An important recent legislative activity of many state medical and dental societies has been to enact any willing provider legislation, which seeks to ensure that all patients have free choice of any provider. The HMOs and PPOs use closed panels of providers to deliver medical and dental services. Providers included in these closed panels are willing to discount their fees and accept practice guidelines in return for receiving a greater volume of patients. The HMOs and PPOs are thereby able to offer their services to insurers and employers at premiums lower than those prevailing in the area. Providers who are not a part of these closed panels do not have access to the HMO's and PPO's patient populations. Providers in closed panels are engaged in price competition with providers who are not in the closed panels.

By enacting any willing provider legislation, medical and dental societies remove providers' financial incentive to discount their fees in return for more patients. If providers in closed panels have to share their patients with providers who are not in closed panels, providers are unlikely to join closed panels and discount their fees.

To enable dentists to charge what the market will bear, the ADA has favored dental insurance but not the use of insurer fee schedules. The ADA has proposed that the dentist charge the patient, and the insurer reimburse the patient. In this manner the dentist would be able to raise prices. Several years ago, Pennsylvania Blue Shield won an antitrust suit against the Pennsylvania Dental Association on just such an issue. Pennsylvania Blue Shield claimed that the Pennsylvania Dental Association boycotted Pennsylvania Blue Shield because the Blue Shield dental plan paid dentists according to a fee schedule. The Pennsylvania Dental Association wanted dentists to be able to charge the patient an additional amount if they so desired.

Similar to the above, the ADA has also opposed the practice of allowing insurance companies to reimburse patients a lower amount if they go to a nonparticipating dentist. The ADA has called for legislation prohibiting insurance companies from this payment approach. (Dentists are not prohibited from participating with the insurance company. However, they would prefer not to participate, to receive the same amount as participating dentists, and to be able to charge the patient an additional amount.)

The American Nurses Association.

The ANA has been in favor of permitting advanced practice nurses to bill fee-for-service, which has been used with such success by physicians, dentists, and other health professionals. Registered nurses are striving to become independent practitioners, such as nurse practitioners and nurse-midwives, who will then be able to bill patients on a fee-for-service basis. The ANA has attempted to secure such direct reimbursement for nurses through government programs, such as Medicare. Fee-for-service payment to a health professional, which in most cases is reimbursed by the government or private insurance, is the most direct way for a health professional to increase income and work independently of physicians.

Nurse practitioners have been able to work independently and be reimbursed by many state Medicaid programs that serve low-income people and by Medicare for patients in rural areas. The numbers of independent nurse practitioners are likely to increase as a result of a decision in 1997 by the federal Department of Veterans Affairs to formally accept nurse practitioners without links to physicians and of a federal law (effective 1998); this allowed Medicare to make direct payments to nurse practitioners who work in cities and suburbs, not just in rural areas.

Another legislative approach ANA pursued to increase nurses' income was to require that the concept of "comparable worth" be used in setting nurses' wages. Equal pay for equal work has already been enacted into law. Proponents of comparable worth go beyond that; they want equal pay for work of comparable value. If a registered nurse does work that is comparable in value to that of an electrician or a family physician, then the nurse should receive a comparable (the same) income.[17] Comparable worth proponents seek to substitute fact-finding commissions for the marketplace, as the marketplace determines wages through the forces of supply and demand. The only way comparable worth can be implemented is to legislate it.

The American Hospital Association.

The American Hospital Association has favored two concepts in the design of payment systems for its member hospitals. The first was to eliminate any incentive for hospitals to engage in price competition. When hospitals started Blue Cross, the plans were required to offer their subscribers a service benefit plan. Such plans provide hospitalized patients with services rather than dollars, a characteristic of an indemnity plan. By guaranteeing payment to the hospital for the services used by the patient, a service benefit policy removes any incentive the patient (or the hospital) may have regarding the cost of hospitalization. Because the patient does not have to make any out-of-pocket payments, the prospective patient has an incentive to enter the most expensive hospital, which may or may not be the highest-quality hospital. Under a service benefit policy, hospitals cannot compete for patients on the basis of price.

Similarly, when Medicare was enacted, the AHA proposed a method of hospital payment, which was adopted by the government, that paid hospitals for providing care to Medicare patients based on each hospital's costs plus 2 percent. Once patients paid a deductible, they were not assessed any copayments. Not only did this method of payment eliminate any incentive for patients to select less costly, more efficient hospitals, but it provided hospitals with an incentive to increase their costs. (Further, hospitals were not permitted to compete for Medicare patients by offering to reduce the hospital deductible.)

The second concept underlying hospitals' preferred method of payment is to be able to engage in price discrimination, that is, to be able to charge different payers different prices. Hospitals prefer to have several different purchasers, rather than one major purchaser, of their services. With multiple payers, hospitals can charge each a separate price, based on willingness to pay. For example, hospitals gave Blue Cross a 20 percent discount compared to what commercial insurers were charged. This discount enabled Blue Cross to offer a more expensive policy (a service benefit) that was in the hospitals' interest. The discount was also a competitive advantage for Blue Cross and enabled the company to increase its market share over the commercial insurers.

Hospitals did very well financially under the initial Medicare payment policy. The government was anxious for hospitals to participate in Medicare and therefore accepted many of AHA's payment proposals. Not only were hospitals able to negotiate a 2 percent addition to their costs of serving Medicare patients and receive favorable treatment for depreciating their assets, but the manner in which hospital costs were calculated gave hospitals additional payment. Hospitals could not separate the actual costs of serving Medicare patients from those of other patients. The method used to calculate Medicare costs was to use the ratio of what hospitals charge for Medicare patients to the charges for non-Medicare patients. That ratio was then used to determine the portion of the hospitals' total costs that should be paid by Medicare. The effect of this policy was to provide hospitals with an incentive to raise charges on those services used predominantly by the elderly, such as bed rails. By raising the proportion of their charges for the aged, a greater portion of the hospitals' total costs were paid by the government. The hospital would then be able to make a higher profit on its charges to commercial insurers.

Hospitals were also able to price-discriminate by setting a higher price-to-cost ratio for those services for which there was a greater willingness to pay, that is, services that were less price-elastic. Ancillary services, such as lab tests and x-rays, had higher price-to-cost ratios than the hospital's basic room charge. Once patients were hospitalized they had little choice on the use or price of ancillary services. Patients who paid part of the hospital bill themselves could, before they entered a particular hospital, more easily compare charges for items such as obstetric services and room rates. The charges for these services were much closer to their costs.

The Association of American Medical Colleges.

Medical and dental schools, as discussed above, seek unrestricted federal and state subsidies rather than charge their students the full cost of their education. Charging tuition that is below actual costs and limiting the number of admissions results in an excess demand.

The method by which public medical and dental schools receive their subsidies is also very important. Subsidies go directly to the school, as do government funds distributed for loans and scholarships. Under this arrangement, the student receives a subsidy (tuition less than costs) only by attending a subsidized school. This method requires students to compete for medical and dental schools. If government subsidies went directly to the student, then the schools would have to compete for students. As with subsidies, medical and dental schools prefer to distribute loans and scholarships themselves rather than have students apply directly to the government for such financial assistance. If the students received the subsidies and loans directly, then they would have an incentive to shop and select a school based on its tuition rates and reputation. The current system provides a competitive advantage to schools receiving subsidies. Needless to say, private schools would prefer that the subsidies go directly to the students

The methods health professionals and health institutions use to price their services has enabled these providers to maximize their revenues. In negotiating with the government, in establishing their own insurance organizations, and in proposing legislation, the health associations representing each provider group have had a clear appreciation for which pricing strategies are in their members' economic interest. As a result, it is difficult to believe the distinction between profit and not-for-profit has any meaning with regard to which group can provide services at a lower price.

Legislation to Reduce the Price and/or Increase the Quantity of Complements

A registered nurse may be a substitute or a complement to the physician. It is difficult to determine when an input, such as a nurse, is a complement or a substitute based only on the task performed. A nurse may be as competent as a physician in performing certain tasks. If the nurse works for the physician and the physician receives the fee for performing that task, then the nurse has increased the physician's productivity and is a complement. If, however, the nurse performs the same task and is a nurse practitioner billing independently of the physician, then the nurse is a substitute for the physician providing that service. The essential element in determining whether an input is a complement or a substitute is who receives the payment for the services provided by that input. Whoever receives the payment controls the use of that input.

State practice acts are the legal basis for determining which tasks each health professional can perform and under whose direction health professionals must work. A major legislative activity for each health association is to ensure that the state practice acts work to their members' interests. Health associations that represent complements, such as nurses and denturists, attempt to have their members become substitutes. Health associations whose members control complements seek to retain the status quo.

In the past, almost all the health professions and health institutions were complements to the physician. That situation has changed. The physician is no longer the sole entry point to the delivery of medical services. For example, HMOs may use nurse practitioners to serve their enrollees. The AMA has continued to oppose the use of independent nurse practitioners and has lobbied against state laws that allow advance practice nurses to provide medical care without the supervision of a physician. The American Academy of Family Practitioners (who would be most adversely affected by independent nurse practitioners) has stated that such nurses should only be paid by insurers when they work in a "collaborative" relationship with physicians.

Providers can increase their incomes if an increase in demand for their services is met through greater productivity than through an increase in the number of competing providers. The providers' income can be increased still further if their productivity increases are subsidized and they do not have to pay the full cost of the increased productivity.

Following are several examples of legislation that has subsidized providers' productivity.

The American Hospital Association.

The American Hospital Association lobbied for passage of the Nurse Training Act in the belief that federal educational subsidies would increase the supply of registered nurses available to hospitals. With a larger supply of nurses, nurses' wages would be lower than they otherwise would have been. For similar reasons, the AHA favored educational subsidies to increase the supply of allied health professionals. The AHA was a strong proponent of the Hill-Burton Act, which provided capital subsidies to modernize hospitals. The AHA opposed legislation that would have increased the cost of inputs to hospitals. It opposed extending minimum wage legislation to hospital employees and has called for a moratorium on the separate licensing of each health professional. (Separate licensing limits the hospital's ability to substitute different health professionals in the tasks they perform and to use such personnel in a more flexible manner.) Conversely, each health professional association demands separate licensing so as to increase the demand for its members' services by restricting the tasks that other professions can perform.

The AHA has opposed proposals for a flat-rate income tax, which would reduce marginal tax brackets by eliminating a number of deductions. The AHA was concerned that eliminating the charitable contribution deduction might adversely affect hospitals. The AHA was also concerned that lowering income-tax brackets would make hospitals' tax-exempt bond financing less attractive to investors.

The American Medical Association.

The AMA has also favored subsidies to hospitals. When a patient demands a treatment for a medical problem, the physician decides on the combination of resources and settings to use in providing that treatment. Hospital care is often the most costly component of that treatment. Before hospital insurance was so widespread, the physician was concerned over the cost of hospital care. The more the patient paid for hospital care, the less there would be available to pay for the physician's services. Similarly, the AMA favored subsidies to increase the supply of nurses, because it lowered hospitals' costs of inputs. The AMA has, however, opposed the increased educational standards that the ANA wanted to impose on nursing institutions as a condition for receiving funds under the Nurse Training Act. Higher educational standards for nurses do not necessarily increase the productivity of nurses, but they do limit the supply of nurses. Financial support for graduate-level training of nurses also increases the nurses' qualifications to be a physician substitute for some tasks.

The AMA has favored internship and residency programs in hospitals. Interns and residents are excellent complements for physicians; they can take care of the physician's hospitalized patients and relieve the physician from serving in the hospital emergency department and from being on call. The more advanced the resident is, the closer the resident is to being a potential substitute for the physician. Residents, however, are complements as the physician bills for the service. For this reason the AMA has favored the use of foreign medical graduates to serve as interns and residents. Once they graduate, however, they become substitutes to existing practitioners. The AMA has, therefore, favored the return of foreign medical graduates to their home country once their residencies are completed. (The AMA advocated a time limit on how long foreign medical graduates can remain in the United States as well as requiring that they be out of the country two years before returning.)[18] The AMA has also favored increased training times for U.S. medical graduates. Not only does longer training time increase the time each graduate serves as a complement but it also delays the time when they become competitors.

A telling example of the AMA's attitude toward new health professionals was its position on physician assistants (PAs). If PAs practiced independently, they would become a substitute to some physicians (family practitioners). Thus, AMA's main concern about emerging health professionals is ensuring that these types of personnel become complements to, not substitutes for, physicians. Thus, whether there is direct or indirect supervision of the PA by the physician is less important to the AMA's political position than who gets the fee for the PA's service.

Another important determinant of the AMA's position toward PAs was whether PAs would create excess capacity among physicians in the community. Excess capacity causes increased competition among physicians for patients. If physicians faced insufficient demand for their services, then increased productivity, through the introduction of new types of personnel, would make it even more difficult for those physicians who would like to be busier. Indicative of this concern by its membership was the AMA's 1972 recommendation that all states enact legislation to empower state boards of medical examiners to approve, *on an individual basis*, a given physician's request to employ a PA and the proposed functions to be performed by that PA.[19] Unless there was sufficient demand per physician in an area, permission to use a PA would not be granted, regardless of the PA's training.

Particularly during the late 1950s, 1960s, and early 1970s, when demand for physicians and dentists was increasing, state practice acts were relaxed to permit greater delegation of tasks. As excess capacity among physicians and dentists increased in the 1980s, medical and dental societies began to oppose further delegation of tasks (for example to expanded function of dental auxiliaries). Growth in productivity among health professionals, paid fee-for-service, was related more to demand conditions facing physicians and dentists than to the competency of the new personnel.

One legislative attempt by physicians and dentists to lower the cost of their inputs has been action at both the federal and state level to limit increases in malpractice premiums. The AMA's preferred approach to reducing malpractice premiums has been to place a $250,000 limit on noneconomic damages, such as "pain and suffering," with no limit on economic damages, such as lost wages, medical expenses, and other costs. The AMA has been successful in having its proposal pass the House of Representatives but not the U.S. Senate. Malpractice premiums have risen for many reasons.[20] One important reason is the incompetency of some physicians. "There have been estimates that as many as 5 to 15 percent of doctors are not fully competent to practice medicine, either from a deficiency of medical skills or because of impairment from drugs, alcohol, or mental illness."[21] Professional associations have been more willing to seek legislation to place limits on the size of malpractice awards than to make a concerted effort to eliminate unqualified practitioners.

Blue Cross plans.

Up until the mid-1980s (at which time large employers pressured insurance companies to reduce their premiums), the Blue Cross premium consisted almost entirely of the costs of hospital care. Its main cost therefore has been the cost and quantity of hospital care used by its subscribers. Commercial insurers had broader coverage (although it included deductibles and cost sharing), so hospital care was a smaller portion of the total premium. Thus, to remain competitive against commercial insurance companies, Blue Cross had to keep the cost of hospital care (both hospital use and cost per unit) from rising so rapidly. Under the service benefit policy, however, patients, their physicians, and the hospital had no incentive to be concerned with cost or use. In fact, it was in the hospital's interest to add facilities and services and pass the costs on to Blue Cross. As more hospitals added facilities and services in a race to determine who could be more prestigious, there was a great deal of duplication of costly facilities and services and, consequently, low use. Blue Cross, however, was committed to pay. To limit the increase in these costly facilities, Blue Cross favored legislative restrictions on hospital investment.

Given the control hospitals had over Blue Cross, Blue Cross was not aggressive in trying to limit the rapid rise in hospital costs, such as by limiting what it would pay hospitals. Blue Cross and the major hospitals favored an indirect approach that prevented smaller hospitals from expanding their beds and facilities and the entry of new hospitals. To receive Blue Cross (and Medicare) reimbursement for capital expenditures, a hospital had to receive the approval of a planning agency for its investment. Existing large hospitals either had the latest facilities or were the likeliest candidates to receive approval from the planning agency, whose criteria favored large, full-service hospitals. These large institutions also favored the development and strengthening of planning agencies because it limited competition.

Blue Cross preferred to rely on controls rather than payment incentives to hold down hospital investment and rising Blue Cross premiums. Hospitals, however, had different objectives and cost control was not one of them. Studies have consistently shown that controls on capital investment were not effective in holding down hospital investment or the rise in hospital costs.[22] It was not until Blue Cross began to experience strong competitive pressures from commercial insurers, sufficient to affect its survival, that it finally undertook more direct means of lowering the costs of its major input. Blue Cross then included lower-cost substitutes to hospitals as part of its benefits, instituting utilization control programs, and changing the method by which it pays hospitals.

Legislation to Decrease the Availability and/or Increase the Price of Substitutes

Health associations try to increase the price of services that are substitutes to those provided by their members. (Similar to increasing the price of a substitute is decreasing its availability.) If the health association is successful in raising the price of a substitute or a competitor, then the demand for its members' services will be increased.

Health associations use three general approaches to accomplish this. The first is simply to have the substitute declared illegal. If substitute health professionals are not permitted to practice, or if substitutes are severely restricted in the tasks they are legally permitted to perform, then there will be a shift in demand away from the substitute service. The second approach, typically used when the first approach is unsuccessful, is to exclude the substitute service from payment by any third party, including government health programs. This approach raises the price of the substitute to those with government or private insurance. If patients go to the substitute provider, they must pay the provider's fee in full, but if they go to a provider covered by their insurance, they pay a small fraction of the fee. The third approach is to try and raise the costs of the substitutes who must then raise their own prices if they are to remain in business. The following examples illustrate the behavior of health associations for each of these approaches.

The American Medical Association.

For many years the AMA regarded osteopaths as "cultists." It was considered "unethical" for physicians to teach in schools of osteopathy. Unable to prevent their licensure at a state level, the AMA tried to deny osteopaths hospital privileges. (A physician substitute is less than adequate if that substitute cannot provide a complete range of treatment.) As osteopaths developed their own hospitals and educational institutions, medical societies decided the best approach to controlling the increase in supply of these physician substitutes was to merge with the osteopaths, make them physicians, and then eliminate any future increases in their supply. An example of this approach, which was used in California until it was overturned by the state Supreme Court, was to allow osteopaths to convert their D.O. degree to an M.D. on the basis of 12 Saturday refresher courses. (By 1966, 15 states had similar merger agreements between the medical and osteopathic societies.) After the merger between the two societies occurred in California, the Osteopathic Board of Examiners was no longer permitted to license osteopaths.

The AMA has been very successful at the state level in defining the tasks that different health professionals can perform. By establishing exclusive control over the tasks permitted to physicians, physicians have been able to obtain a scope-of-practice monopoly. Organized medicine has successfully eliminated substitutes to its practitioners' services. The AMA has not been alone in its efforts to influence state legislatures. Each health association competes with other health professional associations over the tasks its members are permitted to perform while excluding other health professionals from performing those same tasks. When equally capable health professionals are excluded from performing similar tasks, medical care delivery is less efficient, as a greater quantity of care could be produced if all capable provider's skills were used.[23]

Medicare has been the vehicle for much legislative competition. The AMA has lobbied for only covering physician services under Medicare Part

B while excluding nonphysician services. By including only physician services the prices of substitute providers to the aged are effectively increased relative to those of physicians. For example, optometrists and chiropractors are potential substitutes for ophthalmologists and family physicians. By including physician services under Medicare, but excluding payment for nonphysicians, the price of nonphysicians is increased relative to that of physicians. An aged person with Medicare Part B pays less for a physician's services, because the out-of-pocket price of physician services has been lowered for the aged. Anesthesiologists have similarly opposed direct payment of nurse anesthetists under Medicare.[24]

In one case the intervention of the courts prevented physicians from artificially raising the price of a substitute. In Virginia, Blue Shield did not reimburse psychologists as providers of psychotherapy. Psychiatrists' services were therefore less expensive than psychologists' to a patient with Blue Shield. The psychologists brought a successful antitrust case against Blue Shield in 1980 claiming discrimination of nonphysician providers.

Other examples of the AMA's attempts to adversely affect substitutes was to oppose payment for chiropractic services under veterans' benefits and under the CHAMPUS program (the Civilian Health and Medical Program of the Uniformed Services, which provides health benefits for dependents of military personnel). The AMA has also opposed federal funding for advanced nurse training for fear that nurses would become independent nurse practitioners. The AMA's House of Delegates approved a resolution to recommend to all hospital staffs that only physicians take histories and perform physicals. The floor debate indicated that the resolution was directed at PAs, registered nurses, and dentists.

One medical society effectively eliminated competition from two independent nurse-midwives when the malpractice insurance of the backup obstetrician was cancelled. The insurance company was controlled by the medical society. The backup obstetrician had to leave the state to get new insurance.

An increasing problem among physicians is that different physician specialties have come in conflict with other specialties in performing certain tasks. For example, previously radiologists primarily performed diagnostic imaging services. In more recent years, however, medical advances in imaging equipment has led orthopedic surgeons and cardiologists to place sophisticated imaging equipment in their offices; these specialties have become substitutes to radiologists. The American College of Radiology has complained that these other specialties are overusing diagnostic imaging, driving up healthcare costs, and compromising quality. The American College of Cardiology has responded that radiologists are more concerned about competition and with their loss of market share. The American College

of Radiology has started to enlist insurers in regulating which practitioners would receive payment for high-cost imaging services, such as com-
puted tomography (CT), magnetic resonance imaging (MRI), and
positron-emission tomography (PET), performed in a nonhospital setting.[25]

The American Dental Association.

An example of the legislative behavior of dental societies toward substitute
providers is illustrated by dentistry's actions toward denturists. "Denturism"
is the term applied to the fitting and dispensing of dentures directly to
patients by people not licensed as dentists. Independently practicing denturists are a threat to dentists' incomes because they provide dentures at
lower prices. Denturists are legal in most of Canada. As a result of their
political success in Canada, denturists in the United States became bolder
by forcing referendums on the issue and lobbying for changes in state practice acts. Until the 1970s, dental societies had been successful in having
denturism declared illegal nationwide. Since 1977, however, seven states
have legalized denturism.[26]

Occasionally denturists have sold dentures directly to patients ille-
gally. To eliminate this competition and to prevent its increase, local dental societies, such as in Texas, have responded in two ways: first, they offered
to provide low-cost dentures to low-income persons; second, they pressured state officials to enforce the state laws against illegal denturists.

A special ADA commission studied the threat of denturists and
reported that the number of persons who are edentulous is much greater
in the lower-income levels. It is among this population that denturists have
met with great success in selling low-cost dentures. An ADA editorial com-
menting on this special study commission's report proposed the following:

> Organized dentistry should set up some system for supplying low-
> cost dentures to the indigent or the near indigent all over the
> country, but especially in those states where the legislatures are
> considering bills that would allow dental mechanics to construct
> dentures and deliver them directly to the patient . . . this is the
> type of program that would have a favorable impact on the pub-
> lic—not to mention legislators. . . . The supplying of dentures to
> low-income patients by qualified dentists at a modest fee (or even
> at no fee in special cases) and in quantities meeting the public
> demands would go a long way toward heading off the movement
> of legalized denturists.[27]

It was only the threat of competition that resulted in the dental profession's offer to provide low-cost dentures to the indigent or near-indigent.
If the denturist's competitive threat had been eliminated through den-

tistry's successful use of the state's legal authority, the net effect would have been to cause the public, particularly the poor, to pay higher prices for dentures.

The ADA is also concerned that dental hygienists remain complements to, not become substitutes for, dentists. Several state dental hygienist associations have attempted to change the state practice act to permit hygienists to practice without a dentist's supervision and to become independent practitioners. In 1986, the hygienists were successful in achieving this goal in Colorado. The ADA viewed this activity by hygienists as a "war"[28] and challenged the constitutionality of the Colorado legislation. Further, the ADA filed a friend of the court brief against individual hygienists who challenged their state's requirements that they must be supervised by dentists.

The American Nurses Association.

One of the most important substitutes for registered nurses are foreign-trained registered nurses. Nurses' salaries are considerably higher in the United States than in other countries, providing a financial incentive for foreign nurses to enter the country. The ANA has been successful in decreasing the availability of a low-cost substitute for U.S. RNs by making it more difficult for foreign-trained RNs to enter the country. The ANA has proposed that foreign RNs desiring to enter the United States be screened by examination in their home country before being allowed to immigrate. Once a foreign-trained RN enters the United States, the nurse is screened again by taking a state board exam. Since 1996, U.S. immigration law requires foreign nurses to complete a screening program before receiving an occupational visa. The screening exam includes an assessment of the nurse's education, demonstrated by earning a certificate from the Commission on Graduates of Foreign Nursing Schools, which is the organization offering this federal screening program, to ensure that the nurse's education is comparable to that of a U.S. graduate. In addition, it includes licensure validation and English language proficiency.[29]

The ANA's position on entry screening is consistent with a policy of reducing the inflow of foreign nurses. If the screening exam were administered only in the United States, then foreign-trained RNs could still work in some nursing capacity in this country, even if they did not pass the exam. The foreign-trained nurse could then retake the exam in the future. As it is, the screening exam is an additional barrier for foreign nurses to pass before they can enter the United States; if they do not pass the exam, they are unlikely to emigrate.

The ANA has used two additional legislative approaches to raise the cost of substitutes for RNs. The first is to favor increases in the wages of other health professionals. A great deal of substitution for RNs by licensed practical nurses (LPNs) has occurred. The larger the wage increase of LPNs, the less likely it is that LPNs will be used instead of RNs. The disparity between RN wages and those of other health professionals would be diminished.

The second legislative approach ANA uses is to prevent other personnel from performing tasks performed by the RN. The ANA has opposed permitting physicians to decide which personnel can perform nursing tasks; the ANA has opposed permitting LPNs to be in charge of skilled nursing homes, otherwise there would be substitution away from RNs (who receive higher wages) currently performing such functions. The California Nurses Association opposed a bill that would have authorized firefighters with paramedic training to give medical and nursing care in hospital emergency departments. As a means of preventing PAs from assuming a role that the RN would like, the ANA has favored a licensing moratorium. A moratorium would prevent any new health personnel from being licensed to perform tasks that RNs do or would like to perform.

The American Hospital Association.

The AHA opposed the growth of freestanding ambulatory surgicenters.[30] Surgicenters are low-cost substitutes for hospitals; performing surgical procedures in a surgicenter decreases the use of the hospital, and its revenues. To limit the availability of these low-cost substitutes, hospital associations have argued that surgicenters should be permitted only when they are developed *in association* with a hospital. The hospital would then be able to control the growth of this competitive source of care. Denying Blue Cross reimbursement to freestanding surgicenters and including surgicenters under certificate-of-need (CON) legislation were approaches hospital associations favored. Hospitals have had a great deal of influence in the CON process. If approval was to be given for a surgicenter, it was more likely to be given to a hospital wishing to start one than to a freestanding one. (Previously, when hospitals were reimbursed according to their costs by both Blue Cross and Medicare, Blue Cross opposed surgicenters on the grounds that surgicenters raised the cost of care because hospitals are left with excess capacity, which third-party payers then have to cover.)

Health maintenance organizations were also included in state CON legislation for the same reason, as they decrease the use and revenues of hospitals. Several large HMOs were able to persuade Congress that CON legislation was inhibiting their ability to compete and were able to receive an exemption from the federal CON legislation in 1979. (Many states, however, still use CON to limit entry by new health facilities, even by home health agencies, which have virtually no economies of scale and could not be considered to raise costs by duplicating existing medical services.)

In recent years, hospitals have been concerned by the growth of physician-owned specialty hospitals. Physician specialists, such as cardiovascular and orthopedic surgeons, while remaining on the staff of an acute care general hospital, have invested in a specialty facility and referred some of their patients to their own facility for surgery. General hospitals have claimed that these specialty hospitals decrease the demand for their own facilities and take the more profitable, less severely ill patients. Hospital associations were successful in eliminating competition from these specialty hospitals by including in the 2003 Medicare Prescription Drug Act a provision placing an 18-month moratorium on the development of new physician-owned specialty hospitals.

The federal moratorium only restricts the ability of physicians to refer Medicare and Medicaid patients to specialty hospitals in which they have an ownership interest. The AHA has been lobbying to make the moratorium permanent and to also have their state hospital associations lobby state legislatures to prohibit nongovernment patients from being referred to such specialty hospitals.

State hospital associations are also attempting to ban physician self-referral to ambulatory surgery centers. These efforts, such as by the Texas Hospital Association, are opposed by state medical societies, who do not want any limits being imposed on the ability of physicians to own specialty hospitals or ambulatory surgery facilities.[31] Another legislative tactic state hospital associations have used to decrease the availability of a substitute was demonstrated by the New Jersey Hospital Association's success in persuading the governor and state legislature to impose a tax on surgery centers not owned by hospitals of 3.5 percent of gross revenues to fund charity care.[32]

Blue Cross plans.

Blue Cross plans opposed state rate regulation of hospitals that would enable all insurers to pay the same price for hospital care ("all payer" systems). Such policies would have removed the cost advantage Blue Cross had over commercial insurers, because they received a hospital discount. Commercial insurers similarly favored the removal of Blue Cross's federal tax exemption (enacted in 1987), a political success for commercial insurers seeking to increase Blue Cross's costs.

The Association of American Medical Colleges.

Substitutes for U.S. medical and dental schools are foreign schools whose graduates (who may be U.S. citizens) want to practice in the United States.

To reduce the likelihood that foreign medical schools will substitute for U.S. medical schools, the Association of Medical Colleges has been a strong proponent for eliminating Medicare graduate medical education payments to teaching hospitals for residents trained in foreign medical schools. This reduction to teaching hospitals would be a strong incentive for those hospitals not to accept foreign-trained residents. (In 2005, 8,343 of the 24,012 entry-level resident positions in U.S. hospitals were filled by foreign-trained residents.)[33]

The Association of American Dental Schools.

The ADA and the Association of American Dental Schools have been more successful in reducing the attractiveness of a foreign dental education. Practicing dentists do not use residents as do physicians. Therefore, their interest is solely with decreasing the supply of dentists. Increased time requirements have been imposed on foreign-trained dentists desiring to practice in the United States. A minimum number of years of training in the foreign country is required, as well as a license to practice in that country. (For a U.S. citizen, this would mean learning a different language.) And once foreign-trained dentists enter the country, additional requirements are then imposed on them. They are required to take the last two years of dental school in an accredited U.S. dental school. They may also be required to take additional examinations before taking the licensing exam.[34] To date, such restrictive practices have raised the cost of a U.S. dental license for foreign-trained dentists (both U.S. and non-U.S. citizens). The consequence has been a decreased demand for foreign dental education as a substitute for U.S. dental education. The measure of how successful the dental profession and the dental schools have been is that fewer than 5 percent of all practicing dentists in the United States are foreign-trained.

Large employers and their unions.

The concept of interest groups seeking political action to increase the price of substitutes is not reserved solely for providers and insurers of medical services. Large companies and unions, for example, have lobbied state and federal legislatures to enact mandated employer health insurance, whereby the employer must pay a majority of the employees' health insurance premium. Large firms and their employees typically have health insurance; thus, small firms and their employees would be primarily affected by such legislation. Mandated employer health insurance would increase the cost of low-wage labor to small firms and would cause these firms to increase their prices, thereby increasing the demand for substitute suppliers, namely large firms and their union employees.

Legislation to Limit Increases in Supply

Essential to the creation of a monopoly are limits on the number of providers of a service. Health associations, however, have justified supply-control policies on grounds of quality. Restrictions on entry, they maintain, ensure high quality of care to the public. These same health associations, however, oppose quality measures that would have an adverse economic effect on existing providers (their members). *This apparent anomaly—stringent entry requirements and then virtually no quality assurance programs directed at existing providers—is only consistent with a policy that seeks to establish a monopoly for existing providers.*

If health associations were consistent in their desire to improve and maintain high-quality standards, then they should favor all policies that ensure quality of care, regardless of the effect on their members. Quality-control measures directed at existing providers, such as reexamination, relicensure, and monitoring of the care actually provided, would adversely affect the incomes of some providers. More importantly, such "outcome" measures of quality assurance would make entry or "process" measures less necessary, thereby permitting entry of a larger number of providers.

A test of the hypothesis that entry barriers are primarily directed toward developing a monopoly position rather than improving quality of care would be as follows: Does the health association favor quality measures, regardless of the effect on its members' incomes or does it only favor those quality measures that enhance members' incomes? If the health association only favors those quality measures that have a favorable impact on its members' economic position, then it can be concluded that the real intent of those quality measures is the improvement of its members' competitive position rather than the assurance of quality care in the most efficient manner.

The following examples illustrate health associations' positions on quality. Quality programs that are in its members' interests are expected to be favored while those that would have an adverse impact are expected to be opposed.

Health associations always favor state licensure. The profession is the group that lobbies for and demands licensure laws. The profession then controls the licensure process by having its own members appointed to the licensing board and by having them establish the requirements for licensure. Licensure, by itself, is not a sufficiently strong barrier to entry, so additional requirements are then imposed. The major additional requirement is educational. Before any person can take a licensing exam he must have had a specified education, for a minimum number of years. (The number of years is continually increased.) Further, the specified education must take place in an educational institution approved by the profession or by its representatives. The number of educational institutions is kept limited so that, as in medicine and dentistry, there is a continual excess demand for admission. (Medical and dental schools, as well as optometric, veterinary, and similar schools, favor such supply-control policies as it provides them with an education monopoly.) Limiting the number of educational spaces and specifying educational requirements in excess of the skills necessary to practice reduces the number of persons who can take the licensing exam.

If the licensure requirements merely specified passing an examination, then potential applicants for the exam could receive the necessary knowledge in number of ways, in different institutions, and in different lengths of time. Under such circumstances, the number of persons who could potentially take the exam and pass it would be much greater than if those applying were limited by the number of approved educational spaces.

The American Medical Association.

The above approach to quality has been used by both the AMA and the ADA, as well as other health professions. In 1904 the AMA formed its Council on Medical Education. Its purpose was to upgrade the quality of medical education. To receive greater public acceptance of its work, the council induced the Carnegie Foundation to survey existing medical schools. The result was the Flexner report, which recommended closing many medical schools and upgrading educational standards. "Flexner forcefully argued that the country was suffering from an overproduction of doctors and that it was in the public interest to have fewer doctors who were better trained."[35]

As a result of the Flexner report, state medical licensing boards imposed the requirement of graduation from an approved medical school before a person could take the licensure examination. Medical schools were to be approved by the AMA's own Council on Medical Education. The number of medical schools steadily declined from 162 in 1906 to 69 in 1944. The graduates of schools that were closed continued to practice; they were not required to rectify their educational deficiencies. *Whenever standards are raised, grandfather clauses protect the rights of existing practitioners, regardless of their abilities.*

The American Dental Association.

The ADA followed in the footsteps of organized medicine. A licensure requirement, followed by an educational requirement, still left dentistry with "too many" practitioners. Dental schools were effectively able to license their own graduates. The number of dental schools grew, from 10 in 1870 to 60 by 1902.[36] Many of these new schools were for-profit businesses.

Limits were placed on for-profit schools to control the growth in the supply of new graduates. State and local dental societies, as well as nonprofit dental schools, lobbied state legislatures to change the dental practice acts. Under the new state practice acts, the state board of dental examiners mandated that all dental graduates would have to take a licensing examination, and that only graduates from approved schools would be permitted to take the exam.

In 1926, the ADA produced the Gies report, its own version of the Flexner report. Approval of dental schools as a requirement for licensure was to be determined by the ADA's Council on Dental Education. Indicative of the control the ADA has had on its Council on Dental Education is one of the duties of the council, according to the ADA's bylaws: ". . . to accredit on behalf of this association dental schools and schools in related fields of dental education *in accordance with requirements and standards approved by the House of Delegates*" (italics added).[37] The result of these requirements was that the number of schools and spaces declined and the educational requirements for becoming a dentist increased. Educational requirements became standardized and the for-profit dental schools went out of business. As with physicians, practicing dentists, whose interests were served by the ADA, were always grandfathered in as requirements increased.

In the 1990s, there was a growing concern among dentists (as well as among other health professions) that there were too many practitioners. As would be expected, rather than relying on market forces to determine the number of dentists, the ADA approach was to reduce the number of dental school spaces. Indicative of this approach was the following ADA statement, "Resolved, that public statements made by the American Dental Association . . . include the recognition that a surplus of dentists does exist to meet the current demand for dental services, . . . [and that] the ADA encourage and assist constituent societies in preparing legislation that may be used to petition state legislatures and governmental bodies with respect to private schools to adjust enrollment in dental schools."[38]

The American Optometric Association.

Optometrists have also followed the same supply-control policies as medicine and dentistry. By the early 1900s, optometrists were able to secure licensure in all states. However, there were many private schools for training optometrists. By the 1920s the American Optometric Association was successful in disqualifying 20 of the 30 optometric schools and raising educational requirements. Optometry requires six years of education in an approved optometric school and at least three years (most applicants have completed four years) of traditional undergraduate college education.[39] Increasing educational requirements for a profession involves not just increasing the number of years of professional training but also requiring more years of undergraduate training. (It is not intuitively obvious why a professional must also have a full four years of a traditional college education.)

The American Nurses Association.

Nursing also tried to impose stringent educational requirements. Previously, most nurses graduated from diploma schools of nursing (90 percent in 1955). These programs were operated in conjunction with hospitals and generally lasted two years. By the mid-1990s, the number of RNs graduating from a diploma school was about 10 percent, while 60 percent were graduating from associate degree (AA) programs from a two-year college, and about 30 percent were graduating with a four-year BSN degree.[40] The growth in demand for an AA degree was related to their high rate of return; a nurse with a BA received a similar income but was required to take an additional two years of education. The marketplace did not place a sufficiently high return on the additional two years of education to make it worthwhile for most nurses to seek a four-year degree. Because the four-year degree did not meet the market test, the profession decided to impose it.

The ANA has proposed and has lobbied their state legislatures that nursing education take place only in colleges that offer a BA.[41] Only four-year nurse graduates would be referred to as professional nurses; otherwise, the nurse would be a technical nurse. By proposing an increase in the educational requirement of two-thirds of the nurse graduates, the ANA must be well aware that the result will be a decrease in the number of nurse graduates. Any increase in an educational requirement increases the tuition that students must pay as well as the forgone income a student could have earned during those additional years. The consequence of this policy, however, will be a much smaller increase in the supply of RNs, increased wages for RNs, and higher costs of healthcare. With an increased educational requirement, the ANA will also try to justify an increase in tasks that nurses are able to perform. The effect of increased education and an increase in nursing tasks would be an increase in the incomes of existing nurses, who would be grandfathered in as professional nurses.

It is unlikely one would ever observe a health association proposing increased educational requirements that are then applied to its existing members. Only to forestall more stringent requirements proposed by others would a health association favor additional training requirements for its existing members. Health associations typically do not favor relicensure or reexamination requirements for their current members, even though increased knowledge is the basis for requiring additional training for those entering the profession. Reexamination and relicensure would lower the incomes of their members, as they would have to take the time to study for the exam. Current practitioners also may not be able to pass the exam. No health association proposes that the time required to prepare a person to enter their profession be reduced.

Several medical school deans have suggested that one way to reduce the rising cost of a medical and dental education is to reduce the number of years required, for example, one less year of college and/or professional school.[42] People would be willing to pay higher tuition levels for the years they are in school if they could enter practice one to two years earlier. However, the only direction with regard to the number of years of education required was the ADA's proposal that each dental graduate take an *additional* one-year postdoctoral program, which includes hospital experience.[43]

As knowledge increases and educational requirements for new graduates lengthen, the public is led to believe all persons in a profession are equally (or at least minimally) qualified. This is unlikely to be the case, particularly for those practitioners who were trained 30 years ago and have not maintained their knowledge.

At times the profession has imposed requirements on new entrants that are blatant barriers. For example, foreign medical and dental graduates were once required to be U.S. citizens before they were allowed to practice in some states.[44] Further, a dentist desiring to practice in Hawaii, for example, no matter how well-trained or how long in practice in another state, is required to complete a one-year residency requirement before being allowed to practice.[45] Forgoing income for a year before they can practice is a high cost for entering a new market. Such requirements cannot be remotely related to the profession's concern with quality.

If the members of a profession are concerned with quality, then they should favor monitoring quality among themselves. Yet associations have opposed any attempts by others to review the quality of care practiced by their members. Health associations that have proposed continuing education for their members have done so in response to demands by those *outside* the profession. These requirements are made easy to achieve and at low cost to the members of the profession.

An indication of the lack of quality control in the health professions is provided by evidence over time of the number of disciplinary actions taken against physicians by state licensing boards. One such study, conducted in 1969, found that in the preceding five years a total of 938 formal actions had been taken. These disciplinary actions varied from revocation of licenses to simple reprimands. Given the number of physicians involved in patient care during those years, these disciplinary actions amounted to 0.69 per 1,000 physicians per year. Another study through 1972 resulted in an annual disciplinary rate of 0.74 per 1,000 physicians. These numbers include a number of states that had taken no disciplinary actions. Over the period 1980 to 1982, the disciplinary rate rose slightly to 1.3 per 1,000 physicians. The author of these studies, Dr. Robert Derbyshire, asks, "Does organized medicine adequately discipline unethical physicians? The answer is no."[46]

The Florida Board of Medical Examiners was reorganized in 1979 and a layperson appointed as director. The impetus for this change was a belief that the Florida medical licensing board was not performing its function. There was widespread media coverage of Florida physicians who had harmed their patients, violated the law, and yet were found to still be in practice. As a result, Florida strengthened the regulatory process. (A new governor was elected at that time and the state's medical practice act came up for renewal under the state's sunset law provisions.) In 1982, there were 147 disciplinary actions against physicians in Florida. This included revoking and suspending licenses. These actions represented a threefold increase from a prior period. Because there were more than 20,000 physicians in Florida, these disciplinary actions amounted to 7.4 per 1,000 physicians.

Other states had widely varying rates of disciplinary actions. In 1982, Pennsylvania recorded only 0.5 disciplinary actions per 1,000 physicians; New York had 1.1; California 2.8. Seventeen states reported 3.0 or greater. The author of the above study, Dr. Richard Feinstein, states, "It is difficult to believe that in any given year any state or territory would not have at least one physician per thousand who posed a threat to the health and safety of its citizens, and yet in 1982, 14 states reported less than that number of disciplinary actions. Has the balance of interests in these states tipped too far in the direction of protecting the profession to the detriment of its citizens?"[47]

In more recent years there has been an increase in the number of disciplinary actions against physicians. During 2004, 6,265 physicians, less than 1 percent (.9 percent) of approximately 705,000 physicians were disciplined (8.89 per 1,000 physicians). The increase in the number of disciplinary actions has most likely resulted from increased publicity about the inadequate performance by state medical licensing boards. The performance of state licensing boards still varies greatly among the different states. As of 2004, the number of actions per 1,000 practicing physicians was 5.85 in Michigan, 7.08 in California, 8.39 in Pennsylvania, 8.96 in New York, 12.47 in Colorado, 14.74 in Wyoming, 15.13 in Missouri, 16.08 in Alaska, and 25.54 in Florida. (In several states these rates are much greater than they were five years ago; in Florida, for example, the rate is 3.5 times greater than in 1999.)[48]

It is also unfortunate that physicians who lose their license in one state can then move to another state and practice again. Only six states (as of 2003) permit their licensing boards to take action solely on another state's findings.[49] And the Government Accounting Office has recommended that physicians who lose their license in one state should not be able to collect from Medicare and Medicaid as they move from state to state.[50]

In 1986, the AMA acknowledged that physician peer-review programs have not been performing as well as they should. "Because of the fear of personal liability, physicians are reluctant to report colleagues to state medical boards, and adverse hospital review determinations too often stay within the hospital. Peer review can be more careful, vigorous, and uniform."[51] A likely reason for this acknowledgment by the AMA's Board of Trustees of its plans to improve self-regulation among its members is that both government and business are demanding an accounting on quality assurance. Stan Nelson, Chairman of the AMA's Board of Trustees, stated, "Some big businesses, as payors for care, are realizing that they cannot only look at cost. They have to look at quality and they are demanding that the information be available to them."[52]

The current method of quality assurance for health professionals is aimed solely at entry into the profession rather than at monitoring the quality of care given. The inadequate performance of state licensing boards in disciplining their members is evidence of this practice. Further, little communication exists between state licensing boards to check the credentials and status of a physician moving from a different state.

The public is less protected against unethical and incompetent practitioners than it has been led to believe. *The public will become better protected, not as a result of the good intentions of the profession, but when the health professions are forced to respond to the demands for quality from those outside the professions.*

The American Hospital Association.

Hospitals have also been advocates of supply-control policies. These institutions have realized that the first step in achieving monopoly control is to limit entry. Large hospitals have favored CON legislation and bed-reduction programs and have used CON to limit investments by smaller hospitals and prevent entry by potential competitors, such as for-profit hospitals. In the late 1980s, as hospital occupancy rates fell and price competition increased, large hospitals favored government-sponsored bed-reduction programs. Eliminating excess beds reduces incentives for hospitals to compete among themselves.

Blue Cross plans.

Blue Cross plans were established so as not to compete with one another. They were required to sign up 75 percent of the hospitals and beds in an area. This requirement precluded more than one Blue Cross plan from being established within any one market, so Blue Cross had a virtual monopoly over the type of product it was selling, a service benefit policy for hospitalization. (No other insurance company could have competed with Blue Cross on a similar product because they would not have received the hospital discount given to Blue Cross.)

To compete with Blue Cross, commercial insurance companies had to offer a different product, such as payment of a fixed dollar amount for hospital care. To offset the Blue Cross hospital discount, the commercial insurers also had to include lower-cost substitutes to hospital care. The result was that commercial insurance companies innovated the concept of major medical insurance. Major medical did not cover all the costs of hospital care, but it provided medical insurance against large expenditures, both in and outside the hospital.

As the health insurance market has become more competitive, other types of insurance plans, such as HMOs, have taken market share away from the traditional health insurers. Blue Cross plans have had to adapt to this new environment. They have changed their product, offering care in settings other than just the hospital; they have established their own HMOs; and some Blue Cross plans are entering other Blue Cross plan's markets. The Blue Cross monopoly over its brand name within a geographic area has been eroded.

Since the 1980s, much of the diminished political power and economic benefits enjoyed by organized medicine has been the result of the rise of opposing concentrated interests, in part because diffuse costs increased to where they became concentrated, and antitrust laws were applied to the health field. The federal and state governments have developed a concentrated interest in reducing the rise in Medicare and Medicaid expenditures. Unless the rise in the expenditures was reduced, taxes would have to be raised or politically popular programs cut back. Large employers and their unions have similarly developed a concentrated interest in reducing the rise in their employees' health insurance premiums, otherwise their product prices must be increased and employee wages reduced.

Implications of the Legislative Success of Health Associations

Health professionals and health institutions do not exhibit characteristics of a natural monopoly, that is, large economies of scale for a given size of market sufficient to preclude entry of competitors. Because these professionals and institutions cannot achieve a monopoly position through the normal competitive process, they seek to achieve it through legislation.

The first step toward increasing their monopoly power is to erect barriers to entry. The next is to limit competition among their members. They then attempt to improve their monopoly position by further demanding legislation that will increase the demand for their services, permit them to price as would a price-discriminating monopolist, lower their costs of doing business, and disadvantage their competitors by either causing them to become illegal providers or forcing them to raise their prices.

Health professionals, particularly physicians and dentists, have been successful in the legislative marketplace, as evidenced by the design of public programs to pay for their services and by their relatively high incomes. However, three types of "costs" are imposed on the rest of society as a result of the restrictions that cause a redistribution of wealth to members of health associations that have achieved legislative success.

The first is higher prices. The more successful a health association is in achieving its members' goals, the higher will be the price of their members' services. However, once price competition occurs between members of different health associations, the prices of both groups' services will be lower. The establishment of low-cost denture clinics by state dental societies is an example. When competition is reduced, as when state dental societies apply pressure to have the laws against denturists enforced, the price of dentures will once again increase. Allowing freestanding surgicenters to compete with hospitals lowers the cost to the patient for minor surgical procedures (through reduced insurance premiums). Other tactics health associations have used to prevent price competition among their members included prohibiting advertising, limiting productivity increases to prevent excess capacity, preventing physicians in HMOs from having hospital privileges, and requiring free choice of provider under both public and private insurance plans (thereby disadvantaging HMOs and PPOs). These restrictions have resulted in healthcare prices that are higher than they would be otherwise.

The beneficiaries of restrictive policies that maintain high healthcare prices are, of course, the healthcare professionals themselves. These higher prices, which are not visibly attributed to these legislative policies, are borne by patients and by taxpayers who finance government programs.

The second implication of successful legislative behavior by health associations is that the public is provided with a false assurance with respect to the quality of the medical care it receives. The state has delegated its responsibility for protecting the public to the individual licensing boards, which in turn have been controlled and operated in the interests of the providers themselves. The approach toward quality assurance used by both the profession and by licensing boards is needlessly costly and inefficient. It has been more concerned with the process of becoming a health professional, such as entry into the profession, than with monitoring the care provided. As such, state licensing boards have devoted too few resources to investigating complaints against and removing incompetent or unethical providers. Too rarely do state licensing boards take disciplinary action against their members.

The movement toward a competitive market in medical services has resulted in a new emphasis on quality of care. Large employers are pressuring HMOs to provide information on their enrollees' medical outcomes, preventive measures undertaken, and health status indicators of their subscriber population. Through such actions by large purchasers, HMOs are developing "report cards." Employer emphasis on "outcome" measures is forcing HMOs and medical groups to reexamine how medical care is provided. Hospital rankings are now posted on the Internet. It is doubtful that these new approaches toward quality would have occurred had market competition not developed.

The third effect of legislative success by a health association is that innovation in the delivery of medical care has been inhibited. Innovation provides benefits to consumers: greater choice, higher quality, and lower costs. Innovation, however, threatens the monopoly power of a protected provider group, and is therefore opposed. Medical and dental societies have been protectors of the fee-for-service delivery system. These organizations have delayed the introduction of alternative delivery systems, such as HMOs and PPOs.

Rather than being pro-competitive, professions have used any willing provider laws and "free choice of provider" to eliminate competition from "closed" provider panels. Neither HMOs nor PPOs can negotiate volume discounts with closed panels of providers if they have to offer their subscribers free choice of any provider. In addition, HMOs and managed care organizations are able to offer lower premiums than traditional insurance because they are able to impose restrictions on participating providers and by instituting medical management programs. Legislative restrictions against closed panels, such as requiring free choice of provider, prevents managed care organizations from successfully competing against traditional insurance plans.

Concluding Comments

Medical and dental societies have inhibited the development of new types of health personnel, such as nurse midwives, nurse practitioners, and expanded-function dental auxiliaries, because they might become substitutes. The determination of which tasks a health professional is able to perform is related more to their economic effects on another health profession than to the professional's qualifications and training.

Hospital associations have sought, through CON legislation, to stifle innovations such as the growth of freestanding surgicenters. It was the commercial insurance companies that introduced major medical insurance, a distinct innovation that also increased their share of the health insurance market. The process of receiving a professional education (medical, dental, and optometric) has changed little over time (except for an increase in years required) because it has remained under the auspices of accredited schools and their professions. It is highly likely that the necessary knowledge could be provided to students in a shorter period of time, thereby decreasing the total cost of such an education.

Innovation offers the hope of greater productivity, lower costs, and an increase in quality. The political activities of health associations should be viewed in their proper perspective, namely, to benefit their members while imposing a cost on the rest of society. To the extent that the public benefits from actions undertaken by health interest groups, those benefits are a by-product of measures primarily designed to benefit the profession itself. Past reliance on professional regulation to protect the patient has reduced incentives for innovation.

The movement toward market competition in the delivery of health services does not, however, negate the need to be concerned with quality. Large employers and business coalitions wield sufficient purchasing power to force managed care organizations to monitor quality of care within their organizations and to compete on such measures. It is, however, among those population groups not monitored by large employers, such as those on Medicaid and Medicare, that concerns remain over the quality of care received. State and federal authorities do not have the same incentives as large employers (on behalf of their employees) to be as vigilant in monitoring the care of their beneficiaries. Only by including the aged and poor in the same insurance plans as used by large employee groups (such as providing the aged and poor with vouchers to buy health insurance) will the monitoring of care for all population groups be similar.

Study Questions

1. Provide examples of the types of "demand-increasing" legislation favored by different health associations.
2. What do you expect would be health insurers' and the ADA's political position on proposals to limit the amount of employer-paid health insurance that is excluded from taxes?

3. What methods has the AMA used in the past to discourage price competition among its members?

4. How did the initial benefit structure that hospitals designed for Blue Cross eliminate any possibility of hospitals engaging in price competition for patients?

5. Explain why health professionals (e.g., a nurse practitioner), can either be viewed as a complement or a substitute, depending on who receives the fee for the service (e.g., the nurse practitioner or the physician).

6. What are some different approaches medical associations have used to decrease competition from substitute providers?

7. Did hospital and RN associations favor an increase in the number of foreign-trained registered nurses to alleviate nurse shortages?

8. With reference to specific approaches that have been used to increase the quality of health professionals, such as graduation from an approved medical school and increased educational requirements, discuss the following statement, "Health associations only favor those quality measures that enhance their members' incomes, not all quality measures regardless of the effect on their members' incomes."

9. How has quality assurance of health professionals changed with the increase in managed care competition?

Notes

1. In 1975, the FTC charged that the AMA, the Connecticut State Medical Society, and the New Haven County Medical Association restricted the ability of their members to advertise. The AMA claimed that the FTC did not have jurisdiction over them because they were a not-for-profit organization. The approach used in this chapter and in an earlier book by the author, *Health Associations and the Demand for Legislation: The Political Economy of Health*, (Lexington, MA: Ballinger Publishing Company, 1977), with its applications to the AMA, was the basis for testimony by the author on the jurisdictional issue to demonstrate that the AMA acted in the economic interests of its members. The administrative law judge found in favor of the FTC on both the advertising and jurisdictional issues. These decisions were upheld on appeal, and in 1982, the U.S. Supreme Court, by a tie vote, upheld the lower court rulings.

2. A more complete discussion of the change to market competition, as well as the reasons for this change, is provided in Chapter 6: "The Emergence of Market Competition in the U.S. Healthcare System."

3. The antitrust laws were also used to ensure that the interests of Blue Shield and medical societies were kept separate. The FTC investigated physician control of Blue Shield plans and brought a successful suit against the Michigan State Medical Society. The Michigan State Medical Society bargained with Blue Shield on behalf of its physician members. Medical societies are no longer permitted to do this as a physicians' boycott against Blue Shield would be illegal.

4. It has been estimated that the income elasticity of demand for dental services is approximately two; that is, a 10 percent increase in income would lead to a 20 percent increase in expenditures on dental services. Charles Upton and William Silverman, "The Demand for Dental Services," *Journal of Human Resources* 7 (1972): 250–261.

5. John Sheils and Randall Haught, "The Cost of Tax-Exempt Health Benefits in 2004," *Health Affairs*. February 25, 2004. [Online article] http://content.healthaffairs.org/cgi/reprint/hlthaff.w4.106v1.

6. One demand-increasing proposal is reputed to have had an adverse effect on patients' oral health. In 1974, the Federal Social Court in Germany ruled that false teeth should be included in the country's compulsory health insurance programs. "Fillings went out of fashion and prevention was ignored as vast quantities of teeth were pulled and replaced. By 1980, German dentists were using 28 tons of tooth gold a year, one third of the world total." Dentists' incomes soared, exceeding those of physicians by 30 percent. The sickness funds reported a huge deficit, forcing them to raise the level of compulsory contributions. "Dentists Gnashing Teeth in West Germany," *The Wall Street Journal*, December 26, 1985, 11.

7. "Nurses Decry Cost-Cutting Plan That Uses Aides to Do More Jobs," *Wall Street Journal*, January 20, 1994, B1.

8. "Doctors Group Denounces Nurses' Demand for Power." *Washington Post*, December 7, 1993, A3.

9. Fee splitting occurs when a physician refers a patient to a surgeon and in return receives part of the surgeon's fee. Fee splitting is an indication that the surgeon's fee is in excess of her cost; the surgeon can still make a profit though rebating part of the fee. If the fee was not in excess of the costs (including the opportunity cost of the surgeon's time), the surgeon would be unwilling to split the fee. State practice acts permit surgeons to act as a cartel by preventing any one surgeon from engaging in this form of price competition. Fee splitting is a way of eroding the surgeons' monopoly power. Surgeons opposed to fee splitting consider it unethical because the referring physician has a monetary incentive to select the surgeon. Any con-

cern the medical profession has with the quality of surgeons or with the ethical behavior of physicians should be addressed directly through examination and monitoring procedures and not by prohibiting price competition. Unfortunately, as will be discussed, the medical profession has not favored reexamination or monitoring. For a more complete discussion of fee splitting, see Mark V. Pauly, "The Ethics and Economics of Kickbacks and Fee Splitting," *Bell Journal of Economics* 10 (1979): 344–52.

10. Reuben Kessel, "Price Discrimination in Medicine," *Journal of Law and Economics* 1 (1958): 20–53.

11. See, for example, Lee Benham and Alexandra Benham, "Regulating Through the Professions: A Perspective on Information Control," *Journal of Law and Economics* 18 (1975): 421–47.

12. John E. Kwoka, Jr., "Advertising and the Price and Quality of Optometric Services," *American Economic Review* 74 (1984): 211–16.

13. The physician's fee for Medicare, Blue Shield, and private-pay patients was supposed to be the same. The fee was based on the physician's "usual, customary, and reasonable" fee. Blue Shield and Medicare maintained physician fee schedules in their computers. However, Blue Shield paid physicians' fees if they were under a certain percentile limit, whereas Medicare limited the annual increase in physicians' fees for a number of years. Therefore, the physician's fee to a private patient was usually higher than the fee paid by Medicare and Blue Shield.

14. Kessel, "Price Discrimination in Medicine."

15. Group Health Association in Washington, D.C., was one such case cited in the Kessel article.

16. The FTC brought a case against the Indiana Federation of Dentists on grounds of boycotting an insurer for requiring submission of radiographs by dentists. In 1986, the U.S. Supreme Court upheld the FTC by unanimous decision, thereby agreeing with the FTC that the Indiana Federation of Dentists had engaged in an illegal conspiracy. Other state dental boards have undergone similar FTC review. "The Federation argued that if insurers are allowed to determine whether they will pay a claim for dental treatment on the basis of x-rays, they might decline erroneously to pay for necessary treatment and deprive the patient of fully adequate care. The court strongly objected to this argument, likening it to the argument, also rejected in a separate case, 'that an unrestrained market in which consumers are given access to the information they believe to be relevant to their choices will lead them to make unwise and even dan-

gerous choices.'" "U.S. Supreme Court Upholds FTC Order," *ADA News*, June 16, 1986, 2.

17. For a discussion of comparable worth as it applies to nursing, see Joanne Disch and Paul Feldstein, "An Economic Analysis of Comparable Worth," *Journal of Nursing Administration* 16, no. 6 (1986): 24–31.

18. For a review of immigration policies toward foreign medical graduates during this time period, see Alfonso Mejia, Helena Pizurki, and Erica Royston, *Foreign Medical Graduates*, (Lexington, MA: Lexington Books, 1980), Appendix, "Immigration and Licensure Policies."

19. *AMA House of Delegates Proceedings*, 121st Annual Convention, June 20–24, 1972, Report Z (Chicago: American Medical Association), 115. For an excellent study of state legislation authorizing and regulating the practice of PAs, see Stephen C. Crane, "The Legislative Marketplace: A Model of Political Exchange To Explain State Health Regulatory Policy," (doctoral dissertation, School of Public Health, University of Michigan, 1981). In his extensive study of the determinants of state policy regarding PAs, Crane states, "It is clear that the single variable that best accounts for PA policy restrictiveness is the policy preferences of special interest groups" (332).

20. Patricia M. Danzon, "Liability for Medical Malpractice," in *Handbook of Health Economics*, vol. 1b, eds., A. Culyer and J. Newhouse (New York: North-Holland Press, 2000), 1341–1404. The Henry J. Kaiser Family Foundation, Medical Malpractice Policy reference section includes many sources of additional information on recent developments in medical malpractice: http://www.kaiseredu.org/topics_im.asp?id=226&parentID =59&imID.

21. Richard J. Feinstein, "The Ethics of Professional Regulation," *New England Journal of Medicine* 312 (1985): 801–804.

22. David S. Salkever and Thomas W. Bice, *Hospital Certificate-of-Need Controls: Impact on Investment, Costs, and Use*, (Washington, DC: American Enterprise Institute, 1979). For a recent summary of the findings on CON, see Michael A. Morrisey, "State Health Care Reform: Protecting the Provider," in *American Health Care*, ed. Roger Feldman (Oakland, CA: The Independent Institute, 2000), 229–268.

23. Barbara J. Safriet, "Closing the Gap Between Can and May in Health-Care Providers' Scope of Practice: A Primer for Policymakers," *Yale Journal of Regulation* 19, no. 2 (2002): 301–334.

24. *Statements of the American Medical Association*, Compendium of Statements to the Congress and Administrative Agencies, Department of Federal Legislation (Chicago: American Medical Association, 1983, 1984).

25. Cinda Becker, "Imaging Imbroglio: Battle Over Self-Referrals Is Pitting Doc Against Doc," *Modern Healthcare*, December 6, 2004, 16.

26. The seven states are: Maine (1977), Arizona (1978), Colorado (1979), Oregon (1980), Idaho (1982), Montana (1984), and Washington (1994), http://www.international-denturist.org/index.html. Colorado also enacted a bill permitting the independent practice of hygienists. The Colorado Dental Association's executive director attributed this unprecedented action to the state's sunset laws, which gave an opportunity for the bill's proponents to lobby for it. The proponents were feminists (as most hygienists are women), consumer advocates, and a large number of deregulators in the state legislature. The political influence of these groups also changed the composition of the state dental board, making dentists a minority. *ADA News*, May 19, 1986, 5.

27. "Action Urgently Needed on 'Denturist' Movement," editorial, *Journal of the American Dental Association* 92 (1976): 665.

28. Dale F. Redig, "Which Side of this War Are You On?" *ADA News*, November 17, 1986, 4.

29. Commission on Graduates of Foreign Nursing Schools. [Online information, 2005] http://www.cgfns.org/sections/prog/visa.shtml.

30. "AHA Board of Trustees policy statement," *Hospitals, Journal of the American Hospital Association* 47(15) August 1, 1973: 132.

31. Michael Romano, "Taking it to the States: Bills Would Increase Restrictions on Niche Facilities," *Modern Healthcare*, March 21, 2005, 10.

32. Michael Romano, "Community Crackdown: Focus Moves from Specialty to ASCs," *Modern Healthcare*, July 19, 2004, 20.

33. Association of American Medical Colleges, National Resident Matching Program, 2005, http://www.nrmp.org/res_match/tables/table5_05.pdf.

34. "In the [American Dental] Association's view, testing alone cannot provide adequate assurance of competence. Therefore the Association recommends that a foreign-trained dentist be required to complete supplementary education programs in an accredited dental school of at least two-years duration as a precondition to

licensure." Information on Education and Licensure, in *Dentistry in the United States* (Chicago: American Dental Association, 1985), 27.

35. Kessel, "Price Discrimination in Medicine," 27.

36. Kenneth C. Fraundorf, "Organized Dentistry and the Pursuit of Entry Control," *Journal of Health Politics, Policy and Law* 8 (1984): 759–81.

37. *Constitution and Bylaws*, revised to January 1, 1963 Bylaws Section 1110B, 29 (Chicago: American Dental Association).

38. 1984 House of Delegates resolution, October 25, 1984. This resolution follows a previous one (124H-1981) where the ADA was to encourage its "constituent dental societies to utilize these reports (on dentist supply) in petitioning their legislative bodies to consider by lawful means the number of dentists that should be trained." *Transactions*, 125th Annual Session, October 20–25, 1984 (Chicago: American Dental Association, 1984), 537.

39. James W. Begun, *Professionalism and the Public Interest: Price and Quality in Optometry* (Cambridge, MA: The MIT Press, 1981). See also, James W. Begun and Ronald C. Lippincott, "A Case Study in the Politics of Free-Market Health Care," *Journal of Health Politics, Policy and Law* 7 (1982): 667–85.

40. Data from National League for Nursing, *Nursing Data Book*, (New York: National League for Nursing), various years.

41. For a more complete discussion of this proposal, see Andrew K. Dolan, "The New York State Nurses Association 1985 Proposal: Who Needs It?" *Journal of Health Politics, Policy and Law* 2 (1978): 508–30.

42. Robert H. Ebert and Eli Ginzberg, "The Reform of Medical Education," *Health Affairs* 7 (supplement, 1988): 5–38. The authors state, "We believe it is feasible to reduce significantly the time it takes to prepare a primary care physician (or a specialist) without sacrificing quality." (22)

43. "Dentistry's Blueprint for the Future," *Journal of the American Dental Association* 108 (1984): 20–30.

44. Many states adopted the citizenship requirement for foreign medical graduates after the AMA's House of Delegates passed such a resolution in 1938. Five states continued such a requirement as late as 1975. Although citizenship is no longer required in any state, all foreign medical graduates, excluding those from Canadian schools, are required to take an exam before entering a residency program.

45. Another entry barrier used in dentistry is restrictions on interstate mobility. Various studies have shown that dentists graduating from a

dental school within a state have a greater chance of passing that state's licensing exam than dentists from other states. Unlike medicine, most states do not permit reciprocal licensing for dentists. See, for example, Lawrence Shepard, "Licensing Restrictions and the Cost of Dental Care," *Journal of Law and Economics* 21 (1978): 187–201. See also, B. Friedland and R. Valachovic, "The Regulation of Dental Licensing—The Dark Ages," *American Journal of Law and Medicine* 17 (1991): 249–270. Additional studies on licensing restrictions are in the footnotes section of the article by M. Kleiner, http://www.ftc .gov/ogc/healthcarehearings/docs/030610kleiner2.pdf.

46. Robert C. Derbyshire, "Medical Ethics and Discipline," *Journal of the American Medical Association* 228 (1974): 59–62. See also, Robert C. Derbyshire, *Medical Licensure and Discipline in the United States* (Baltimore, MD: Johns Hopkins University Press, 1969), and Robert C. Derbyshire, "Medical Discipline in Disarray: Offenders and Offenses," *Hospital Practice*, 19, no. 3 March 1984: 98a–98v.

47. Feinstein, "The Ethics of Professional Regulation," 803. In view of the poor record of state medical boards in disciplining physicians, the comments by Dr. James Sammons, executive vice president of the AMA, were all the more revealing. In opposing mandatory reevaluations for relicensing, Dr. Sammons stated, "There are better ways to measure competency. [Reviews in hospitals and state medical boards] are best able to weed out incompetent physicians." "Cuomo's Plan for Testing Doctors Is Part of Growing National Effort," *New York Times*, June 9, 1986, 1, 19.

48. The Federation of State Medical Boards, Summary of 2004 Board Actions, http://www.fsmb.org. Data on the number of actions per 1,000 population was calculated by the author based on the data from The Federation of State Medical Boards, Summary of 2004 Board Actions, http://www.fsmb.org.

49. Drew Carlson, The Federation of State Medical Boards, personal correspondence with the author, August 9, 2005.

50. Government Accounting Office, *Expanded Federal Authority Needed to Protect Medicare and Medicaid Patients from Health Practitioners Who Lose Their Licenses*, May 1, 1984, http://archive.gao.gov/d5t1/124032.pdf (most recent information from Congressional Budget Office as of August 10, 2005).

51. "AMA Adopts New Self-Regulation Plan For MD Profession," *ADA News*, November 17, 1986, 18. See also, "AMA Initiative on Quality of Medical Care and Professional Self-Regulation," *Journal of the American Medical Association* 256 (1986): 1036–37.

52. Ibid.

THE REASONS FOR DEREGULATION

After completing this chapter, the reader should be able to

- contrast the public interest and economic theory in explaining why regulated industries are deregulated,
- explain the role of the courts in leading to industry deregulation,
- discuss the consequences of deregulation on labor unions in the previously regulated industry,
- explain why the railroad industry eventually sought deregulation,
- use the economic theory of regulation to explain the deregulation of industries, and
- discuss the factors that determine whether an industry remains regulated or becomes deregulated.

It is clear why existing firms in an industry would want to be regulated. They can achieve through regulation rewards that would be unattainable in a competitive market. Yet starting in the 1970s, a number of industries were deregulated: railroads, trucking, airlines, banking, telecommunications, and the securities industry. The health sector also changed in the 1980s from a heavily regulated industry to one characterized by market competition.

Was deregulation brought about because it was in the public interest? Did legislators recognize that the costs of regulation, in terms of higher prices and a smaller output to consumers, exceeded its benefits? The economic theory of regulation, as an approach for explaining legislative outcomes, must be able to explain not only why industries seek regulation and are able to control the regulatory process but also why some of those same industries are deregulated. Deregulation presumably destroys the economic wealth of regulated firms, so those firms would be expected to oppose it. Regulated industries are likely to offer an amount of political support up to the value of their regulatory benefits. Who would be able to offer more?

Although deregulation occurred among some industries during the 1970s and early 1980s, other industries maintained their regulatory protection. And in some industries government regulation actually increased.

The following discussion attempts to explain why deregulation occurred in some industries and not others. It is shown that the reasons for deregulation are consistent with the hypotheses of self-interest and that legislators seek to maximize their political support. First, a brief discussion of several deregulated industries is presented. Second, the similar characteristics of deregulated industries are examined to suggest reasons for deregulation. The reasons for deregulation are then used in the next chapter to explain the change to market competition in the health industry.

Examples of Deregulated Industries

Railroad Freight Transportation

The classic case of a regulatory agency that serves the economic interests of those being regulated is the Interstate Commerce Commission (ICC). Federal regulation of railroads began in 1887 with the passage of the Interstate Commerce Act, which established the ICC. The two interest groups favoring this act were shippers and the railroads themselves. The railroads wanted to end the frequent rate wars and secret concessions some railroads gave to shippers. The shippers also wanted less rate instability but were concerned because they were being charged more to ship freight short distances than long distances. (Prices were higher for short hauls because there was less competition.)

Subsequent federal legislation empowered the ICC to set maximum rates, control entry and exit into the industry, and perform many of the tasks necessary for operating the industry. This resulted in the industry performing as a cartel.[1] The method the ICC used to establish fixed rates was to set rates generally proportional to the distance traveled, rather than to cost. This resulted in raising long-haul rates rather than lowering short-haul rates as the shippers wanted.

With federal regulation, investment returns in the railroad industry improved and investor risk was reduced. Employee wages were also increased. Federal regulation enabled the railroads to achieve rates of return above those achievable in a competitive environment.

In the 1920s, two new unregulated competitors came on the scene, buses and trucks, which decreased the benefits of regulation to railroads. Bus and trucking companies were not subject to large economies of scale and the number of bus and truck firms increased rapidly. The profitability of railroads declined as trucks undercut the high, fixed rail rates for short hauls. Railroads countered this competitive threat by bringing trucking and buses under state regulation. In the late 1920s, however, two Supreme Court decisions negated the states' authority to regulate interstate trucking and buses. As a result, the railroads sought federal regulation to protect their interests. Shippers, on the other hand, opposed the extension of the ICC's jurisdiction over these low-cost alternatives. Truckers, however, favored federal regulation. Existing truckers saw regulation as a means of protecting themselves from newcomers.

Both railroads and truckers achieved what they had sought. The Motor Carrier Act of 1935 set minimum prices and established entry controls on trucks. Railroads were protected from price competition by low-cost substitutes (trucks), and truckers received the benefits of a cartel, that is, control over prices and entry into their industry. Including another producer group, common-carrier trucks, under the ICC's jurisdiction, however, would eventually result in a decline in the relative political influence of railroads.

Railroads began to lose their profitability by the 1950s. Rates proportional to distance resulted in railroad rates that were below cost for short hauls (and low-density markets) and above cost in long-haul, high-density markets. Railroad rates were set so high in long-haul markets that truckers, whose costs were generally higher than railroads for long-haul freight, found it worthwhile to compete. A number of railroads went into bankruptcy, including the Penn Central (in 1970), in large part because of losses in the short-haul market and increased competition in the long-haul market.

Regulation was no longer working to the benefit of the railroads. Despite rate regulation, they were losing their market share to the truckers. Improved technology and the interstate highway system benefited the truckers; trucking costs were reduced and motor carrier service became faster and more reliable. As a cartel for establishing rates, the ICC was now hurting rather than helping the railroads. The Association of American Railroads complained that unless the ICC granted greater rate and route flexibility to the railroads, they would end up "dead in the water."[2] Other special interest groups, such as the truckers' association, the Teamsters, and users of regulated services were representing their interests before the ICC and offering political support to legislators. The ICC had other concentrated interests (and the political support they provided) to consider when making decisions.

The railroads saw their salvation in greater price flexibility so they could compete with the truckers. Railroad profitability was also adversely affected by their being required to provide money-losing services, such as passenger service, and the requirement that they serve certain passenger and freight routes. Railroads had to receive ICC approval to drop these services. However, those benefiting from these services wanted them continued. Regulation had given these beneficiaries a valuable right, which they did not want to lose. To return to profitability, the railroads needed greater flexibility in both prices and services.

On the side of the railroads were the major shippers. Greater price flexibility meant lower prices to shippers. The National Association of Manufacturers was in the forefront of the deregulation movement.

In the 1970s several railroads went bankrupt. The political choices were to nationalize the railroads and subsidize them or permit deregulation. The administration favored greater flexibility for the railroads; they were concerned that the bankruptcy of more railroads would mean continued large government subsidies. (Conrail lost $1.4 billion in its first four and one-half years.)[3] The railroads also preferred deregulation to nationalization.

Several changes were made in railroad regulation in the 1970s, such as providing railroads with limited pricing flexibility. The trend toward deregulating the railroads culminated in the Staggers Rail Act of 1980, which permitted greater price and service flexibility.

As a result of partial deregulation, railroads were able to compete favorably against truckers. They raised their short-haul rates and lowered their long-haul rates. Railroads, which are very efficient, that is, low cost, in transporting large volumes of freight over long distances, were able to increase their market share over truckers in the long-haul market by lowering prices. Rates for some products, such as grain, declined by more than 30 percent.[4] Piggyback methods, which combine the flexibility of trucks in local pickup and delivery with the long-haul efficiency of railroads, and previously prohibited by the rate structure of the ICC, were introduced. The result was an integrated transportation system. Market share of railroads, compared to truckers, increased; for example, shipping of fruits and vegetables by rail nearly doubled between 1979 and 1983.[5]

Service quality on the railroads also improved. Accidents on poorly maintained tracks, which had been increasing before deregulation, were reduced. From the shipper's perspective, their costs of maintaining inventories (logistic costs) were reduced as rail service became more reliable. Railroads were now able to negotiate delivery times and other services with shippers, whereas formerly were prohibited from doing so by the ICC because it was viewed as a form of price cutting.[6] Railroads were now permitted to abandon unprofitable branch lines. Rather than reducing service on these lines, new railroads operated them using nonunion labor; with lower operating costs. Service continued and these lines served as feeder traffic into the larger railroads.

The consequence of these actions was that railroad profitability increased. Profits more than doubled between 1978 and 1981.[7] Federal subsidies to railroads declined from more than $500 million in 1980 to $66 million in 1985. And railroad rates, which had been 4.2 cents per ton-mile in the 1970s declined to 2.6 cents by 1988; rates have continued to fall, saving shippers $30 billion in 1999 alone.[8]

Labor, however, was a big loser in deregulation. Previously, railroads faced detailed labor work rules and labor protection provisions. After deregulation, railroads were able to make sizable reductions in their workforce—a decrease of 40 percent between 1980 and 1985.[9] Because of these adverse effects, in 1986 labor attempted, unsuccessfully, to subject the railroads once again to regulation.

The Trucking Industry

In 1980, the Motor Carrier Act was passed. This act replaced earlier legislation governing the trucking industry, allowing for ease of entry and removal of pricing restrictions. There was, however, an important distinction between these two pieces of legislation. Railroads wanted to be free of previous regulatory restrictions; truckers and the Teamsters wanted the restrictions affecting trucking to remain in place. The regulated firms in trucking were in a different situation than the railroads. They were not going bankrupt. In fact, deregulation of trucking was strongly opposed by the Teamsters and by the American Trucking Association, the two beneficiaries of continued regulation. Why then was trucking also partially deregulated?

An important reason for this change was a court case. The ICC turned down a request from the PC White Truck Line to permit it to enter new markets. The applicant then appealed its case to the District of Columbia Court of Appeals. In 1977, the court ruled in favor of the applicant, stating that in deciding on entry requests the ICC should not only consider whether existing trucking services are adequate, but take into account the beneficial effects that increased competition might have on the public.[10] The significance of this case was that unless the ICC considered the beneficial effects of competition when judging new applications, the courts would reverse their decisions.

In subsequent decisions, the ICC placed greater emphasis on the beneficial effects of competition to the public. In the Liberty Trucking Co. case (1979) the ICC found that increased competition outweighed any harm that might occur to existing carriers. As a result of these decisions, the number of applications to enter trucking markets expanded by tenfold over the previous decade. The entry barriers were being removed as a result of the 1977 District of Columbia Court of Appeals judicial decision.

During this period, the ICC commissioners were slowly being replaced with market-oriented commissioners. Presidents since Kennedy had favored some form of trucking deregulation, although all were unsuccessful. In the 1970s President Ford again raised the visibility of deregulation as a political issue, promoting it as a means of reducing the rate of inflation, an important concern at the time. Oil prices had increased sharply and there was opposition to passing on these cost increases in the form of higher shipping costs. President Ford, however, was unsuccessful in deregulating trucking or any other industry. President Carter also saw deregulation as a partial means to combat high oil prices and stagflation in the economy; he continued to raise the visibility of deregulation as a political issue. (He was also attempting to establish his leadership on deregulation and thereby preempt his political rival, Senator Edward Kennedy, from receiving credit for this issue.) The initial success that either administration had was to appoint regulatory commissioners who were more market-oriented. These new appointees were in favor of the court rulings (PC White and Liberty) that liberalized entry into trucking.

When the new appointees achieved a majority in the ICC, the ICC announced (in 1979) that it was going to reevaluate the method that had been used in establishing trucking rates (rates were set collectively, not competitively). At this point, the trucking association and the Teamsters decided it would be in their own best interest to push for legislation that would stop the movement toward competition in both entry and pricing.

The trucking industry was successful in introducing anticompetitive legislation favorable to their interests in the House of Representatives. Trucking companies operate in all congressional districts; and the Teamsters and truckers' association were providing political support to many legislators. However, the administration opposed the bill, as did the press, which made this restrictive legislation very visible. The press emphasized the waste and inefficiency resulting from trucking restrictions, such as truckers not being able to carry full loads both to and from their destinations. The Teamsters were also receiving bad publicity during this period; the president of the Teamsters went to jail for attempting to bribe Senator Howard W. Cannon, the Chairman of the committee with jurisdiction over the deregulation bill, and the issue had become too visible. President Carter threatened to veto the House bill if it became law.

The Senate passed a bill that permitted the reforms in trucking to continue. Senators do not need campaign funds as frequently as representatives. Further, the size of a political contribution to a senator or representative from any one political action committee was limited by law. Senate races require a great deal more money than races for the House; political contributions from any one group are a small percentage of a senator's total contributions. Given their broader constituencies and their needs for greater amounts of money, senators are generally less responsive than representatives to the demands of small special-interest groups. With respect to trucking legislation, however, senators up for reelection were more likely to vote for three restrictive amendments desired by the truckers and Teamsters than those senators not running for reelection.[11] Once the restrictive amendments were defeated, those senators running for reelection also voted for passage of the final bill. In this way they could say they were "pro-consumer," because they had voted for deregulation.

The House went along with the Senate, and the Motor Carrier Act was passed. Because 1980 was also an election year, the president, in signing this legislation, used it as an indication of his political leadership. It was believed to be important to consumers.

The big losers under partial deregulation were the Teamsters; they had been earning approximately 50 percent more than they would in a competitive environment: in the first year after deregulation they lost half that amount.[12] Another loser was the regulated trucking firms. There was a tremendous increase in the number of new trucking firms; between 1980 and 1982, the number of firms increased by 42 percent.[13] Price competition by the new firms, some that were owner-operated and others that used nonunion labor, reduced the profitability of the previously protected trucking firms. One indication of the monopoly profits received by a trucking firm during regulation was the value of a trucking license, which was $530,000 in 1977 and subsequently declined to $13,000 in 1981 with increased entry. As competition increased, prices declined by approximately 25 percent between 1977 and 1982. As prices and profitability declined, the percentage of firms going bankrupt increased. As shipping prices declined because of increased entry, Teamsters' wages declined as well. In their opposition to deregulation, the Teamsters clearly foresaw its consequences.

These consequences of competition, however, did not result in any decline in quality. According to surveys of shippers, quality either improved or stayed the same. Further, complaints by shippers to the ICC declined.[14]

The opponents of deregulation, the trucking firms and their unionized employees, continued their battle at the state level, where they had more influence than at the federal level. The federal act deregulating interstate trucking did not preempt state laws regulating intrastate trucking. Thus, only six states fully deregulated trucking during 1980 to 1991. Most states continued to regulate the movement of intrastate goods, thereby maintaining artificially higher intrastate rates. Large shippers, however, such as Federal Express, continued to press for federal legislation ending state regulation. The large shippers did not have the political advantage at the state level that the trucking associations had.

As occurred with interstate deregulation, the impetus for federal legislation deregulating intrastate trucking evolved from court decisions. Circuit courts in Texas and California deregulated Federal Express intrastate trucking operations, which placed other air/ground operators, like United Parcel Service and Roadway Package Service, at a competitive disadvantage. Further, if, as was likely, United Parcel Service and Roadway Package Service were similarly deregulated, then trucking companies would be competitively disadvantaged. These companies could consolidate small shipments into truckload lots, offering strong competition to traditional less-than-truckload carriers. Thus, deregulation of intrastate trucking would be the only solution for truckers. The lobbying organization for truckers, the American Trucking Associations, agreed to deregulation of intrastate trucking by saying they would no longer oppose deregulation.[15] The truckers realized they would be at a major disadvantage to the air/ground carriers if truckers were not deregulated as well. Thus, intrastate deregulation of trucking was enacted at the federal level in 1994.

Deregulation results in an estimated savings of about $100 billion a year.[16] Manufacturers are able to reduce their inventories, move their products more quickly, and be more responsive to consumers, all of which has enabled U.S. industry to become more competitive internationally.

Airlines

For many years, domestic air transportation policy was based on the Civil Aeronautics Act of 1938 and the Federal Aviation Act of 1958. Regulation of the industry was placed in the hands of the CAB.[17] The CAB controlled entry into the industry, not permitting a single new trunk carrier from 1938 through the 1970s. It also determined the routes each airline could fly; regulated airfares; and exercised control over the airlines' service competition, even to the extent of regulating the amount of meat that could be served in a sandwich.[18] The CAB's primary concern in setting airfares was airline profitability. Any carrier seeking to enter another market had to prove it would not harm the carrier currently serving that market.

Some of the consequences of airline regulation were as follows: (1) fares were approximately 50 percent higher than fares in unregulated markets, such as, intrastate travel within California and Texas, which was free of federal control; (2) there was extensive nonprice competition between the airlines, such as frequency of flights and the rapid introduction of new equipment, leading to higher operating costs; and (3) fares were set proportional to distance traveled, when in fact cost per mile was lower on long-distance flights than on short-distance flights. Cities that were less frequently traveled were subsidized by the busier routes.

In the late 1960s, the airlines had converted their fleets to jet aircraft. In addition, the airlines competed among themselves on frequency of flights. The consequence was that airline capacity increased faster than the growth in demand. Faced with rising costs and declining profits, the airlines kept asking the CAB for increased fares.

In 1975, at the recommendation of new staff member Stephen Breyer (now a Supreme Court justice), Senator Edward Kennedy decided to hold hearings on airline regulation. It was believed that deregulation would be a visible consumer issue that would provide Senator Kennedy with political support.[19] Media coverage of the hearings showed that consumers were being denied the benefits of airline competition, such as lower prices. During the 1975 hearings, the airlines were opposed to any form of deregulation. However, the hearings performed an important service.

The hearings made clear that regulation was not really working for two of the major proponents of continued regulation, small cities and the airlines themselves. Certain small cities (and consequently their legislators) were concerned that air travel to their cities would be sharply curtailed under deregulation. At Senator Kennedy's hearings it was determined that few cities would actually lose their air service, and most cities did not require subsidies to have continued air service. Small aircraft, less than 30 seats, had been exempt from CAB entry limits. Exempt firms had been increasing the number of flights, and scheduling them at more convenient times, to small communities just as the CAB-regulated major airlines, with their larger planes, were decreasing service to small communities.

The hearings also showed that regulation was not working for the airlines. The protected airlines were not making monopoly profits. They had been using up the excess profits they made on their most profitable routes because of nonprice competition. Therefore, the industry did not have much to lose under deregulation. At the same time, the deregulated airlines, those flying in the intrastate markets of California and Texas, were quite profitable. At the hearings, evidence of the benefits of lower airfares to the airlines was presented. Intrastate airlines were shown to have higher load factors and increased profitability as a result of reduced fares.

In late 1975 another important event occurred. The District of Columbia Court of Appeals overturned an earlier CAB decision on the denial of a route to Continental Air Lines. After almost nine years of litigation, the court stated that the CAB's rejection of competition was not in accord with the public interest. (This was the same court that in 1977 would rule in favor of competition in trucking in the PC White case.) Although the court's decision was not a signal for unlimited entry, it was the beginning of the elimination of barriers in the airline industry's profitable cartel markets.

Faced with this criticism of its policies (and the subsequent appointment of Alfred Kahn, an economist who became chairman of the CAB, and more competitively oriented board members), over the next several years the CAB permitted a little more flexibility for air charters as a low-cost substitute to scheduled air service. American Airlines, recognizing the threat of low-cost charters serving the New York-to-California market, offered discount fares. The results were surprising: air traffic surged. The success of this fare flexibility, and its profitability for the airlines, encouraged the CAB to continue and expand fare flexibility. The airlines' profitability increased dramatically. Fares declined (adjusted for inflation), air traffic increased at a faster annual rate than in the previous ten years, and public support for airline deregulation grew.

As a result of increased information, opposition to deregulation among the airlines changed. The industry was split over the benefits of continued regulation. United, the largest domestic carrier, favored deregulation because it believed it would have a greater chance to grow and gain market share. Under regulation it was unlikely to be awarded new routes. Pan Am, an international carrier, also favored deregulation because it wanted domestic routes but had not been able to receive any under CAB regulation. Other airlines that had competed vigorously in intrastate competition with the major airlines, Pacific Southwest Airlines (California) and Southwest Airlines (Texas), believed their only chance to compete in interstate markets was in a deregulated industry.

The association representing airline interests had members with conflicting interests. Within the association, large carriers had different economic interests than the smaller carriers. Each airline provided its own political support to legislators; the association itself was able to provide very little. In subsequent hearings before the House, the carriers were split in their opposition to deregulation, and the association did not testify.

Indicating the importance of information in changing the airlines' perceptions of the profitability of deregulation was the comment by Frank Borman, chairman of Eastern Airlines: "I think I was most surprised by how much traffic is generated by cutting fares. Deregulation saved the industry. It turned it from what would have become a moribund, stagnant industry like the Europeans' into a vibrant, growing industry."[20]

As this perception of potential profitability spread, opposition to deregulation within the industry decreased. To alleviate the concerns of some small communities, the only potential losers under deregulation, a separate subsidy program was proposed. Legislators therefore had little to lose by supporting deregulation; they could be pro-consumer. Airline opposition was no longer an important concern, and small communities would not be hurt. It was not until after all this had occurred that a deregulation bill was feasible.

In October 1978, Congress passed the Airline Deregulation Act and the airline industry was deregulated. (The CAB itself was abolished at the end of 1984.) The congressional action continued what the CAB had started. The flexibility CAB showed, and the resulting increase in air traffic and airline profits, limited the airlines' opposition to legislation officially deregulating the industry. There were no large monopoly profits to be protected by returning to the previous heavily regulated system. The public favored lower fares. Several of the major carriers (and the intrastate airlines) saw opportunities in deregulation. And the small cities, and their representatives in Congress, realized they would not be hurt by deregulation. By the time the bill came before Congress in the fall of 1978, "there was little opposition and the bill passed by a large majority."[21]

The deregulation of the airlines led to a complete reversal in the structure of the industry; after being a regulated cartel the industry felt the full force of market competition within a relatively short time.

As a result of airline deregulation, the structure of fares changed. Prices more closely approximated costs of service. Thus, airfares in long-distance and high-density markets declined up to 40 percent.[22] The average price to fly one domestic mile has dropped by more than 50 percent (inflation adjusted) since deregulation.[23] As fares declined, airline load factors increased. Long-distance air travel proved to be very responsive to lower prices; nonbusiness travel increased substantially. (As load factors increased, passenger comfort has decreased. Passengers, however, have apparently chosen lower prices over comfort as first-class travel has fallen sharply.) An important reason for the reduction in airfares in high-density markets has been the entry of new and regional airlines. These carriers offered large discounts, created price competition, and increased their market share, which went from 12 to 30 percent between 1978 and 1982.[24]

Those airlines initially protected by the CAB had higher operating costs than their new competitors and found it difficult to transform themselves into lower-cost carriers. Labor contracts with their unionized employees kept their labor costs higher than those of new carriers that entered the market. The new entrants did not use unionized labor, paid their pilots perhaps one-third as much as the established airlines, and did not have restrictive work rules. To compete on price, the older airlines had to reduce their labor costs so that they were comparable to those of their new competitors. However, the older airlines had difficulty renegotiating their labor contracts; their unions fiercely resisted changing employee wages, benefits, and work rules. The airlines were reluctant to push their unions too hard in fear that they would strike, with the consequence that their passengers would go to other airlines and it would be too costly to recover, if they were in fact able to recover. Several of the original trunk carriers had financial difficulties; of the 10 major carriers operating in 1978, five either went out of business or merged with other airlines. Some airlines, such as Continental, declared bankruptcy, enabling them to hire nonunion employees and to change their work rules.

Unionized labor in the airlines industry had, with good reason, opposed deregulation. Airline employees faced difficult times; as the lower-cost airlines grew and increased their market share, airline employees from the older airlines lost their jobs or were forced to renegotiate their wages downward.

Throughout deregulation, quality, as measured by airline accidents and fatalities per passenger mile, improved.[25] Further, economists have estimated that consumers save about $20 billion per year due to lower fares resulting from a competitive airline marketplace.[26]

The structure of the industry changed after deregulation. The major airlines developed a hub-and-spoke method of delivery. The major airlines encouraged regional and local airlines to serve smaller cities (the spokes), to feed more traffic into the hubs. The effect of the hub-and-spoke system was that consumers had more choices in departure and arrival times and a far greater choice of destinations. Those who lived in a hub city had access to a much larger number of destinations, while residents on the spokes of the hub also gained access to many destinations via the hub. Discount airlines, however, found that flying a large number of planes into an airport at the same time and then departing in a mass rush (the hub-and-spoke method) was inefficient. Instead, the discounters relied on direct flights between non-hub cities.

In recent years, all of the major airlines have run into financial difficulty. Consumers are very price sensitive, and the rise of the Internet made it easier for them to shop for lower fares. With their high-wage labor contracts and their cost structure compared to the discounters, the major airlines could no longer charge the high fares to cover their higher costs. Rising fuel costs in the past several years were an additional financial burden to the airlines. As a result, more of the major airlines entered bankruptcy. To survive, the major airlines are attempting to further reduce their labor costs and emulate the lower-cost airlines.

Even with the benefits of deregulation to consumers, there are still proposals for the government to reregulate the airlines and exercise greater federal control. One complaint has been the higher fares at hub airports. Hub airports are dominated by one or two airlines, which means higher fares than those at airports where there is greater competition. However, fares at hub airports are still about 20 percent lower than if the industry had still been regulated. The other major complaint by consumers has been about congestion and delays and that start-up airlines cannot compete effectively.

The problems concerning congestion, delays, and limited entry by start-up airlines are not the result of too much competition but the result of restraints on market forces. When the airlines were deregulated, the government kept control (and ownership) over the airports and the air traffic control system. As airline traffic soared, airports (unlike an investor owned utility) were unable to levy fees on takeoffs and landings to finance capacity for additional airline spots, upgraded landing equipment, and more controllers. The Department of Transportation must request funds from Congress for capital investments and personnel. Thus, given the large increase in demand at airports, the Federal Aviation Authority (FAA) rations airline "slots." The FAA also runs the air traffic control system. Numerous congressional hearings have been held to pressure the FAA bureaucracy to modernize the air traffic control system, which uses outdated computers and radars. Changes in the air traffic control system could enable airports to accommodate more traffic.[27]

By allowing airports to be freed of governmental control, greater use could be made of market forces; airports would have an incentive to raise the revenues to expand the number of runways, increase the number of airline slots, add additional controllers, and adopt new technology to increase air traffic volumes. Introducing market forces in these areas (i.e., deregulation of the air traffic control system, with the FAA maintaining oversight of airline safety) would enhance the benefits of deregulation, namely, increased safety, greater choice of airlines, and lower fares.

New York Stock Exchange

The New York Stock Exchange (NYSE) was founded in 1792 and was operated as a cartel until 1975. The NYSE had a fixed number of members, and it fixed the prices members could charge for selling and purchasing stocks. The Securities and Exchange Commission was the government regulatory agency that enforced the economic interests of the NYSE. The monopoly power of the NYSE was based on the fact that it handled more than 80 percent of all stock trading. The NYSE also undertook a number of regulatory functions to minimize the financial irresponsibility of its members and to set minimum standards before a company could list its stock for trading on the exchange.[28]

The commission (price) charged for the purchase and sale of stock was fixed and did not reflect the actual costs of the transaction. For small orders, the commission was below the actual cost; for large orders the commission was greatly in excess of costs. Thus, there was a cross-subsidy from the large-volume traders to the small traders.

Before 1960, less than 2 percent of the volume on the NYSE was attributed to large block sales by institutions. By 1976, large institutional firms accounted for 44 percent of the NYSE volume (and 54 percent of the dollar value) of shares traded.

A new group of traders had arisen: large institutional traders with a definite economic interest in paying the lowest commissions for their trades. NYSE member firms, with fixed commission rates set by the exchange, were not permitted to engage in price competition for the business of these large traders. Instead, they engaged in nonprice competition (such as conducting "free research") for large institutional traders, which increased their costs and thereby decreased the profitability of regulated prices. In response to the search by these large institutional traders for lower commissions, nonmember firms appeared to arrange large block sales and purchases. Such a firm would match large buy-and-sell orders for institutional traders, and the sale would be consummated off the NYSE, at a lower commission. The NYSE cartel began to collapse. Large institutions also started using regional stock exchanges to place their orders. As the volume of large trades on the NYSE fell, the NYSE allowed its member firms to give discounts for large trades.

The Securities Acts Amendments of 1975, which eliminated fixed commissions, was a recognition of economic realities; fixed commissions were no longer economically viable.

The rise of large institutional traders, the development of (lower-cost) substitute exchanges to serve the large traders, the loss of volume by the NYSE to these substitute exchanges, and the decline in profitability of NYSE member firms that did not compete for the business of large traders, led to de facto deregulation. The change in the securities laws merely ratified what was occurring. No longer could member firms receive monopoly profits through fixed commission rates; therefore, there was little economic value left to protect by maintaining fixed commissions.

Deregulation brought increased volume back to the NYSE and, as in a competitive market, commissions became more closely related to the cost of executing trades. Commissions on small trades increased by approximately 12 percent, while for large institutional traders commissions were reduced by more than 50 percent.[29] And as the cost of trading declined, volume increased. In addition, the lower cost of large trades was believed to increase the growth of institutional ownership of stocks through mutual funds.[30]

As price competition increased, brokerage firms that could only survive in a regulated environment had to merge. The firms were forced to take advantage of economies of scale in their operations. Previously, larger, more efficient firms had to compete at the same price as smaller firms. Larger brokerage firms favored deregulation because they believed their economies of scale would enable them to reduce their prices and increase their market share at the expense of small brokerage firms. The other effect of deregulation was the emergence of discount brokers. Brokers began to unbundle their services. Previously, because large trades were so profitable, brokers competed on nonprice factors, such as research services to clients. With the rise of price competition, some customers decided to purchase their research services separately and pay just for the trading services they used. Discount brokers have captured an increasing share of the retail sales market.

Brokerage firms have also diversified as revenues from commissions account for a smaller percentage of their total revenues, down from 50 percent in 1975.[31] Brokerage firms have established related businesses in insurance, money market funds, and real estate operations.

Banks and Savings Institutions

Banking and savings and loan institutions (S&Ls) are among our most heavily regulated industries. Limits are placed on the amount of interest these institutions can pay to their depositors, on the interest they can charge on some types of loans, on who can establish new banks, and on the activities in which these institutions can engage. However, particularly since 1980, there has been a great deal of change. Some of these changes permit banks to engage in branch banking, to operate in other states, and to pay market interest rates to customers. Although the industry continues to be quite heavily regulated by federal and state authorities, deregulation has been occurring. To illustrate the reasons for partial deregulation in this industry, only one regulatory change will be examined, namely, interest paid on savings accounts.[32]

In 1933, the Federal Reserve Board promulgated Regulation Q, which established maximum interest rates (2.5 percent) that commercial banks could pay to depositors on savings accounts. These maximum rates were permitted to rise to reflect market rates until 1966. As inflation increased in the 1960s, interest rates rose (so as to provide lenders with a "real," that is, an inflation-adjusted, rate of return). The S&Ls had their assets in long-term mortgages that paid low rates of interest to the S&Ls. To attract and keep depositors, the S&Ls would have had to raise their interest rates on deposits. However, this policy would result in the S&Ls paying more to their depositors than they were receiving on their mortgages. The solution was for Congress to extend Regulation Q to S&Ls.

Since 1966, the maximum rates paid depositors had been set below the market rate of interest. The effect of doing so was to provide S&Ls with a source of funds at a price that was below the price at which they could loan these funds. Profitability of savings and loan associations increased. (A reason S&Ls gave for setting rates to depositors below market rates was that by making S&Ls more profitable, they would increase their housing loans at lower than market rates of interest. In fact, this did not occur.

Two-thirds of mortgages were written by mortgage bankers, insurance companies, and others that did not have access to this cheap source of funds. Mortgage rates were determined by the overall market.)[33]

Establishing maximum interest rates adversely affected small savers. Savers with funds of $100,000 or more were exempt from these maximum rates after 1970. (Commercial banks, fearful that they would lose their large depositors, were allowed to pay market interest rates on large deposits.) Savers with smaller sums, $10,000 to $25,000, could invest those funds in Treasury bills and bonds and thereby receive the higher market rates of interest. It was only the small saver who did not have a substitute source for their savings who was adversely affected by having to accept the lower rates. To ensure that small savers did not withdraw their funds from S&Ls and invest in Treasury bills, the regulators increased the minimum size of Treasury bills, from $1,000 to $10,000 in 1970.

There were an overwhelming number of small savers and so the cost of this regulatory policy was diffuse; the foregone interest each saver lost was small and spread out over many individuals. The cost of organizing and representing their interests was not worth the effort.

As market interest rates continued to rise and the spread between those interest rates and the amount paid to S&L depositors increased, S&Ls had to engage in nonprice competition to attract savers. S&Ls offered radios, television sets, and other prizes to depositors. Because this policy raised the cost to the S&Ls of attracting depositors, which had the same effect as increasing interest on new deposits, it was in the S&Ls' combined interest to limit such competition. The regulators responded by setting limits on such prizes.

As a result of increasing market interest rates and regulated bank rates, money market mutual funds were formed in the early 1970s and expanded rapidly. The development of these money market mutual fund accounts drew savings from the savings and loan associations. However, as was initially the case with railroads, rather than rid themselves of regulations and compete, the savings and loan associations sought to have the money market funds placed under the same maximum rates. They were unsuccessful in overcoming the opposition of the commercial banks and money market firms. The money market funds increased their market share as smaller depositors began to leave the S&Ls in search of higher rates of interest.

In 1978 some deregulation over maximum rates occurred. Credit unions were permitted to pay market rates to their depositors, and new types of savings accounts were established that permitted higher rates of interest. Yet complete deregulation did not occur until years later, in 1986.

The savings and loan associations favored continuing maximum rates because, although they lost savers to competitors, maintaining the maximum rates was still very profitable. Even though they were losing business, in 1982 S&Ls still held almost $500 billion in savings accounts, while paying below-market rates of interest. These funds were being loaned out at market rates of interest.

The effect of partial deregulation clearly benefited the small savers; they could now receive increased interest rates on their savings. "It was estimated that decontrol would increase interest payments to depositors by at least $20 billion per year."[34] The big losers were the savings and loan associations. To compete, they now had to pay more for their money. They also lost customers to substitute savings sources.

The economic value of interest rate regulation to the S&Ls decreased as small depositors were able to receive higher interest rates by switching to unregulated competitors that had developed, such as mutual funds.

The gap between regulated interest rates and market rates provided an incentive for innovation to occur outside the regulated market. These competitors grew as they were able to exploit this difference in interest rates. Money market mutual funds and commercial banks also had a sufficiently strong economic interest to be able to compete successfully in the political as well as economic arena with S&Ls.

Telecommunications

Through the 1950s, AT&T was a fully regulated monopoly. Large economies of scale existed in the provision of local telephone service and the Federal Communications Commission (FCC) prevented entry into the market. Local telephone services were provided by AT&T or by other local telephone companies with no effective competition. Long-distance service provided by AT&T also had the characteristics of a natural monopoly, namely, large economies of scale. Local and long-distance service used common equipment. AT&T also had a monopoly on telephone equipment, even though this market lacked the characteristics of a natural monopoly. The breakup of AT&T occurred because of technological changes in the equipment and long-distance markets and subsequent court decisions.[35]

There was no economic reason why the equipment segment of the industry could not have been competitive. However, AT&T had the monopoly and wanted to keep it. Competition began only as a result of a successful court case against AT&T.

Hush-A-Phone was a nonelectrical, cuplike device that could be placed on the telephone to provide greater privacy. AT&T informed distributors and customers of Hush-A-Phone that this device was illegal because AT&T prohibited the attachment of any non-AT&T devices to telephones. On appeal by Hush-A-Phone, the FCC upheld AT&T's claim that the device could not be used with AT&T equipment. Hush-A-Phone then appealed the decision to the Appeals Court and won. The court stated that as long as the device did not harm telephone subscribers it was permissible.

As a result of that court precedent, another innovation, Carterfone, was marketed. Carterfone connected mobile radiotelephone systems to the telephone network. When AT&T objected, the FCC, following the court-established precedent, permitted it. Once these decisions had been made, the precedents were established that ultimately severed the terminal equipment market from the rest of the AT&T monopoly.

AT&T's pricing structure and the development of new technology led to deregulation of long-distance rates. AT&T was the only provider of long-distance service. Large economies of scale existed in providing this service. Telephone rates were regulated so that the price of a call was approximately proportional to the distance of the call. (The ICC and CAB used a similar pricing principle.) The cost of serving telephone users, however, was not proportional to the distance of their calls. The actual costs for long-distance calls fell sharply as distance increased. Thus, charges were much higher than costs for long-distance calls, while local calls were priced much closer to cost and, in some cases, less than cost. This uniform pricing strategy, price being proportional to distance rather than cost, resulted in long-distance users subsidizing local service users. (Regulators were able to reassure concerned politicians that residential users would object to higher-priced local phone service.)

By the mid-1970s, new technology resulted in competition for AT&T's long-distance markets. The costs of microwave and satellite communications were below the costs of AT&T's traditional technology for providing long-distance telephone service. Because the price-to-cost ratio was highest in the long-distance market, this was also the most profitable market for the use of the new technology. Microwave technology was not subject to large economies of scale; thus, private firms could have their own long-distance service. Using subsidized local calls to connect their microwave system, private firms could have lower long-distance costs than AT&T's high long-distance rates. Large users of long-distance service had an incentive to purchase microwave systems given the high (price-to-cost) regulated long-distance rates.

AT&T vigorously opposed competition in their long-distance market, and the FCC protected AT&T's position by denying entry to new competitors. The courts, however, said that the FCC had to show that protecting AT&T's monopoly position was in the public interest. Unable to do so, the FCC was forced to allow competition for long-distance telephone service.

AT&T, however, controlled 80 to 85 percent of the country's local telephone lines, which were still a natural monopoly. All long-distance telephone users had to be connected to the local telephone company. AT&T used its ownership of local telephone companies to deny its long-distance competitors access to AT&T's customers. As long as AT&T was able to maintain monopoly power in any one of the three necessary components of telephone service—that is, equipment, long-distance service, or local service—it could maintain its monopoly position in any of the three markets. (A monopolist in any one of these markets has as much power as a monopolist of all three markets.) Although there was now competition in the equipment and long-distance markets, long-distance users had to be connected to local service, and AT&T's control over local telephone service gave it monopoly power over all three markets. AT&T could charge a sufficiently high price to its long-distance competitors for access to local subscribers to make it unprofitable for long-distance competitors.

In 1975, the Justice Department filed a major antitrust suit against AT&T on the grounds that AT&T had monopolized each of the three interrelated markets. The Justice Department wanted AT&T to divest itself. In that same period, thirty-five private antitrust suits were filed against AT&T. AT&T's competitors claimed that they could not get equal access to AT&T's local service, thereby placing them at a competitive disadvantage.

AT&T was concerned that if it lost the antitrust suit, it would then be liable for triple damages in all the private antitrust suits that were (and that might potentially be) brought against them. (The private plaintiffs would not have to bear the expense of proving an antitrust violation but merely prove the size of their damages.) In 1982, therefore, AT&T decided to settle the case by separating the ownership of the competitive markets from the monopolized market. To avoid losses, local telephone services were to become a separate business. AT&T was to continue in the competitive long-distance and telephone equipment businesses. (The local telephone service was spun off into seven "Baby Bells," whose rates continued to be regulated. Consolidation occurred among these local companies. In addition to having their regulated rates set artificially low [relative to cost], they were prevented from entering the long-distance telephone market.)

Once the courts permitted firms using new technology to compete with AT&T in its most profitable markets, it was inevitable that long-distance charges would decline. Conversely, the price of local service, which was heavily subsidized, increased.

The introduction of new technology in long-distance markets changed prices for users and produced winners and losers.[36] Users of long-distance service benefited, while users of local service paid increased charges. As the cross-subsidy between local and long-distance service disappeared, and even though regulators kept local rates relatively low (to costs), local prices increased sharply, approximately 100 percent higher than before deregulation, while long-distance rates similarly declined.

Another loser under deregulation has been management and labor. In the period immediately preceding divestiture, AT&T reduced its workforce by 6 percent and manager salaries were frozen; after divestiture, AT&T continued to reduce its employees by the tens of thousands. The number of employees per manager at AT&T was only half those of its competitors (4 to 1 versus 9 to 1). Pay for AT&T employees was also twice as high as its major competitors.[37] To become price-competitive, AT&T had to reduce the number of employees, increase productivity, and renegotiate its labor contracts so that wages were comparable to those of its major competitors.

The regulated pricing structure for long-distance service provided large users of such services with an incentive to adopt new technology, which was not subject to large economies of scale. These users and the eventual application of this technology to smaller users would have ultimately eroded the economic value of AT&T's monopoly using more costly traditional long-distance equipment. The intervention of the courts, however, made deregulation occur much more rapidly.

Technology is continuing to change the market for telecommunications.[38] In 1993, to reduce the federal budget deficit, Congress required the FCC to begin auctioning spectrum, which created the wireless market, adding additional competitors to both the local and long-distance phone markets. Wireless services are an almost perfect substitute to ordinary wire line voice and low-speed data calls. The number of wireless subscribers is now about equal to the number of wire line subscribers. Stimulating this dramatic growth in wireless usage has been sharp declines in its price. In addition to wireless competitors, cable television companies have entered the telephone service market.

The rapid rate of technical change in telecommunications has eliminated differences between voice, video, and data transmission. Although the long-distance market was opened to competition, local telephone companies were initially restricted from entering the long-distance market and, because of their monopoly status, were required to share their networks and services with long-distance carriers at regulated, cost-based rates. This meant that only local phone companies could complete local calls, only long-distance carriers could connect people from remote locations, and only cable companies could offer cable television. Changes in technology and the courts led to the Telecommunications Act of 1996, which, together with subsequent FCC rulings, eliminated restrictions on entry into both local and long-distance markets.[39] There is now a blurring of previously distinct product and service areas. The barriers between industries have been removed. In addition to each of the above companies being able to offer services previously sold by the others, new industries are entering the business, such as electric utilities that have fiber-optic wires that can carry voice and video as well as broadband services for delivering content over the Internet, which enables computer users to make inexpensive long-distance calls using voice modems.

Reasons for Deregulation

Regulated industries are characterized by limited entry and fixed prices that benefit the regulated firms. In addition, employees receive higher wages than in a competitive industry and politically important constituencies benefit from cross-subsidies. These three groups favor continued regulation: the regulated firms that receive monopoly prices and, presumably, monopoly profits; the users of subsidized services whose cross-subsidies would disappear if prices were to reflect their costs of service; and union members in the regulated industry, whose wages would be reduced if they were in a competitive industry.

Not all regulated industries have been deregulated, and some of the industries that have been deregulated have been only partially deregulated. There are, however, certain similarities among those industries that have experienced deregulation.

Increased Regulatory Costs to Groups with a Concentrated Interest

An industry may lose regulatory benefits for the same reasons they were able to achieve these benefits. Regulatory policies that affect a group will change when a change occurs in the relative political support offered by opposing groups. Regulation imposes costs on others. As these costs increase and become substantial (concentrated), they provide an incentive for others to organize and provide political support so as to lessen these costs. Those bearing the costs of regulation face a simple cost/benefit calculation. For an industry adversely affected by regulation, there are costs of ascertaining the effects of regulation on their profitability, organizing their members (and of overcoming any free rider problems), and providing political support. The benefits are the lessened costs of regulation.

An increase in regulatory costs imposed on others is not a sufficient condition to set in motion the forces to overturn the costs of regulation. If imposed on the public in a diffuse manner, it is unlikely that individuals will find it in their interest to learn about these costs, bear the costs of organizing, and raise political support. An example of these large regulatory costs are federal agricultural price supports. Maintaining high farm prices costs many billions of dollars in taxes; further, the prices paid by consumers for farm products are greater than what they would be without such regulation. The cost per consumer or per taxpayer, however, is relatively small. Import restrictions (tariffs or quotas) on items such as textiles also raise the price; however, the cost to consumers is not sufficiently high to cause them to lobby Congress.

Before change can come about, large regulatory costs have to be imposed on groups that have a concentrated interest in having them reduced. It is less costly to organize firms in an industry than large numbers of individuals. Firms are also more aware of policies that affect their costs and revenues. When regulatory costs become sufficiently large, it will then be worthwhile for a group to organize and raise the political support to overcome them. Money market funds and commercial banks would not have been able to raise large sums of savings had they not opposed the S&Ls on maximum interest rates. Institutional traders could not have achieved large savings on their commission rates if they had not bypassed the NYSE and developed alternative trading sources, such as, regional exchanges. These concentrated interests saw the benefits of deregulation in terms of increased profitability or reduced costs.

The federal government itself develops a concentrated interest when the financial commitments imposed on it require cutbacks in other politically popular programs or necessitate a tax increase. It was for this reason that the Administration proposed greater rate and service flexibility for the railroads; it wanted to forestall additional railroad bankruptcies. The government would have had to bear large costs if they had to provide subsidies to railroads in financial difficulty. During the 1970s, when inflation was increasing, various administrations proposed deregulation as a means of reducing the rise in prices; otherwise more politically costly measures to reduce inflation would have had to be used.

Erosion of Monopoly Profits

Another reason for deregulation is a decline in the regulated firm's profitability. Regulation was meant to achieve what the regulated firm was unable to achieve in a competitive market, namely, monopoly profits. If monopoly profits are no longer attainable through regulation, then the regulated firm has little economic incentive to support continued regulation. This was particularly true in the case of railroads, airlines, and the NYSE. As the economic value of regulation declines, so does the necessary political support offered by the firms to maintain regulation. In fact, some regulated firms actively promoted deregulation in their belief that their economic returns would be improved. (The value of regulatory benefits also declined for certain constituents of airline regulation, thereby leading to their loss of support for its continuance. Small communities became less concerned that they would lose air service if deregulation occurred.)

The decline in the economic value of regulation may occur for several reasons. One reason is entry by new firms. Because the number of firms in regulated industries is limited, substitute industries arise to take away the regulated industry's monopoly profits; new firms typically enter by introducing new technology. In the case of railroads, trucking was one such innovation; with regard to the commissions on securities, regional exchanges and off-floor trading eroded the volume and profitability of the NYSE; money market mutual funds grew rapidly at the expense of the savings and loan associations; and microwave and satellite technology enabled new firms to enter AT&T's profitable long distance markets.

The incentives for entry and innovation are greatest in those regulated markets where profitability is greatest, that is, where prices are highest in relation to cost. In regulated industries prices are not set proportionate to cost; instead, prices are often established proportionate to distance, volume, or some other criteria. Because unit costs in regulated industries decline as distance or volume increases, profitability is highest in long-distance or large-volume markets. With railroads, airlines, and telecommunications, profitability was greatest in the long-distance markets; in the NYSE it was large trades; in banking it was large deposits.

The regulated industry's initial response to innovation is to reduce competition by encompassing the new competitors within the regulatory agency's jurisdiction. This occurred with railroads and was attempted with telecommunications and banking. The truckers' association accepted regulation because it was seen as a means of limiting entry to new truckers. In telecommunications, the FCC tried to exclude new competitors but was unable to do so as a result of court intervention. In some instances, the competitors are sufficiently organized and the economic advantage of deregulation so large, that they are willing to invest the necessary political support to bring about deregulation. This was the case in banking (the commercial banks) and in securities trading (the large institutions desired lower commissions).

When new competitors enter the regulated firm's markets, they decrease the regulated firm's market share and profitability.

The other reason for erosion of monopoly profits in regulated industries is intensive nonprice competition. Because prices are fixed and above costs, regulated firms compete for market share by offering additional services or amenities. For example, the airlines introduced jet aircraft and increased the number of scheduled flights, the S&Ls offered prizes to new depositors, and securities firms offered research services to attract customers. Eventually, the regulatory agency has to establish limits on nonprice competition, which increases the regulated firm's costs and reduces its profitability. Profitability of airlines and railroads increased when price flexibility became permissible.

Courts and Antitrust

The antitrust laws are another important reason why industries have been deregulated. The federal judicial system is less in need of political support, hence less subject to political pressures, than Congress or the regulatory agencies. Consequently, the federal courts are more likely to act without regard to a specific industry's economic interest when applying the antitrust laws. Although it is possible for a concentrated interest group to receive congressional exemption from the antitrust laws, it has been very difficult to do so. (There are a few exceptions—labor unions are one.) For an industry to receive an exemption requires a much higher degree of political support, that is, a higher cost, than is required to achieve regulatory benefits for an industry where those costs are diffuse and less visible.

The prospect of losing an antitrust case, with its consequent economic losses, was what convinced AT&T that it should settle with the government. Previously, competitors had undertaken several successful court appeals, which enabled them to enter AT&T's protected markets. Had it not been for the judicial system and the applicability of the antitrust laws, AT&T would have been able to retain its monopoly power. The courts were also important in permitting increased entry in trucking and airlines.

The basis of the antitrust laws is that competition will achieve economic efficiency and is therefore in the public interest. Nevertheless, the development of new technology that provides a low-cost substitute to the service provided by a regulated industry threatens the regulated industry's revenues. The regulated industry will at first try to include that technology under the regulatory agency's jurisdiction. In that way the regulated industry can control the introduction of low-cost substitutes. However, if antitrust suits are brought against the regulated industry, it is likely that the courts will rule that competition is in the public interest. At that point the regulatory agency will have to accommodate the new competitors. The ultimate effect, which usually takes a number of years to play out, will be a loss of revenues for the regulated industry and its eventual deregulation. The federal judicial system may be society's best method of ensuring the introduction of new technology.

Deregulation is most likely to occur in circumstances where low-cost substitutes erode the market share and profitability of the regulated firms. There is then little economic value remaining for the regulated industry to protect. As profitability decreases, so does the amount of political support firms are willing to provide to maintain regulation. When the courts become involved because of antitrust claims, then the regulated firms are unable to prevent erosion of their profits.

When the courts are not involved, as in those cases where Congress provides explicit mandates to the regulatory agency, then attempts at deregulation are less certain. The power of opposing interests will determine the outcome. If the regulated firms still receive large economic benefits from regulation, then they will strongly oppose deregulation. For example, the truckers' association and the Teamsters were able to maintain regulatory benefits at the state level long after interstate trucking was deregulated.

When the regulated firms continue to receive large economic benefits and the costs of regulation are diffuse, opposing interest groups are unlikely to arise, and deregulation is unlikely to occur. For these reasons, many industries retain their regulatory benefits, for example, dairy and farm price supports and maritime shipping rates.

The economic theory of regulation provides a more accurate explanation for the deregulation that has occurred than the public interest theory. The deregulation trends of the 1970s occurred because of the rise of opposing interest groups and lower-cost substitutes, the decline in profitability of the regulated firms, and the jurisdiction of the federal courts. It was not because legislators believed the public would benefit or that it was an idea whose time had come.

Study Questions

1. What would the public interest and economic theory predict would be the legislative position of regulated industries toward attempts to deregulate their industry?
2. Based on the economic theory of regulation, what strategies might a regulated industry try when technology creates a lower-cost substitute to the regulated industry?
3. Why did the railroad industry eventually seek deregulation?
4. What is the economic theory of regulation explanation for the deregulation of industries that occurred during the 1970s and 1980s?
5. What information would you require to determine why an industry has remained regulated and, similarly, why an industry has been deregulated?

Notes

1. The discussion in this section is based on the following articles and books: Sam Peltzman, "The Economic Theory of Regulation After a Decade of Deregulation," *Brookings Papers: Microeconomics 1989*

(Washington, DC: The Brookings Institution, 1989), 1–41. (See also the comments by Roger Noll on Peltzman's paper, 48–59.) The above paper by Peltzman was also reprinted in Sam Peltzman, *Political Participation and Government Regulation* (Chicago: The University of Chicago Press, 1988), 286–323. Marcus Alexis, "The Political Economy of Federal Regulation of Surface Transportation," in *The Political Economy of Deregulation*, eds. Roger G. Noll and Bruce M. Owen (Washington, DC: American Enterprise Institute, 1983), 115–31; Marcus Alexis, "The Applied Theory of Regulation: Political Economy At The Interstate Commerce Commission," *Public Choice* 39, no. 1 (1982): 5–27; Thomas G. Moore, "Rail and Trucking Deregulation," in *Regulatory Reform: What Actually Happened*, eds. Leonard W. Weiss and Michael W. Klass (Boston: Little, Brown and Company, 1986), 14–39; Theodore E. Keeler, "Theories of Regulation and the Deregulation Movement," *Public Choice* 44, no. 1 (1984): 103–45; Ann F. Friedlaender, "Equity, Efficiency, and Regulation in the Rail and Trucking Industries," in *Case Studies in Regulation: Revolution and Reform* eds., Leonard W. Weiss and Michael W. Klass (Boston: Little, Brown and Company, 1981), 102–141; and Martha Derthick and Paul J. Quirk, *The Politics of Deregulation* (Washington, DC: The Brookings Institution, 1985).

2. Moore, "Rail and Trucking Deregulation," 20.

3. Ibid., 22.

4. Christopher C. Barnekov, "The Track Record," *Regulation* 11, no. 1 (1987):19–27.

5. Elizabeth E. Bailey, "Price and Productivity Change Following Deregulation: The U.S. Experience," *The Economic Journal* 96, no. 381 (1986): 1–17.

6. Ibid., 22.

7. Thomas G. Moore, "Rail and Truck Reform—The Record So Far," *Regulation* 7, no. 6 (1983): 33–41. See also, John C. Taylor, "Regulation of Trucking by the States," *Regulation* 17, no. 2 (1994): 37–47; and Thomas G. Moore, "Clearing the Track: The Remaining Transportation Regulations," *Regulation* 18, no. 2 (1995): 77–87.

8. Barnekov, "The Track Record," 19. See also, Thomas Moore, "Moving Ahead," *Regulation*, 25, no. 2 Summer 2002: 6–13.

9. Ibid., 26.

10. *P.C. White Truck Line, Inc. v. Interstate Commerce Commission and United States of America*, 551 Federal Reporter, 2d Series, 1977: 1326.

11. Derthick and Quirk, *The Politics of Deregulation*, Table, 134.

12. Moore, "Rail and Truck Reform—The Record So Far," 39.

13. Ibid., 37.

14. Ibid., 40.

15. Jim Thomas and Foster Thomas, "A Dynamic Duo on Capitol Hill," *Distribution* 93, no. 12 (1994): 32–6.

16. Moore, "Clearing the Track: The Remaining Transportation Regulations," 82.

17. The discussion in this section is based on Alfred E. Kahn, "Deregulation and Vested Interests: The Case of Airlines," in *The Political Economy of Deregulation*, eds. Roger G. Noll and Bruce M. Owen, (Washington, DC: American Enterprise Institute, 1983) 132–151; Daniel P. Kaplan, "The Changing Airline Industry," in *Regulatory Reform: What Actually Happened*, eds. Leonard W. Weiss and Michael W. Klass (Boston: Little, Brown and Company, 1986), 40–77; Theodore E. Keeler, "The Revolution in Airline Regulation," *Case Studies in Regulation: Revolution and Reform*, eds., Leonard W. Weiss and Michael W. Klass (Boston: Little, Brown and Company, 1981) 53–85; and Derthick and Quirk, *The Politics of Deregulation*.

18. Noll and Owen, *The Political Economy of Deregulation*, 156.

19. Derthick and Quirk, *The Politics of Deregulation*, 40–1.

20. "Frank Borman on Deregulation, Unions, Managing—and Borman," *Wall Street Journal*, June 11, 1986, 33.

21. Leonard W. Weiss, "Introduction: The Regulatory Reform Movement," in *Regulatory Reform: What Actually Happened*, eds. Leonard W. Weiss and Michael W. Klass, (Boston: Little, Brown and Company, 1986), 10: 1–13.

22. Bailey, "Price and Productivity Change Following Deregulation: The U.S. Experience," 6. See also, Thomas G. Moore, "U.S. Airline Deregulation: Its Effects on Passengers, Capital, and Labor," *Journal of Law and Economics* 29, no. 1 (1986): 10.

23. Susan Carey and Scott McCartney, "How Airlines Resisted Change for 25 Years, and Finally Lost," *The Wall Street Journal*, October 5, 2004, A1.

24. Bailey, "Price and Productivity Change Following Deregulation: The U.S. Experience," 12.

25. Although airline traffic has more than doubled since 1978, safety has continued to improve both in aircraft miles flown as well as in absolute numbers. See: http://www.airlines.org/econ/d.aspx?nid=1036.

26. Robert W. Poole and Viggo Butler, "Airline Deregulation: The Unfinished Revolution," *Regulation* 22, no. 1 (1999): 44–51.

27. Ibid. See also, Thomas Moore, "Moving Ahead," 12.
28. This discussion is based on Gregg A. Jarrell, "Change at the Exchange: The Causes and Effects of Deregulation," *Journal of Law and Economics* 27, no. 2 (1984): 273–312; and Hans Stoll, "Revolution in the Regulation of Securities Markets: An Examination of the Effects of Increased Competition," in *Case Studies in Regulation: Revolution and Reform* eds., Leonard W. Weiss and Michael W. Klass (Boston: Little, Brown and Company, 1981), 12–52. For a broader discussion of securities regulation, including regulation of derivatives and insider trading, see Craig Pirrong, "A Growing Market," *Regulation*, 25, no. 2 Summer 2002: 30–37.
29. Bailey, "Price and Productivity Change Following Deregulation: The U.S. Experience," 5.
30. Ibid.
31. Ibid., 11.
32. The discussion in this section is based on Andrew S. Carron, "The Political Economy of Financial Regulation," in *The Political Economy of Deregulation*, eds. Roger G. Noll and Bruce M. Owen (Washington, DC: American Enterprise Institute, 1983), 69–83; and Lawrence J. White, "The Partial Deregulation of Banks and Other Depository Institutions," in *Regulatory Reform: What Actually Happened*, eds. Leonard W. Weiss and Michael W. Klass (Boston: Little, Brown and Company, 1986), 169–209.

    A broader review of bank deregulation is provided in Charles W. Calomiris, "Banking Approaches the Modern Era," *Regulation* 25, no. 2, Summer 2002: 14–20. For an explanation of deregulation of branch banking using the public interest theory versus the economic theory, see Randall S. Kroszner, "The Motivations Behind Banking Reform," *Regulation* 24, no. 2, Summer 2001: 36–41.
33. Carron, "The Political Economy of Financial Regulation," 71.
34. Ibid., 73.
35. The discussion in this section is based on Gerald W. Brock, "The Regulatory Change in Telecommunications: The Dissolution of AT&T," in *Regulatory Reform: What Actually Happened*, eds. Leonard W. Weiss and Michael W. Klass (Boston: Little, Brown and Company, 1986), 210–33; Keeler, "Theories of Regulation and the Deregulation Movement," 103–45; and Sam Peltzman, *Deregulation: The Expected and the Unexpected*, Selected Paper No. 61, (Chicago: Graduate School of Business, University of Chicago, 1985).
36. In their empirical study testing which theory, the economic theory

or the public interest theory, provides a more accurate explanation for the deregulation of intrastate interLATA services, Kaserman, Mayo, and Pacey comment that because all states maintain some regulatory control over AT&T and not its competitors (MCI and Sprint), AT&T favored deregulation while its competitors favored continued regulation of its major rival. This legislative strategy of AT&T's competitors is consistent with the discussion in Chapter 4 of how firms attempt to disadvantage their competitors (substitute providers). David Kaserman, John W. Mayo, and Patricia L. Pacey, "The Political Economy of Deregulation: The Case of Intrastate Long Distance," *Journal of Regulatory Economics* 5, no. 1 (1993): 49–63.

37. Bailey, "Price and Productivity Change Following Deregulation: The U.S. Experience," 8.

38. Lenore Tracy, "The Relentless March of Market Forces," *Telecommunications* 33, no. 10 (1999): 107–110. See also, Lawrence Gasman, "The Telecommunications Act of 1996," *Regulation* 19(3) (Summer 1996): 49–55. See also, Robert W. Crandall, "A Somewhat Better Connection," *Regulation* 25, no. 2 (Summer 2000) 22–28.

39. Jerry Ellig, "What's Next for Telecom?" *Regulation* 28, no. 1 (Spring 2005) 8–9.

THE EMERGENCE OF MARKET COMPETITION IN THE U.S. HEALTHCARE SYSTEM

After completing this chapter, the reader should be able to

- list examples of anticompetitive practices that existed in healthcare before price competition occurred,
- describe a change in purchaser and supplier conditions in the 1970s and 1980s that made it likely that price-based competition in healthcare would occur,
- explain the necessity for antitrust laws to apply to healthcare for price competition to occur,
- name which federal health policies indirectly contributed to the conditions that enabled price competition to start,
- discuss why employers and government developed a "concentrated" interest in limiting the rise in health expenditure,
- identify why "any willing provider" laws are anticompetitive, and
- contrast the public interest and economic theories with the predicted effect of CON legislation on reducing increases in hospital expenditures.

Since the mid-1980s, the delivery of medical services in the United States has changed dramatically. Rather than moving in the direction of increased regulation, which was the trend during the 1970s, market competition became the dominant force affecting hospitals and health professionals.

Why did market competition occur? The U.S. healthcare system was highly regulated and there was apparently no reason to assume a change in trends. The economic motivation of existing providers was to maintain the status quo; market competition threatened their economic well-being. In such circumstances change is unlikely to occur.

Once many of the regulatory constraints on the medical care system have been removed, what are the implications of market competition for healthcare providers? And is the public likely to be better or worse off as a result of market competition?

U.S. Medical System Before Market Competition

Goal of Increased Access to Medical Care

In 1966 the Medicare and Medicaid programs began. Medicare is a federal program to finance the medical costs of the elderly. The benefits and beneficiaries are well defined. Under Medicaid certain minimum benefits and classes of beneficiaries are defined; however, individual states have the flexibility to increase those benefits and expand eligibility for those considered to be medically indigent. The federal government helps states pay for the programs.

To ensure that hospitals and physicians participated in these public programs, the federal government required hospitals to accept Medicare patients (but not Medicaid patients). In addition, the federal and state governments generously paid hospitals according to their costs (plus 2 percent under Medicare) and paid physicians a fee for service, according to their usual and customary fees. These financial inducements resulted in high participation rates by hospitals and physicians in both programs. As a result of Medicare and Medicaid, the aged and the medically indigent increased their use of hospitals and physicians.[1]

Rising inflation during the late 1960s (to finance the Vietnam War) served to further stimulate the private demand for health insurance. As incomes increased due to inflation, employees moved into higher income-tax brackets and unions bargained for increased health benefits. Employees preferred to receive health insurance as a fringe benefit, because employer-paid health insurance is tax-exempt. The tax advantages of employer-purchased health insurance increased as employee incomes rose and they moved into higher marginal tax brackets. (In 1965, the highest federal marginal tax bracket was reduced from 91 percent to 70 percent [until 1981] and added to that were state income taxes.)

As insurance coverage in the private sector increased, consumers' out-of-pocket costs for medical services decreased and their concern over rising medical costs diminished. Employers often paid the entire insurance premium for their employees. Price competition among third-party payers, such as Blue Cross and commercial insurers, in the private sector was limited as employers and their employees became less price sensitive. Blue Cross had a competitive advantage over commercial insurers in that they received large discounts from the hospitals (which provided their initial capital and controlled them). And certain unions, the largest of which was the UAW, would not contract with commercial insurers. Commercial insurers did not use aggressive cost-containment methods, such as utilization review, in part because of concern that physician organizations would boycott their plans.

With the increase in insurance coverage, from both the private and government sectors, an "erosion of the medical marketplace" began.[2] Out-of-pocket medical prices to consumers diminished, and providers sharply increased their prices with little fear of diminished demand. (Figure 6.1 illustrates the rapid increase in healthcare expenditures after the mid-1960s.) With increased demand for medical services and rising medical prices, health insurance premiums increased rapidly. Part of the increased cost of health insurance premiums was paid by employees in the form of lower wage increases, and the remaining cost was passed on by employers in the form of higher prices for their goods and services. (Import competition was minimal during this period.) In a growing economy with increasing inflation, higher prices and lower wage increases due to higher insurance premiums were less noticeable to both the worker and the public.

There was a great deal of satisfaction with the healthcare system during this period. The aged and the poor received increased access to mainstream medical care. Congress consistently voted for increased health expenditures, more medical research, increased benefits under Medicare, inclusion of new beneficiary groups under Medicare (renal dialysis), and expansion of health manpower training programs. Health programs were politically popular with consumers and health providers.

During this period, physicians had medical responsibility for the care of their patients, but were not fiscally responsible for the costs of treatment. Each provider was paid separately by the third-party payer. Patients had limited financial incentive to be concerned with their use of services or their treatment costs ("moral hazard"). Physicians had the financial incentive to provide more services since they were paid a fee for each service ("supplier-induced demand"). Hospitals were being reimbursed, for the most part, according to their costs, and this gave them a strong incentive to expand their services. Hospitals competed, but it was for physicians and prestige. Given cost-based hospital payment systems, even small hospitals attempted to add the facilities and services available in major medical centers. Blue Cross and Medicare did not pay for out-of-hospital services, thereby providing patients with the incentive to have all their medical needs attended to in the most expensive setting, the hospital.

The determination of the number of health providers and the size of their practices was not based on which size firm was most efficient, as is the case in price-competitive industries. Instead, provider preferences and state regulation were the determining factors. Small and large hospitals, whose facilities and services were little used, were able to survive and even grow. Physicians were able to remain as solo practitioners or join groups according to their preference. State practice acts limited the tasks permitted to different health professions. Advertising was considered to be

FIGURE 6.1
Annual
Percentage
Changes in
National
Health
Expenditures
and the
Consumer
Price Index
1965–2003

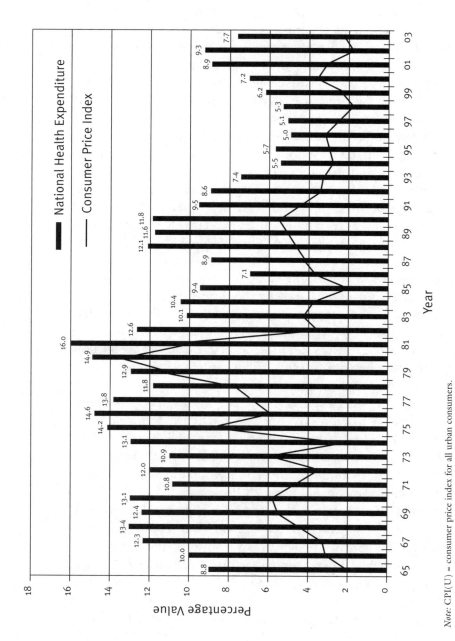

Note: CPI(U) = consumer price index for all urban consumers.
Sources: 1. Data from Department of Labor, Bureau of Labor Statistics. 2005. http://www.bls.gov. 2. Data from U.S. DHHS, Centers for Medicare and Medicaid Services. 2005. http://www.cms.hhs.gov/states/nhe-oact/.

unethical and was banned by medical societies or by state practice acts. Information on physicians and hospitals from accrediting agencies was unavailable to the public. And many states had enacted laws making it very difficult for prepaid healthcare (currently called HMOs) to organize and compete against traditional insurers relying on fee-for-service medicine.

Pressures for Change

The large increases in demand from both the public and private sectors, together with the declining portion of the bill paid for by the patient, led to rapidly rising prices and expenditures for medical services. The prices of those services most covered by insurance, such as hospital care, increased fastest. Out-of-pocket payments by the public for all medical services declined from 52 percent in 1965 to 17 percent in 1998. For hospital care the decline in the portion of the bill paid out-of-pocket was more significant, falling from 17 percent in 1965 to 11 percent in 1981 to about 3 percent in 2003. In 1965 patients paid 62 percent of the bill for physician services themselves; in 1985 they paid less than 20 percent of the bill, and in 2003 about 10 percent.[3]

As a consequence, federal expenditures for Medicare and Medicaid increased enormously, from $3.6 billion in 1965 to $31.4 billion by 1975, to $112 billion by 1985, and to more than $440 billion in 2003. State and local expenditures under Medicaid also increased sharply, from $0.7 billion in 1966 to $109 billion in 2003. Expenditures in the private sector went from $31 billion a year in 1965 to $913 billion in 2003. Public expenditures (federal and state) for Medicare and Medicaid increased more rapidly than private health expenditures, thereby increasing the overall portion of the health sector that was paid for by public funds, from 22 percent in 1965 to 46 percent in 2003.[4]

These massive increases in health expenditures from both the public and private sectors greatly exceeded the economy's rate of inflation. Healthcare as a percentage of gross domestic product went from 5.9 percent in 1965 to 15.2 percent in 2003. *These expenditures were equivalent to a huge redistribution program, from the taxpayers to those working in the health sector and to the beneficiaries of these public programs.*

Early attempts to reduce the rise in health expenditures came from the federal government. Original expectations were that Medicare would cost only $2 billion a year initially and would reach $9 billion per year by the early 1990s. However, Medicare was a defined-benefit program and its benefits and beneficiaries were defined by law; no limit was placed on its overall expenditures. Unless the rise in Medicare expenditures was reduced, the Medicare Trust Fund, which funded hospital care for the aged, would be bankrupt. Successive administrations developed a concentrated interest in halting Medicare's rapidly escalating expenditures. However, any administration asking Congress to change the law by imposing a greater contribution on the aged would have lost a great deal of political support from the aged and their supporters. Thus, the federal government had only two alternatives for limiting the increase in Medicare expenditures, which were rising by approximately 15 percent a year: (1) increase the Medicare payroll tax on employee wages and the wage base to which it applied and/or (2) limit payments to providers.

Both choices, increasing the Medicare payroll tax and paying providers less, were (politically) troublesome for an administration, but less so than reducing benefits or increasing contributions from the aged.

The federal government started chipping away at the cost-based reimbursement of hospitals in 1969, when it removed the plus 2 percent from the cost-plus formula. In 1971, because of rising inflation, President Nixon placed the entire U.S. economy under a wage and price freeze (the Economic Stabilization Program). The rest of the economy was removed from this freeze after one year. However, the health sector remained under price controls until April 1974. In the first year after their removal, physician and hospital expenditures increased very rapidly, 17.5 percent and 19.4 percent, respectively.

Additional regulatory methods were used to limit these rapid expenditure increases. Each one failed. Physician fee increases under Medicare were limited by the Medicare fee index. As a result, increasing numbers of physicians declined to participate in the Medicare program, while physicians who did participate charged for additional services, thereby negating the effect of the fee freeze. Congress passed the National Health Planning and Resources Development Act CON in 1974, which limited hospitals' capital expenditures. The CON was supposed to limit both the number of hospital beds and the number of expensive, but little used, facilities and services in an area. Researchers have since shown what many expected, that the CON legislation had no effect on decreasing the rate of increase in hospital expenditures.[5] Congress passed utilization review programs (Professional Standards Review Organizations, or PSROs) for Medicare patients in 1972. Again, empirical studies failed to find significant savings in hospital use or expenditures as a result of these programs.[6]

In 1979, President Carter made hospital cost-containment his highest legislative priority. His proposed legislation would have placed limits on the annual percentage increase in each hospital's expenditures. The regulatory approach moved from the use of indirect methods, such as limits on capital expenditures (CON) and utilization (PSROs), to placing direct controls on hospital expenditures.

President Carter suffered an important legislative defeat. The AMA and hospital associations were instrumental in providing political support to defeat the proposed legislation.[7] The proposed cost-containment legislation was too direct a threat to hospitals' goals and revenues. Previous regulation, such as CON, was not only ineffective in preventing hospitals from expanding but it was also used to protect those same hospitals from competition.[8] Federal efforts to control the rise in federal health expenditures were stymied.

Meanwhile, a number of states began implementing their own rate-review programs. These programs were, in many cases, assisted in implementation and design by the state hospital associations themselves. Rather than imposing stringent rate controls at the federal level, many hospital spokespersons believed their influence would be greater at the state level and that state rate-review programs would be more considerate of individual hospital differences.[9]

By the late 1970s, it appeared that pressures to contain the rise in health expenditures would result in increased regulation. Rather than eliminating previous regulations (such as CON), which had proven to be ineffective, additional regulations were proposed. Hospitals were to be subject to controls on their use, on their capital and operating expenditures, and on their ability to enter other hospital markets. At this point, hospitals began to be talked about as if they were "public utilities."

Emergence of Market Competition

A number of events provided the preconditions for market competition: (1) federal legislation unintentionally created excess capacity among physicians and hospitals, and (2) businesses developed a concentrated interest in holding down their employees' health insurance premiums. However, it was the application of the antitrust laws that made it possible for competition to occur.

Federal Initiatives

Increased supply of physicians.

For approximately 15 years, through the 1950s and early 1960s, the supply of physicians in relation to the population remained constant, at 141 physicians per 100,000 people. During this period physicians' incomes were rising (compared to those of other occupations) as were the number of applicants to medical schools.[10] As the demand for physicians' services continued to grow, stimulated by the passage of Medicare and Medicaid and the growth of private health insurance, an increased number of foreign medical graduates came to the United States.

During this period there was constant talk of a physician shortage. Many qualified U.S. students who could not gain admission to medical school went overseas to receive their education. Many middle-class families were concerned that their sons and daughters would not become physicians while, at the same time, there was increased immigration by foreign medical graduates. Congress responded to these constituent pressures and passed the Health Professions Educational Assistance Act. Senator Ralph Yarborough stated the reasons for the passage of the act in 1963: "It was when we were trying to give more American boys and girls a chance for a medical education, so that we would not have to drain the help of other foreign countries." And again, "To me it is just shocking that we do not give American boys and girls a chance to obtain a medical education so that they can serve their own people."[11] It took a number of years before the full magnitude of this act took effect. New medical schools were built, and existing schools were given financial incentives to increase their spaces. (The same occurred for other health professions.)

By 1980 the supply of physicians had reached 200 per 100,000 people, almost a 50 percent increase from the early 1960s. Continuing to rise rapidly, the supply of physicians exceeded 250 per 100,000 by the mid 1990s, reaching 300 per 100,000 in 2003.[12]

Contrary to what many believed, the market for physicians does follow the laws of supply and demand. With the rapid increase in the supply of physicians, physicians developed excess capacity. As a result, an increased number of physicians participated in Medicare, more physicians relocated to areas previously short of physicians,[13] and more physicians were willing to discount their fees to insurers in return for greater volume.

In response to their constituents' interests and over the objections of the AMA, Congress enacted legislation that eventually created excess capacity among physicians. It was not the intent of Congress to create competition among physicians. However, their actions in passing the Health Professions Educational Assistance Act set the stage for it.

The HMO Act.

In the early 1970s, President Nixon wanted a health initiative that would not be very costly to the federal government. His proposal (developed by Paul Ellwood) was to stimulate the growth of prepaid health plans, renamed HMOs.

When Congress passed the HMO Act in 1973, it included two provisions helpful to the development of HMOs and one that was a hindrance. First, firms with 25 or more employees had to offer their employees an HMO option if a federally qualified HMO was available. Second, federally qualified HMOs were exempt from restrictive state practices, such as being unable to advertise, having to be nonprofit, and needing to have a majority of their board members be physicians. These anticompetitive restrictions, enacted with the support of state medical societies, lessened the like-lihood of an HMO's success and decreased the incentive for entrepreneurs to invest their capital in starting an HMO. A reason often mentioned by survey respondents for not choosing an HMO was a lack of information about how such an organization delivers care.[14] Mandating an HMO option through the workplace enabled a federally qualified HMO to provide this information in a low-cost manner.

In the initial HMO legislation, federally qualified HMOs were required to offer a set of benefits that generally exceeded the benefits offered by their competition, such as the traditional Blue Cross plans, thereby rais-ing their premiums. This requirement proved a hindrance in that few exist-ing HMOs opted to become federally qualified. This restriction was eased in subsequent amendments to the HMO Act.

HMOs initially had a small competitive effect. They represented a small percentage of the market, and premium competition was limited. HMOs generally set their premium equal to that of Blue Cross (which was the amount employers were willing to pay on behalf of their employees) and tried to attract enrollees by offering additional benefits. By not offer-ing lower premiums, employers did not save when their employees joined an HMO. The HMOs, however, achieved their savings by decreasing the use of hospitals. As more people joined HMOs, the decreased hospital usage of HMO subscribers contributed to hospitals' excess capacity.

1979 amendments to the CON legislation.

The initial CON legislation established planning agencies whose purpose was to limit the increase in hospital capital expenditures. The HMOs needed access to a hospital to provide a full range of medical services. Some HMOs had hospitals they wanted to expand, while other HMOs wanted to con-struct hospitals. HMOs began to complain to Congress that CON legisla-tion was being used to block their growth, because physicians and existing hospitals viewed them as a competitive threat. In managing a patient's treat-ment, HMO physicians decreased the use of hospitals and locked patients into the HMO delivery system, thereby making them inaccessible to providers not participating in the HMO. "HMOs were subjected to more extensive controls than fee-for-service providers. Although financing plans and provider organizations of other kinds could be established without government approval, establishment of an HMO was subject to planning agency review.[15]

In 1979, Congress amended the CON legislation so that the act could not be used to inhibit competition. However, these amendments did not grant all HMOs a complete exemption from the CON act. It loosened the restrictions. The large HMOs, such as Kaiser, fared better in the legislation than the smaller, newly developing ones. The larger HMOs, located in states with rapid HMO growth such as California, used their political influence to provide themselves with a competitive advantage over the small HMOs, who did not receive the same exclusion from planning agency review.

Even after Congress loosened the anticompetitive restrictions of the CON act, and despite evidence of its ineffectiveness as a cost-control measure, many states continue to use CON in an anticompetitive manner, denying entry to freestanding surgicenters, applying it to equipment used in physician offices, and including HMOs in CON reviews.[16]

Except for the change in the CON legislation and the enactment of the HMO Act and its amendments, it was difficult for Congress to develop a consensus with the various health interest groups as to what legislative approach, if any, should be proposed to resolve the problem of rising federal health expenditures.

Some opponents of President Carter's cost-containment legislation, such as Representatives Richard Gephardt and David Stockman, began to propose an alternative approach—the use of market competition. Various academics, such as Alain Enthoven, wrote on the virtues of market competition.[17] Health interest groups, however, such as the AMA, the AHA, the insurance companies, Blue Cross organizations, and the unions, all testified against competitive approaches.

Elimination of "free choice" of provider under Medicaid.

It was not until several years later, under President Reagan, that additional cost-containment legislation was enacted. In 1981, in return for limiting increases in federal Medicaid expenditures, Congress amended the Medicaid Act to provide states with greater flexibility in how they pay providers. States were no longer required to offer the medically indigent "free choice" of medical provider. This meant states could take bids and negotiate contracts with selected providers for the care of the medically indigent. Although states were a potentially powerful market force in the Medicaid program, many moved slowly. By 1994, 24 percent of the Medicaid population was enrolled in managed care, reaching 60 percent by 2004.[18]

New hospital payment system under Medicare.

Then, early in the Reagan administration, a revolutionary method was introduced to pay hospitals under Medicare, that of diagnosis-related groups (DRGs). Hospital and medical associations were powerless against a Republican administration intent on reducing federal expenditures for hospitals.

Payment to hospitals according to DRGs was phased in over a five-year period starting in September 1983. Hospitals were now paid a fixed price per admission for the care of their Medicare patients. The incentives facing hospitals changed. It was now in their economic interest to provide less service rather than more. Lengths of stay for the elderly began to decline. Medicare patients, who represented approximately 40 percent of hospital patient days, began to be discharged earlier. The average length of stay for the aged declined from 9.9 days in 1983 to 6.2 days by 1998. More dramatic than the decline in the length of stay was the decline in total patient days per 1,000 Medicare enrollees. These declined from 3,842 days per 1,000 in 1983 to 1,860 in 2002.[19]

By the time hospitals began to experience the effect of DRGs on their occupancy rates, however, the move toward market competition had already started. The DRGs reinforced the competitive pressures on hospitals stimulated several years earlier by declining occupancy rates.

Private Sector Initiatives

Approximately two-thirds of the population has private health insurance coverage, most of which is purchased through the workplace. The stimulus for competition started in the private sector.

In 1981, the nation was faced with a severe recession. In addition, the automobile and steel industries faced increased import competition from foreign producers. These were also the same industries that had the most comprehensive health insurance programs for their employees. The recession led to unemployment, loss of income, and a decrease in health insurance benefits, which resulted in a decline in elective hospital admissions. The recession also lowered tax revenues for states. Consequently, many states cut back on their Medicaid benefits, reduced payments to healthcare providers, and decreased the eligibility criteria for Medicaid. As a result of these factors, the hospital admission rate for those under 65 years of age started to decline in late 1981.

Once the recession ended, industry was still concerned about labor costs. Those industries engaged in competition with foreign producers found that the strength of the U.S. dollar relative to other currencies forced them to reduce their costs to remain competitive.

Industry began to examine ways they could contain the increase in their employees' health insurance costs. Employers pressured health insurers to hold down their premium increases and to institute new cost-saving programs. Also, an increasing number of business firms started their own self-insurance plans. The firms believed they, rather than insurance companies, would be better able to control their employees' healthcare use. (Also, by being self-insured, employers were exempt from costly state health mandates.) Other firms joined healthcare coalitions in their area. These coalitions collected data on the use rates and charges of different providers to determine which providers were more costly. Employers also imposed deductibles and coinsurance requirements on their employees, who previously paid very little out-of-pocket when they used medical services, thereby increasing their employees' price sensitivity.

One of the most important changes firms (or insurance companies on their behalf) introduced was a change in the benefit package. Insurance coverage for lower-cost substitutes to hospitals was introduced. Previously, even though it was less costly to perform surgery in an outpatient setting, if this service was not covered by insurance it then became less costly to the employee to have the surgery performed in a hospital. Thus, by adding outpatient surgery to the benefit package the insurance premium paid by the employer could be reduced.

Dramatic changes occurred in the private health insurance market in the 1980s. Previously, private health insurers were passive intermediaries, collecting premiums from employers, paying hospitals and physicians, and then merely passing higher provider prices back to the employers in the form of increased premiums. In the early 1980s, large employers, faced with growing import competition and rising employee labor costs, including rising health insurance premiums, pressured their health insurers to control rapidly increasing costs. To survive in a competitive health insurance market, health insurers began to change their role.

To control rising costs, insurers interfered with the traditional physician-patient relationship. Under managed care, insurers questioned physician decision making. Insurers introduced utilization review to determine whether certain hospitalizations were necessary.[20] Patients were financially penalized if they did not receive prior approval from the insurer for a specialist referral or a hospitalization. As competition among insurers increased, so did the type of plans that they offered. Insurers formed PPOs and HMOs, which are closed panels of providers, selecting providers based on their prices and willingness to accept clinical practice guidelines. In return for increased benefits or lower insurance premiums, insured patients could no longer select any physician; they could only select physicians belonging to an insurer's provider network. Insurers established drug formularies that determined the prescription drugs physicians were permitted to prescribe. Insurance benefits were expanded to include treatment settings, such as home health care, that cost less to care for the patient than keeping the patient in the hospital. And insurers changed patient and provider incentives in an attempt to eliminate unnecessary care.

Efforts by managed care insurers to reduce hospital utilization, such as utilization controls, the growth of HMOs, and coverage of care in non-hospital settings, were succeeding. Hospital utilization rates started to decline. As a result, occupancy rates in nonfederal, nonprofit, short-term general hospitals declined from 75 percent in 1980 to 64 percent by 1985.

(Occupancy rates rose slightly in 2003 to 66 percent.)[21] The new approach used by Medicare—paying hospitals by DRGs—and private contracting by Medicaid reinforced the incentives facing hospitals in the private sector to lower their costs. The pressure on hospitals to compete was reinforced as utilization by the elderly and the poor declined. (See Figure 6.2.) As excess capacity increased, hospitals participated with HMOs and PPOs. Providers not participating in HMOs and PPOs had access to a declining population base.

Managed care, which started in California in the early 1980s, spread slowly throughout the country. Hospital use rates fell and use of specialists by managed care plans declined, as did physician incomes. Hospitals and physicians had excess capacity and, although they were opposed to managed care, they had to participate in managed care otherwise they would not have access to patients.

Managed care plans were successful in expanding their market share because their cost-containment methods enabled them to charge lower premiums than traditional health insurers. Employees, when required to choose among competing health plans, were very price sensitive; they were willing to switch health plans if one plan was only slightly more expensive than another. A difference of $5 or $10 a month in an employee's monthly out-of-pocket cost would cause 25 percent of the health plan's enrollees to switch to a lower-cost health plan.[22] Physicians were shocked by the lack of patient loyalty. As managed care plans increased their market share, traditional health insurers adopted the same cost-containment techniques to survive.

Enforcement of Antitrust Laws

Concern by business with employees' healthcare costs and the creation of excess capacity among both hospitals and physicians were important preconditions for competition. However, had it not been for the application of the antitrust laws, it is unlikely that market competition would have occurred.

Medical societies and state practice acts inhibited market competition by threatening to boycott health plans and limiting advertising, fee splitting, corporate practice, and delegation of tasks. Blue Cross and Blue Shield maintained the principle of "free choice"; that is, their subscribers had no incentive to choose between providers on the basis of price. Blue Cross enrollees had a service-benefit policy. Regardless of whether the participating hospital had high or low costs, Blue Cross paid 100 percent of their enrollee' hospital costs. Under Blue Shield, price comparisons by enrollees were also discouraged; Blue Shield reimbursed participating physicians according to their usual fees (up to a percentile limit).

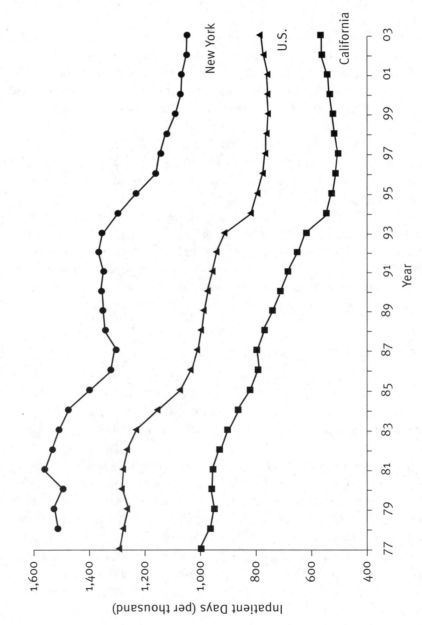

FIGURE 6.2

Trends in Hospital Utilization (per thousand) for the U.S., California, and New York, 1977–2003

Sources: 1. Population data from U.S. Census Bureau, http://www.census.gov. Data as of July 1, except 1980, 1990 and 2000, as of April 1. 2. Utilization figures American Hospital Association. 2005.   Hospital Statistics,   various years.   Chicago: Health Forum LLC, an affiliate of AHA

In the 1930s, during the depression, the same preconditions for market competition existed. Physicians and hospitals had excess capacity; patients and their insurance companies were concerned about the cost of healthcare. And yet market competition did not occur. For example, insurance companies in Oregon attempted to lower their insurance premiums so as to better compete for subscribers. The method used to reduce the cost of the insurance premium was to place restraints on physician utilization by requiring reauthorization of services and monitoring claims. Physicians accepted such constraints on their behavior because they did not have as many patients as a result of the depression and were not sure of their ability to collect from those they did have. Consumers benefited from the lower insurance premiums.

The response by the medical societies in Oregon to a competitive market in medical care was twofold: first, the medical societies threatened to expel any physician who participated in these competitive insurance plans; and second, the medical societies started their own insurance plans. These plans did not use aggressive utilization methods. With the growth of their own insurance plans, physicians were encouraged to boycott other plans. The effect of these policies was to cause other insurance plans to decline. To have physicians participate in their plans, the insurance companies had to drop their aggressive cost-containment efforts. The medical societies were thereby able to determine that the types of insurance programs offered to the public were also those in the physicians' economic interests.[23] Thus, unless the antitrust laws were applicable to the health sector, physician and hospital boycotts and other anticompetitive behavior could have prevented market competition from occurring once again.

Up until 1975 it was believed that the antitrust laws did not apply to "learned professions," which included the health professions. In 1975, the U.S. Supreme Court decided the case of *Goldfarb v. Virginia State Bar*. The local bar association, believing lawyers were not engaged in "trade or commerce," established a minimum fee schedule. The Supreme Court ruled against the bar association, thereby denying any sweeping exclusion of the learned professions from the antitrust laws.[24] In another important precedent, in 1978 the Supreme Court denied the use of anticompetitive behavior by the National Society of Professional Engineers even if it was to prevent a threat to the profession's ethics or public safety. Encouraged by the Supreme Court decisions, the FTC began to vigorously enforce the antitrust laws in the health field. In 1975, the FTC charged the AMA and its constituent medical societies with anticompetitive behavior. In a 1978 decision, the FTC prevailed. The AMA appealed the verdict to the Supreme Court, but was again unsuccessful.

The Supreme Court's decision, rendered in 1982, was a clear signal to health providers that they would now be subject to the antitrust laws.

The AMA led other professional associations in a lobbying effort in Congress to exempt state-regulated professions from the jurisdiction of the FTC. One lobbyist reported that this was the AMA's most important fight since its battle against Medicare in 1965.[25]

The AMA was able to gather 219 cosponsors (a majority) to its bill in the House of Representatives, placing a moratorium on the FTC's jurisdiction. The AMA's stated position was, "The standards of quality established by the American Medical Association and other medical societies . . . are being undermined by a federal agency that possesses no medical qualifications."[26]

The AMA was successful in having its self-interest legislation passed in the House. This was reminiscent of the political influence of the truckers and Teamsters. The AMA and its state societies contribute a great deal more to political campaigns than any other health association.[27]

Although the AMA attempted to portray the legislation as preventing the FTC from "meddling" in quality of medical care, others quickly viewed the legislation as being in the self-interest of its proponents. Although lawyers would also have been one of the state-regulated professions exempted from FTC jurisdiction (and thereby able to prohibit advertising among lawyers and set minimum prices for legal services), the "American Bar Association's antitrust section urged lawyers to oppose exemption, calling it a special-interest ploy that would injure consumers."[28] Still others said that the AMA was more interested in placing "the economic health of its members above the nation's physical health."[29] The press also began to pick up the story. An analysis of campaign contributions by health political action committees prepared by Congress Watch stimulated new articles and editorials around the country, and prompted a commentary by Bill Moyers on the CBS Evening News (May 18, 1982). The opponents of the legislation were able to generate "the rarest of political weapons—public opinion."[30]

Other organizations also opposed the AMA and the bill's proponents. The Washington Businessman's Group on Health, which represents nearly 200 of the Fortune 500 companies, believed the FTC restrictions proposed by the AMA would increase the cost of employee health insurance. An incident affecting the practices of some of their members convinced the American Nurses Association that it needed the FTC's protection. Under the pressure of local medical societies, certain rural clinics, where nurse practitioners were working under the supervision of physicians, were closed when the insurance companies revoked the malpractice insurance of the participating physicians.[31] These and more than 30 other health and consumer organizations formed a coalition opposing the bill restricting the FTC. They stimulated grassroots support through TV programs, newspaper editorials, and articles on the op-ed pages.

Despite the above publicity and grassroots pressure, the bill passed by a large margin in the House of Representatives, 245 to 155. Apparently, representatives' continual needs for campaign contributions carried the day for the bill's proponents. The Senate, however, defeated the bill 59 to 37. The Senate's action was again similar to its rejection of restrictive trucking legislation. The truckers and Teamsters were successful in the House but not in the Senate. The Reagan administration also opposed the bill. The AMA and its allies were able to offer greater political support in the House, and they were successful in that chamber. Once again, however, the Senate did not go along with the House. Perhaps the six-year terms of senators provided some insulation from the constant need for campaign contributions. Senators not up for reelection are more independent than members of the House. Alternatively, newspapers and other media placed so much emphasis on the AMA's contributions and the vote for and against the FTC that a number of senators feared a supporting vote would be used against them at election time.[32]

As a result of the Supreme Court's decision and the defeat of subsequent legislation, professional associations could no longer inhibit competition. The FTC was able to bring suit to prevent physician and dentist boycotts against insurers (Michigan State Medical Society and the Indiana Federation of Dentists); prevent physicians from denying hospital privileges to physicians participating in prepaid health plans (Forbes Health System Medical Staff); enable advertising to be used (*FTC v. AMA*); oppose the per se rule against exclusive contracts (*Hyde* case); and enable PPOs and HMOs to compete.[33]

Consequences of Market Competition in Medical Care

Impact on Health Professionals

The increased ratio of physicians to the general population created excess capacity among physicians. To increase their volume of patients, physicians were more willing to change their organizational affiliations and their practice patterns. As HMOs increased their share of the insurance market, they needed more physicians to care for their enrollees. More physicians were willing to work for HMOs than previously. As competition among HMOs and traditional insurers intensified, both types of insurers attempted to lower their enrollees' medical costs by decreasing hospital utilization. Physicians were required to follow utilization guidelines; they had to receive authorization to hospitalize patients, to extend a patient's length of stay, and to refer patients to specialists. The HMOs and indemnity insurers also developed panels of participating physicians. Insured patients had a financial incentive to use these provider panels, if they did not then they had to pay higher out-of-pocket prices. To be included in these provider panels, physicians typically had to discount their fees to the insurers and not be "high" users of medical services.

As HMOs and insurers decreased hospital use rates, and hospital excess capacity increased, hospitals had to compete on price, offering discounts to HMOs. To be price competitive, hospitals had to increase their efficiency and become concerned with physician practices within the hospital. Hospitals were financially responsible for their physicians' practice styles. Competition provided insurers and hospitals with an incentive to monitor physician practice behavior.

To increase their own market power, physicians joined multispecialty medical groups to better negotiate fees and to be able to receive capitation payments from insurers and HMOs. To be competitive, these large medical groups had to have their own effective monitoring system to ensure that their physicians were practicing quality and cost-effective medicine. To control use of services, these medical groups often required their physicians to refer to specialists associated with their medical group. Specialists who were not part of those medical groups or who were not in insurer and HMO provider panels experienced large decreases in their patient referrals. Their incomes declined.

These were only some of the consequences of market competition to health professionals. Physicians in different specialties also came in conflict with one another. To increase their revenues, physicians tried to expand the services they offered by performing services previously performed by other specialties.

Health professionals are also engaged in intense political competition among themselves. Each health profession attempts to use state practice acts to increase the tasks they are allowed to perform while preventing other professions from encroaching on their tasks. Thus, optometrists are in competition with ophthalmologists, obstetricians with nurse midwives, family practitioners with nurse practitioners, psychologists with psychiatrists, and podiatrists with orthopedic surgeons.

Managed care decreased the economic returns to a career in medicine. The increased supply of health professionals, the applicability of the antitrust laws, and market competition had an adverse effect on the economic outlook and practice styles of physicians. It is not surprising that health associations such as the AMA have been so opposed to market competition.

Impact on the Structure of the Medical Care Delivery System

The main determinant of the number and size of firms in a competitive industry is which size of firm (in relation to the size of the market) is most efficient. This relationship between cost and size is referred to as "economies of scale," and it differs for each industry. If there are no barriers to entering or exiting an industry, then each firm will strive to take advantage of any economies of scale that may exist in order to minimize its costs. If a firm cannot compete at the same price as a more efficient firm, then it will either merge so as to be a more efficient size or go out of business.

In the past, economies of scale played an insignificant role in determining the structure of the healthcare industry. Legal (or regulatory) and cost-based financing methods determined its structure. Many of these regulations negated the importance of economies of scale in the delivery of medical services. Of what use was a lower-cost delivery system, such as an HMO, if it was illegal?

The stated reasons for many of the legal restrictions were to enhance the quality of care and protect the public. *Cynics, however, believed the profession was better protected than the public.* The effects of these restrictions were fewer providers, higher prices, and less innovation in the delivery of medical services.

As many legal restrictions were swept away by the antitrust laws, and as methods of financing medical services have changed, economies of scale became a more important determinant of the industry's market structure. Access to capital markets, lower interest costs on debt, volume discounts on supplies, advertising for all the specialties and services offered by an organization, lower data-processing costs, and lower malpractice premiums are several economies that occur with increased size of a health organization. Both the number and size of medical groups increased.

Initially, hospitals of less than optimal size started taking advantage of economies of scale by forming loose affiliations with one another. As the competitiveness of the industry increased, hospitals began merging and forming large hospital systems. The next step was to go beyond horizontal mergers and vertically integrate. Unfortunately, vertical integration did not succeed as physicians and hospitals were unable to align their incentives so as to minimize the total cost of care. As the demand for hospital care declined, the number of financially viable hospitals also declined. (Hospital consolidation and fewer competing hospitals eventually led to an increase in hospital market power.)

The federal government and private insurers, in their attempts to reduce expenditures, started providing insurance payments for less costly substitutes to hospitals. Hospitals facing a decrease in demand for their inpatient services became providers of these substitute services, for example, outpatient surgery centers. Several physician specialties, searching for new sources of revenue, began competing with hospitals as they started their own outpatient surgery units and even specialty hospitals. To prevent physicians from capturing their high profit margin patients, such as orthopedic, cardiovascular, and renal dialysis patients, hospitals started joint ventures with their physicians.

Consolidation and mergers among insurers also occurred (and are continuing). The larger the health insurer and the greater the number of enrollees, the larger the price discounts it is able to negotiate with providers. Investments in information technology have also become essential, not only for processing claims, but also for analyzing large amounts of data. An insurer that has millions of insured lives is able to collect data on treatments by disease across different regions where physicians have different practice styles. By analyzing different treatment patterns, insurers are able to determine not only which treatments for a given disease are less costly, but also which provide better patient outcomes (this is referred to as "evidence-based medicine"). The most cost-effective treatment patterns can then be disseminated to its participating providers. To be able to have access to such a large data base, insurers must be very large, provide insurance in different regions of the country, and develop an information technology infrastructure to conduct such analyses. Small insurers serving a single location are likely to be at a disadvantage.

Large insurers have additional competitive advantages over their competitors. Those insurers serving a greater number of regions are better able to negotiate national accounts with employers whose employees are located in many parts of the country. In addition, large insurers are able to offer a wider range of insurance products to employers. Given differences in employee preferences and willingness to pay for health insurance, insurers had to offer more than just an HMO product. A large insurer can expand into related product lines. For example, a health plan can sell insurance for a fee-for-service delivery system, an HMO, a PPO option, an administrative services only option to those businesses that self-insure, and a high-deductible plan available to satisfy different consumers. Health plans try and segment the insurance market by offering different products to each segment.

The market for healthcare services is consolidating. More hospitals are becoming part of a hospital system to take advantage of economies of scale and to increase their market power when dealing with insurers and HMOs. (The fewer the hospitals competing for the insurer's patients, the more each hospital is able to increase its prices.) Physicians have also consolidated into larger groups for the same reasons; however, poor management has led some physician groups into bankruptcy. Health insurers offer employers a diversified product line and have continued to consolidate.

Impact on the Public

The introduction of market competition has benefited consumers in a number of ways. The public has a greater choice of insurance products and delivery systems. Previously, traditional fee-for-service insurance plans were the only option available to those purchasing insurance. As long as consumer tastes vary, a variety of insurance products and delivery systems (and types of providers within each delivery system) can be expected to coexist in a competitive market.[34] Consumers have different preferences as to how much they are willing to pay for choice of provider and other health plan attributes. Managed fee-for-service, HMO, PPO, and high-deductible plans are the major options now available for consumers to choose among. Those willing to limit the comprehensiveness of their coverage (by choosing high-deductible plans) or their choice of provider, as with HMOs, can have lower out-of-pocket costs. Price competition also results in a great deal more innovation in methods of delivering medical services. Same-day outpatient surgery and home care are examples of alternative methods of providing care previously provided in the hospital. Insurers (and consequently providers) have become more responsive to the public's preferences.

Second, managed care competition was effective in reducing the rise in health insurance premiums. During the mid-1990s, health insurance premiums rose very slowly and in California, which had one of the most competitive medical environments in the United States, health insurance premiums actually declined for several years.[35] (See Figure 6.3.) The Congressional Budget Office estimated that, because of managed care, healthcare expenditures were almost $400 billion lower by the year 2000 than they had forecast. The introduction of managed care resulted in a redistribution of wealth; lower rates of increase in health insurance premiums resulted in greater take-home pay for employees, while those in the health sector suffered declines in their incomes.

Third, there has always been a concern that quality of care would suffer under a price-competitive system. Some physicians might engage in unethical behavior to increase their incomes or HMOs and other providers might have an incentive to provide fewer services, taking advantage of consumer ignorance. With informed purchasers in a competitive market, it is unlikely that quality could be lower than under the previous, regulated market when the dissemination of information on quality was purposely prohibited and state licensing boards performed very poorly in monitoring and disciplining physicians. Studies indicated that enrollees in managed care plans were more likely to receive preventive services and that there

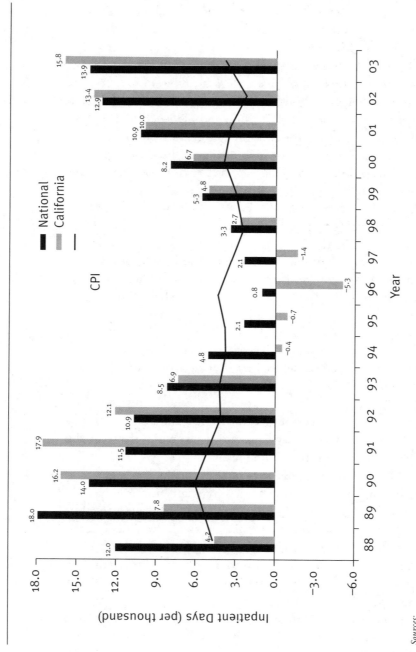

FIGURE 6.3
Annual Percentage Increase in Health Insurance Premiums for the U.S., California, and the CPI, 1988–2003

Sources:
1. National data: 1988–1998, Jon Gabel. KPMG Survey of Employer-Sponsored Health Benefits, HIAA Survey of Employer-Sponsored Health Benefits; 1999–2003. Kaiser/HRET. [Online information], http://www.kff.org/insurance/7148/uploaded/Employer-Health-Benefit-Survey 2004-Chartpack.pdf (accessed on July 27, 2005).
2. California data: CALPERS (California Public Employees Retirement System) and Kaiser/HRET 2004 California Employer Health Benefit Survey. [Online information], http://www.kff.org,
information], http://www.kff.org.
3. CPI data: Bureau of Labor Statistics [2005 Online information], http://data.bls.gov.

was generally no difference in quality of care between HMO enrollees and non-HMO enrollees.[36]

Insurers, businesses, and provider organizations are all using computerized claims-processing systems to monitor costs and appropriateness of utilization and to detect poor quality. A greater emphasis on quality of care is likely for those providers that are part of larger groups or that participate in alternative delivery systems. (Poor quality is also likely to cost HMOs or PPOs their business at that employer. Poor quality of care does not make good business sense.)

Under the previous cost-based system, many hospitals provided complex services, because it was prestigious to do so, without too much concern about the costs. Some of these services, such as open-heart surgery, require surgeons to perform a large number of procedures before they are sufficiently well experienced in the technique. Thus, hospitals that performed few procedures not only had higher average costs, but they also had a higher mortality rate.[37] As insurers have became more price-competitive, they have negotiated contracts for transplant and other high-tech services with hospitals on the basis of price and outcomes. Facilities performing few such complex procedures cannot compete with a consequent reduction in the mortality rate.

Fourth, consumers today have greater access to information than ever before. Under pressure from employers, HMOs and managed care organizations are publishing "report cards," which include measures of their enrollees' health status, patient satisfaction, the percentage of their enrollees provided with preventive measures, and outcomes of medical treatment. In addition to competing on their premiums, health plans are being pressured to compete on patient satisfaction, preventive measures provided, and quality of care, too. This quality dimension provides benefits to enrollees that did not occur under a regulated system.

Also making the consumer better informed is the growth of the Internet, which has increased the availability of health information, including outcome measures on specific medical providers. As consumers begin searching the web for health information on their illnesses, as more providers establish their own web sites, and as web sites become available that evaluate different healthcare providers, consumers are becoming better decision makers.

Competition has, unfairly, been blamed for a decrease in care available to those unable to pay. As hospitals face strong competitive pressures, many have reduced the amount of charity services they provide. Exacerbating this problem is that Medicaid programs have been reducing the amount they pay hospitals for their care of the medically indigent.

The decreased provision of charity care by hospitals and low Medicaid reimbursement rates have resulted in some hospitals trying to shift the indigent to other hospitals. This problem, referred to as "dumping," has received media attention. Public hospitals, including those teaching hospitals operated by state governments, receive more of the patients refused at other hospitals. These hospitals find themselves disadvantaged if they are forced to compete while subsidizing the costs of patients refused by their competitors.

Inadequate care for the poor is *not* the result of a competitive system. Instead, it is the consequence of government unwillingness to fund medical care to the poor. Competition eliminates cross-subsidies. Unless government payments for the aged and medically indigent are sufficient to cover their costs of care, hospitals will be discharging these patients too soon or these patients will be shifted to other providers, namely the public hospitals. Although one outcome of a competitive system is increased efficiency, another is that the manner in which the poor are financed and provided for becomes more obvious and requires society to make explicit choices on how we wish to provide for them.

The Change in Market Competition

By the late 1990s several events occurred that caused healthcare costs and insurance premiums to increase sharply again. Labor shortages began to occur as the economy expanded. Employees wanted less restrictive health plans and fewer restrictions on their access to specialists. To compete for skilled employees, employers accommodated them by offering managed care plans with expanded provider networks and fewer controls on use of services. At the same time, tight restrictions on access to care had created a consumer backlash against HMOs. Further, lawsuits were filed against HMOs for denying patients access to costly experimental treatments. To forestall large financial penalties, HMOs made experimental treatments more readily available to patients whose probability of a cure was low. State and Congressional legislators viewed the backlash as an opportunity to gain political support by enacting laws limiting HMOs' ability to contain costs, such as mandating minimum lengths of hospital stay for a normal delivery.

The initial success of managed care in lowering the rise in healthcare costs was a setback to those who favored a single-payer (Canadian style) healthcare system for the United States. The backlash against HMOs provided those legislators who were ideologically opposed to competitive healthcare markets with an opportunity to impose restrictions on HMOs, thereby increasing their premiums. The failure of the competitive market to control rising costs would, in the opinion of single-payer advocates, eventually lead to public dissatisfaction with the private market and demands for a government takeover of the healthcare system.

Many states also enacted legislation limiting managed care's cost-control efforts spurred on by those with a self-interest in increasing their professional incomes, namely organized medicine. Physicians were opposed to having to compete on price to be included in an HMO's provider network. "Any willing provider" laws were enacted in many states that permitted any physician (or dentist) to have access to an HMO's patients. These laws lessened the incentive for physicians to discount their prices in return for a greater volume of an HMO's patients.

Similarly, under pressure from different interest groups, states enacted legislation that required health insurers to include a broad range of providers as well as a broad range of services, such as acupuncture and hair transplants. There are more than 1,500 such state mandates in the fifty states. The net effect of these mandates is to increase the cost of health insurance.

The cost of health insurance began to increase sharply as managed care's cost-containment techniques were eliminated because of legislation, fear of lawsuits, and employees' demands for fewer restrictions on their access to specialists. Also contributing to rising healthcare costs are advances in medical technology and an increase in hospitals' market power. As their excess capacity declined, hospitals have increased their prices to health insurers.[38] Many hospitals closed in the 1980s and 1990s, and many others merged, decreasing hospital competition.

Once again rising health costs are a major public concern. Given the weakened state of managed care, a greater emphasis is being placed on the consumer, rather than the provider or insurer, to limit medical expenditure increases. "Consumer-driven" healthcare appears to be gaining popularity. Consumer-driven health plans give employees more choices in selecting their providers and level of benefits. The basic cost-control technique, however, is to shift more financial risk to the employee through the use of high-deductible policies in the expectation that greater out-of-pocket payments would make consumers more price sensitive, and hence, they would use fewer services and less costly services.

One version of a high-deductible plan is the health savings account (HSA). The employer annually contributes a fixed amount of money (tax exempt) to an employee's healthcare account (e.g., $1,500) and purchases a catastrophic health insurance policy for the employee. Employees can use the money in their healthcare account to pay for medical services. If they do not use all the funds, the funds remain in the employee's account. If they use all the funds and still require medical services, they must then pay a large deductible (e.g., $2,500) before the catastrophic plan becomes effective. The catastrophic plan relies on a closed panel of providers to provide the required medical services.

Medical costs will continue to increase. The U.S. population is aging and new medical advances extend both the quality of life and life itself. It is unrealistic to expect competitive medical markets to prevent medical costs from rising. Instead, *competitive markets will achieve the rate of increase in costs based on providers and insurers efficiently providing the amount of medical services consumers are willing to spend.*

The public is unrealistic in its demands for healthcare. People want to pay very little and have unrestricted access to all healthcare providers and to the latest medical advances. Unfortunately, many politicians are willing to regulate price reductions on medical services and prescription drugs for short-term political gain, without acknowledging that the eventual trade-off will be decreased access to medical care and to new technology.

Concluding Comments

As a result of the 1981 recession and severe import competition, industry became more concerned with costs and, in particular, with employees' health insurance premiums. As a result, industry developed a concentrated interest in lowering the rate of increase in its healthcare expenditures. One approach businesses used was to self-insure. In this way, a firm could exercise greater control over its employees' utilization of medical services. Up until that time, health insurance companies had not been very aggressive in introducing utilization review programs or monitoring health providers' charges. Consequently, employers found themselves paying successively higher premiums. The trend by business toward self-insurance and the increased emphasis on reducing health insurance premiums in turn stimulated price competition among insurers.

In response to industry demands for lower rates of increase in their health insurance premiums, insurance companies began to introduce cost-saving innovations in their benefit packages. By insuring low-cost substitutes to hospital care, increased cost sharing by employees, and the use of HMOs and PPOs, admission rates and lengths of stay in hospitals were reduced.

The HMOs, which had traditionally been unable to attract sufficient numbers of physicians, now found it easier to do so as a result of the increased supply of physicians. The HMOs also found it easier to market their services as companies offered their employees dual-choice options. Insurance companies started utilization management programs and PPOs as HMOs became more successful and were able to offer employee groups lower premiums. Hospital occupancy rates declined as a result of the cost-saving measures of the private sector.

The federal government had, in turn, developed a concentrated interest in controlling the rise in medical expenditures as a result of rapidly rising Medicare and Medicaid expenditures. The options facing the federal government were to increase the Medicare portion of the Social Security tax, divert more general income taxes to Medicare (Part B) and Medicaid, or reduce Medicare benefits to the aged. Neither option was politically acceptable. The only acceptable alternative, therefore, was to squeeze the providers. From the 1970s on, the federal government, through successive Democratic and Republican administrations, became more aggressive in opposing health associations, such as the AMA and hospital associations. The federal government instituted the DRG program, which led to a decline in hospital occupancy rates.

With declining occupancy rates and excess capacity, hospitals, to survive, had to compete for market share in a declining inpatient market. Consequently, hospitals participated in PPOs and HMOs for fear of being excluded from these markets. They offered increasingly greater discounts to larger purchasers.

The growth in excess capacity among physicians and hospitals, and the change in employer and government incentives, were important preconditions for market competition. However, it is unlikely that market competition would have been possible had it not been for the applicability and enforcement of the antitrust laws. In a previous time, with similar preconditions, anticompetitive behavior by physician associations prevented the emergence of market competition. In the 1930s excess capacity also existed among physicians, but prepaid plans and efforts by insurance companies to institute cost-control measures were thwarted by local medical societies.

The reasons for the emergence of market competition in healthcare were similar to those of other deregulated industries. Employers and the federal government each developed a concentrated interest in holding down the rise in their medical expenditures. Low-cost substitutes to traditional providers developed, namely HMOs and outpatient surgery centers. These new delivery systems decreased hospital and physician revenues. The growing supply of physicians increased competitive pressures among physicians. Declining occupancy rates did the same for hospitals. And the judicial system ensured that market competition would occur when the Supreme Court upheld the applicability of antitrust to the healthcare industry in 1982.

Study Questions

1. What are examples of anticompetitive practices that existed in healthcare before price competition occurred?

2. What purchaser and supplier conditions changed during the 1970s and 1980s that made it likely that price-based competition would occur in healthcare?

3. Why was it necessary for the antitrust laws to apply to healthcare before price competition could occur?

4. Which federal health policies indirectly contributed to the conditions that enabled price competition to start?

5. Explain why employers and government (at both the state and federal level) developed a "concentrated" interest in limiting the rise in health expenditures.

6. Why are "any willing provider" laws anticompetitive?

7. Contrast the predictions of the public interest and economic theories with regard to how effective CON legislation was expected to be in reducing the rate of increase in hospital expenditures.

Notes

1. Karen Davis, "Equal Treatment and Unequal Benefits: The Medicare Program," *The Milbank Memorial Fund Quarterly* 53, no. 4 (1975): 449–488; and G. Wilensky, L. Rossiter, and L. Finney, "The Medicare Subsidy of Private Health Insurance," mimeograph (Washington, DC: National Health Care Expenditure Survey, National Center for Health Services Research, 1983). The above data are published in Paul J. Feldstein, *Health Care Economics*, 6th ed. (Clifton Park, NY: Thomas Delmar Learning, 2005), 465–6.

2. Joseph P. Newhouse, *The Erosion of the Medical Marketplace* (Santa Monica, CA: RAND Corporation, 1978).

3. Data from the U.S. Department of Health and Human Services, Centers for Medicare and Medicaid Services, Office of the Actuary: National Health Statistics Group, 2005, http://www.cms.hhs.gov /statistics/nhe/historical/.

4. Ibid.

5. David S. Salkever and Thomas W. Bice, *Hospital Certificate-of-Need Controls: Impact on Investment, Costs, and Use* (Washington, DC: American Enterprise Institute, 1979).

6. A 1981 update of the Congressional Budget Office's study of PSROs stated, "Although PSROs appear to reduce Medicare utilization, the program consumes more resources than it saves society as a whole." *The Impact of PSROs on Health Care Costs: Update of CBO's 1979 Evaluation*, (Washington, DC: Congressional Budget Office, The Congress of the United States, 1981), xiii.

7. Paul J. Feldstein and Glenn Melnick, "Congressional Voting Behavior on Hospital Legislation: An Exploratory Study," *Journal*

of Health Politics, Policy and Law 8 (1984): 686–701.

8. W. Wendling and J. Werner, "Nonprofit Firms and the Economic Theory of Regulation," *Quarterly Review of Economics and Business* 20, no. 3 (1980): 6–18.

9. David H. Hitt, "Reimbursement System Must Recognize Real Costs," *Hospitals* 51, no. 1 (1977): 47–53; and David H. Hitt, "Reimbursement System Must Recognize Real Costs-Part 2," *Hospitals* 51, no. 1 (1977): 69–70, 72, 75–7.

10. Feldstein, *Health Care Economics*, 340–345.

11. "Health Professions Educational Assistance Amendments of 1965," *Hearing Before the Subcommittee on Health of the Committee on Labor and Public Welfare*, United States Senate, 89th Congress, 1st Session, September 8, 1965: 39–40.

12. *Physician Characteristics and Distribution in the US* (Chicago: American Medical Association, 2005).

13. The physician assignment rate on Medicare claims was 51.8 percent in 1975 and remained constant until 1980 (51.5) at which time it started to increase, reaching 68.5 percent in 1985. Alma McMillan, James Lubitz, and Marilyn Newton, "Trends in Physician Reassignment Rates for Medicare Services, 1968–1985," *Health Care Financing Review* 7, no. 2 (1985): Table 2, 62. For evidence on changes in the geographic distribution of physicians, see William B. Schwartz, Joseph P. Newhouse, Bruce W. Bennett, and Albert P. Williams, "The Changing Geographic Distribution of Board-Certified Physicians," *New England Journal of Medicine* 303 (1980): 1032–38.

14. S. E. Berki and Marie L. F. Ashcraft, "HMO Enrollment: Who Joins What and Why: A Review of the Literature," *The Milbank Memorial Fund Quarterly* 58 (1980): 588–632. For a complete discussion of the background of the HMO legislation, see Lawrence D. Brown, *Politics and Health Care Organization: HMOs as Federal Policy* (Washington, DC: The Brookings Institution, 1983).

15. For a complete discussion of CON and its legislative changes, see Clark C. Havighurst, *Deregulating The Health Care Industry: Planning For Competition* (Cambridge, MA: Ballinger Publishing Co., 1982), 222.

16. Ibid. For reviews of CON, see Michael A. Morrisey, "State Health Care Reform: Protecting the Provider," in *American Health Care: Government, Market Processes, and the Public Interest*, ed. Roger Feldman (Oakland, CA: The Independent Institute, 2000), 229–266; and Christopher Conover and Frank Sloan, "Does

Removing Certificate-of-Need Regulations Lead to a Surge in Health Care Spending?" *Journal of Health Politics, Policy and Law* 23(1998): 455–81.

17. Alain C. Enthoven, *Health Plan* (Reading, MA: Addison-Wesley Publishing Co., 1980).

18. Data from U.S. Department of Health and Human Services, Centers for Medicare and Medicaid Services, 2005, http://www.cms.hhs.gov/medicaid/managedcare/trends04.pdf.

19. Data from U.S. Department of Health and Human Services, Centers for Medicare and Medicaid Services, 2005, http://www.cms.hhs.gov/researchers/pubs/datacompendium /2003/03pg39.pdf.

20. Sherry Glied, "Managed Care," in *Handbook of Health Economics,* vol. 1A, eds. A. J. Culyer and J. P. Newhouse, (New York: North-Holland Press, 2000), 707–54.

21. Author calculations based on data from American Hospital Association, *Hospital Statistics, 2005.* (Chicago: American Hospital Association, 2005), Table 1.

22. Bruce Strombom, Thomas Buchmueller, and Paul Feldstein, "Switching Costs, Price Sensitivity and Health Plan Choice," *Journal of Health Economics* 21, no. 1 (2002): 89–116.

23. Lawrence G. Goldberg and Warren Greenberg, "The Emergence of Physician-Sponsored Health Insurance: A Historical Perspective," *Competition in the Health Care Sector,* ed. Warren Greenberg (Germantown, MD: Aspens Systems Corporation, 1978); Reuben Kessel, "Price Discrimination in Medicine," *Journal of Law and Economics* 1 (1958): 20–53; Reuben Kessel, "The AMA and the Supply of Physicians," *Law and Contemporary Problems* 35, no. 2 (1970): 267–283; and Elton Rayack, *Professional Power and American Medicine: The Economics of the American Medical Association* (New York: The World Publishing Co., 1967).

24. *Goldfarb v. Virginia State Bar, United States Reports,* 423 October Term 1975: 886.

25. *Congressional Quarterly,* 42, January 7, 1984, 15.

26. William Rial, "Should the FTC Regulate American Medicine?" *National Journal* 14 (1982): 1576–77.

27. Paul J. Feldstein and Glenn Melnick, "Political Contributions by Health Pacs to the 96th Congress," *Inquiry* 19, no. 4 (1982): 283–294.

28. *National Journal,* 14, September 18, 1982, 1590.

29. *Congressional Quarterly,* 42, January 7, 1984, 15.

30. *National Journal,* 14, September 18, 1982, 1590.

31. Ibid., 1592.

32. *Congressional Quarterly*, 42, January 7, 1984, 19.

33. For the latest overview of antitrust actions in the healthcare field, see FTC, Bureau of Competition, Health Care Services and Products Division, Overview of FTC Antitrust Actions in Health Care Services and Products, June 2005, http://www.ftc.gov/bc/050802antitrusthealthcareprods.pdf. See also, Deborah Haas-Wilson and Martin Gaynor, "Special Issue on Competition and Antitrust Policy in Health Care Markets," *Health Economics* 7 (1998); and Deborah Haas-Wilson, *Managed Care and Monopoly Power* (Cambridge, MA: Harvard University Press, 2003).

34. In the period before deregulation of the medical care industry, the industry was characterized by fee-for-service payment with many independent providers. If this system was the result of a competitive market, it would suggest that consumers had relatively similar tastes. In a country as large and as diverse as the United States, this would be highly unlikely. Instead, the delivery and payment system that existed was indicative of a noncompetitive market that prevented the exercise of differences in consumer tastes.

35. Paul J. Feldstein, *Health Policy Issues: An Economic Perspective*, 3rd ed. (Chicago: Health Administration Press; Washington, DC: AUPHA Press, 2003), Figure 18.4, 218.

36. Kathryn A. Phillips, Susan Fernyak, Arnold L. Potosky, Helen Halpin Schauffler, and Melanie Egorin, "Use of Preventive Services by Managed Care Enrollees: An Updated Perspective," *Health Affairs* 19, no. 1 (2000): 102–16; Robert H. Miller and Harold S. Luft, "HMO Plan Performance Update: An Analysis of the Literature, 1997–2001," *Health Affairs*, 21, no. 4 (2002): 63–86; Robert H. Miller and Harold S. Luft, "Does Managed Care Lead to Better or Worse Quality of Care?" *Health Affairs* 16, no. 5 (1997): 7–25; Robert H. Miller and Harold S. Luft, "Managed Care Plan Performance Since 1980: A Literature Analysis," *Journal of the American Medical Association* 271 (1994): 1512–19; Feldstein, *Health Care Economics*, 176–7; M. A. Smith, J. R. Frytak, J. I. Liou, and M. D. Finch, "Rehospitalization and Survival for Stroke Patients in Managed Care," *Medical Care* 43 (2005): 902–10; B. E. Landon, A. M. Zaslavsky, S. L. Bernard, M. J. Cioffi, and P. D. Cleary, "Comparison of Performance of Traditional Medicare vs. Medicare Managed Care," *Journal of the American Medical Association* 291 (2004): 1744–52.

37. Harold Luft, John Bunker, and Alain Enthoven, "Should Operations Be Regionalized", *New England Journal of Medicine*

301(1979): 1364–69. See also, Robert Hughes, Sandra Hunt, and Harold Luft, "Effects of Surgeon Volume and Hospital Volume on Quality of Care in Hospitals," *Medical Care* 25 (1987): 489–503.

38. James F. Burgess, Jr., Kathleen Carey, and Gary J. Young, "The Effect of Network Arrangements on Hospital Pricing Behavior," *Journal of Health Economics* 24 (2005): 391–405. See also, Ranjani Krishnan, "Market Restructuring and Pricing in the Hospital Industry," *Journal of Health Economics* 20 (2001): 213–37.

THE CONTROL OF EXTERNALITIES: MEDICAL RESEARCH, EPIDEMICS, AND THE ENVIRONMENT

After completing this chapter, the reader should be able to

- describe why an "externality" can be used to justify government intervention in the marketplace,
- discuss how both producer interests and the public's political support were accommodated in congressional funding for medical research,
- contrast the political response to two different health epidemics: AIDS and swine flu,
- describe the congressional approach of mandating "scrubbers" to reduce air pollution using the public interest and economic theory, and
- explain why legislation promotes the use of "process" measure to reduce air pollution.

Externalities are a rationale for government intervention in the private sector. Externalities occur when an action undertaken by a firm (or individual) has secondary or indirect effects on others, which may be favorable or unfavorable. Within a private market, business only considers its production costs and its selling price in determining how much to produce. Similarly, individuals consider only the price they must pay and the benefits they expect to receive in determining how much of a particular good to purchase. However, as a result of these private decisions, persons and businesses, that are not directly involved in the production or purchase of that good may be affected. When costs are imposed on others who are not market participants, or they receive benefits as a result of someone's private decision, then the level of output produced in the private market will result in either too small a level of benefits (i.e., positive external benefits) or too small a level of costs of production (i.e., positive external costs). For example, private markets generally produce too much environmental pollution and too little medical research.

The role of government is to ensure that external costs are added to the cost of producing the service and/or the external benefits are added to the private benefits consumers receive. Only when all the costs and benefits are included will an optimal output be achieved. The following are examples of externalities.

In producing its product, a chemical company may also produce chemical waste, which it then dumps in a nearby lake. Then the lake may no longer be usable for fishing or recreational purposes. The chemical company has imposed a harmful externality, referred to as an external cost, on all who used that lake. In calculating its costs of production, the chemical company does not include these external costs. The purchasers of those chemicals pay a price that is lower than if all costs, including external costs, were included. The result is that more chemicals are sold than if the selling price reflected both the firm's costs of production and the external costs imposed on others.

Medical research is an example of external benefits being provided to others. If a company undertakes research and discovers a cure for AIDS, many people, other than those purchasing the company's drug, will also benefit. The company calculates the costs of conducting research, the probability of success, and the monetary return of success in deciding whether or not to undertake the research. The individuals purchasing the drug do so based on calculations of their costs and benefits. The external benefits to those who have a lessened chance of contracting the disease are not included in either the producers' or purchasers' calculations. If these external benefits were included in the company's calculations, then the profitability of the research would be increased and it would be worthwhile for the firm to spend additional funds on research.

There are many other examples of externalities, ranging from those that may be trivial in terms of public policy (e.g., a neighbor playing loud music late at night, although this externalitiy is not trivial to enraged neighbors who are trying to sleep) to cases where the external costs and benefits are sufficiently widespread and significant to warrant government intervention.

Both the purchasers and producers of a good only consider their own benefits and costs when deciding how much to buy or produce. Because external costs or benefits are not part of their calculations, the outcome is that either too much (in the case of external costs) or too little (external benefits) is produced. Economists refer to this result as "an inefficient allocation of resources." Technically, an efficient allocation of resources occurs when the marginal benefits (both private and external) are equal to the marginal costs (again, both private and external) of producing the product. As long as the value (marginal benefits) of the output exceeds its costs of production, then an increase in output would be worthwhile; the increased output will result in greater benefits than costs. Alternatively, when the costs of the last units exceed the benefits derived from those units, then those resources should be moved into other uses where they can produce output with a higher value.

The appropriate role of government in cases of externalities is to assess the magnitude of these external costs and benefits and to include them as part of the private decision-making process. For example, in the case of pollution the government should determine the external costs and place a tax (equal to the cost of pollution) on the amount of pollution produced. The production costs and the selling price of the good produced would then include all of the relevant costs. In the case of external benefits, the government should calculate their size and provide a subsidy (equal to the external benefits) to the producers. The subsidy would reduce the cost of production, and, consequently, the selling price, thereby increasing the quantity of the good sold.[1]

A great many difficulties are involved in determining the external costs and benefits of different activities. What are the harmful health effects of air pollution? How should one assess the lost recreational use of polluted lakes? How much weight should be assigned to these external costs so that they may be translated into monetary amounts?

Determining external benefits is also fraught with difficulties. For example, everyone benefits from having the government defend this country, even though the size of the defense budget and the nature of foreign threats may be subject to dispute. No one can be excluded from enjoying the benefits of a secure national defense. However, it is rational for any one individual not to voluntarily contribute, as each will receive the same benefit whether or not a contribution is made. People hope to receive a free ride, that is, to enjoy the benefits without having to pay. If too many people become free riders, then an activity with external benefits will not be undertaken or would be smaller than if all the benefits were included. (Asking people how much the external benefit is worth to them is likely to lead to their understating its value so as to reduce their contribution.)

Unless the government is able to determine the external costs and benefits of various activities and incorporate those externalities in private decision making, either too much or too little of that activity will be undertaken.

When externalities exist, government involvement is generally accepted to be within its proper role. Further, legislation dealing with pollution and medical research is observed. Is this government intervention evidence that at least in this legislative area the self-interest paradigm is not applicable? Unless a theory can explain a wide range of applications, it becomes necessary to explain why a theory is applicable in some cases but not others. The bases of the theory would have to be reexamined.

This chapter provides an explanation of government intervention when externalities arise based on the self-interest of concentrated interests and of legislators, namely maximization of their political support.

Political Support Maximization as a Basis for Government Intervention When There Are Externalities

According to the concept of political support maximization, elected officials also undertake a cost/benefit analysis when deciding which programs to support or oppose. To the elected official, however, the definition of costs and benefits is not related to issues of external costs and benefits. The only relevant costs and benefits for a legislator are the political support gained from taking an action (the benefits) compared to the political support lost (the costs) of that same action. When the benefits exceed the costs, legislators will gain more from their proactive position on an issue than they will lose.

Given the divergence in definitions of costs and benefits legislators and economists use to determine the appropriate role of government when externalities occur, it is not surprising that the outcomes are not similar.

Legislators must perceive the existence of political support before they enact legislation. In nonhealth areas, such as national defense and space exploration, political support from narrow constituencies, as well as from the public at large is essential before Congress will appropriate funds. The debate over the size of the defense budget represents differences of opinion between legislators whose constituencies differ on this issue. National defense is very visible and, unless legislators represent their constituents' views, they are likely to lose political support and face opposition at their party's primary or at the next election. And they are loath to generate opposition to their own reelection.

Separate components of the military budget are also visible, and various constituencies have strong feelings about its appropriate size. Legislators have not favored closing military bases or eliminating military contracts in their own districts, even though such changes might result in a more efficient defense budget. In fact, there are numerous cases where the military has favored closing some bases or shutting down the production of some plants, for example, an outdated plane factory in Texas, but has been opposed by the district's legislators. Legislation in the public interest must not be contrary to the constituents' interest or a legislator is unlikely to vote in favor of it.

When President Kennedy announced in 1961 that the United States would place a man on the moon by the end of the decade, he was responding to the public's desire not to be second to the Soviet Union in space exploration. President Kennedy was also demonstrating leadership on a popular issue. From a political perspective, the space program had all the ingredients for legislative success: the public favored it and there was limited opposition; in other words, the political benefits exceeded the political cost of the action.

Government intervention on issues that involve externalities is based on the degree of political support for those issues. Analyses of what should be done and the optimal amount to spend on such programs are of secondary, if any, importance. The size and composition of the defense budget is, for the most part, a political determination. The military establishment may attempt to develop a budget based on a calculation of the equipment and personnel required to meet various strategic objectives; however, the military also considers its own needs (the size of military pensions) as well as the likely response of Congress. It is no secret or coincidence that military expenditures and military bases are concentrated in those congressional districts where the legislators have the greatest control over the military budget.

When externalities exist, government intervention occurs only when there is a net gain in political support from the government's action. When widespread public support exists, as evidenced by public opinion polls and organized environmental groups, then those programs with little or no opposition will be passed quickly. The only controversy will be over which politician can take credit for the legislation. The legislation may even result in a serious attempt to resolve the concern in a meaningful manner.

When legislative proposals aimed at correcting harmful externalities impose costs on some group, such as requiring certain industries to invest in equipment or reducing the labor force of an industry, then legislators must perceive a net gain in political support by satisfying, if possible, two competing political constituencies. The first constituency is the part of the public that is concerned with these issues. If the public is not well-informed, people are likely to be satisfied by passage of symbolic legislation. The second constituency is the affected industry and union. This group is likely to be appeased if the regulations are written in such a manner that they will either not be harmed (e.g., they will be exempt, or grandfathered, from the new regulations) or they will actually gain a competitive advantage by having the regulatory costs imposed on competitors and/or new market entrants. The concerned public provides the political support necessary to have the legislation enacted, while those industries and unions likely to be directly affected provide political support to ensure that they are not harmed. Because the public does not have information on the details of the legislation, it is unaware of the methods used to achieve the legislation's objectives. For this reason the stated goals of the legislation are so often at odds with its effects.

The following examples of externalities in the health field serve to illustrate these principles.

Federal Support for Medical Research

Before 1940, most medical research was funded by nonfederal sources. Drug companies undertook research in the expectation of earning a profit. Most medical research, however, was funded by private foundations through gifts to medical schools and medical research institutes. These private foundations were started by wealthy businessmen who "hoped for recognition in this world or the next."[2] Several private groups also raised funds for research. For example, the National Tuberculosis Association was very successful in their sales of Christmas seals, which provided the funds for tuberculosis research.[3] These private sources supported medical research for specific diseases, such as cancer and syphilis, because the public was more apt to contribute the greater their fear of the disease.[4]

Approximately one-third of all federal research during this period was undertaken by the U.S. Department of Agriculture. Farmers were early to recognize the economic value of medical research.

> Federal aid was extended in this period to studies on the health of farm animals, while almost no funds were available for direct work on the diseases of man. . . . This was partly because of the nature of medical science . . . and partly because human welfare brought no direct financial return. Hogs did.[5]

The Bureau of Agricultural Economics, which was created in 1922, brought together some of the country's best social scientists. Their goal was to apply their talents to problems of "profitability and productivity" in agriculture.[6]

Federal support of medical research received its impetus from World War II. The prestige of scientists increased with the application of scientific knowledge to the war effort. The atomic bomb is the most notable example. Another example is the development of penicillin in 1941. Although penicillin had been discovered earlier, it took a coordinated effort by scientists to make it usable for American troops. As the war ended, there was a belief that science could do a great deal to alleviate human suffering.

Mary Lasker and Florence Mahoney, who had access to great wealth and a newspaper chain, are given a good deal of credit for the growth in federal support for medical research in the post–World War II period. Although they were certainly influential in the early stages, it is naive to believe Lasker and Mahoney were the primary reason for the vast funding of the NIH. These two women were also very much in favor of national health insurance, and yet despite all their efforts in that regard, they were unsuccessful. To understand why they were so successful in securing federal support for medical research and so unsuccessful in their other endeavors, it is necessary to take a closer look at the differences in political support for these different federal programs.

President Truman's proposal for national health insurance in the late 1940s generated strong opposition. The AMA mounted a national campaign against it and was instrumental in defeating it. The AMA demonstrated that it could help defeat legislators at election time who opposed them on this issue. The AMA's political influence during this period, from the late 1940s through the 1950s, was at its peak.

Medical research, however, was not controversial. In fact, once Lasker and Mahoney were able to enlist the help of certain representatives and senators who, once they recognized that it was in their own political interest to support medical research, then made a career out of doing so. Lasker and Mahoney had the foresight to see the political and societal advantages for supporting medical research.

Lasker and Mahoney were initially able to convince Senator Claude Pepper (as the chairman of the appropriate Senate committee) to hold hearings on medical research and become a proponent of their cause. Senator Pepper, in turn, was rewarded with contributions and newspaper endorsements from the Lasker and Mahoney families in his reelection campaign.[7] When the Republicans gained control of the Senate in the late 1940s, Senator Styles Bridges became the new chairman of the Senate subcommittee, and Lasker and Mahoney persuaded him to take up the cause of medical research, too.[8]

Senator Bridges, as had Senator Pepper before him, realized that support for medical research brought favorable newspaper coverage and visibility as a compassionate legislator. When the Democrats regained control over the Senate, Senator Lister Hill similarly recognized the political advantages of continued support for medical research. Such support made Senator Hill a national figure. Previously known primarily as a Southerner opposed to civil rights legislation, he was able to gain tremendous prestige (and was reelected numerous times) for his support of medical research.[9]

Lasker and Mahoney were equally successful in the House of Representatives in convincing the appropriate subcommittee chairs of the benefits of supporting medical research. In the late 1940s, Frank Keefe, the Republican chairman of the Labor-Federal Security Subcommittee, told Mahoney ". . . that he had only one speech on the campaign trail, and that it was on health and what the federal government must do to advance it. That speech got him elected to five consecutive terms in Congress."[10] When the Democrats took control of the House and the subcommittee chairs changed, support for medical research became a bipartisan issue.[11] Representative John Fogarty was quick to realize the political benefits of supporting medical research and was an ardent proponent until his death in 1964.

The 1971 Cancer Act was motivated by the public's fears about cancer. "The American people fear cancer more than any other disease and they want something done about it."[12] "Senator Yarborough's interest in the matter [cancer] was genuine, but he also hoped his sponsorship of the legislation within the committee would meet with widespread approval and help him secure reelection."[13] Senator Edward Kennedy subsequently proposed a new large-scale effort on cancer. Not to be outdone, President Nixon proposed his own plan to find a cure for cancer in his January 1971 State of the Union Address. The public's fears "prompted politicians to compete for the role of the most compassionate and determined public trustees, by launching a new war against the dread disease."[14]

The AMA's opposition to legislation affecting the financing of personal health services left Congress with few alternative approaches to demonstrate to their constituents that they were compassionate individuals deserving of their support. Members of Congress clearly believed they were responding to the public's desire for increased medical research. Newspaper polls showed that the public was willing to spend more on cancer research, even if they had to pay increased taxes. Public interest in health was also indicated by the very high readership of newspaper articles on health.[15]

When Congress perceived a political advantage in supporting medical research, they responded with a vengeance. Congressional committees appropriated more than was requested by the administration or even by the research agencies. A favorite tactic was for the committee chair to ask the agency director what they could do if they had a few more million dollars. When President Eisenhower budgeted $126 million for medical research in fiscal year 1957, Congress appropriated $183 million. The next year the administration proposed $190 million, Congress responded with $211 million. For fiscal year 1961 the Kennedy administration proposed $400 million and Congress provided $547 million.[16]

Some policy makers were concerned that the research institutes were receiving more funds than could reasonably be spent. A number of times the NIH had to return unspent funds to the Treasury. The NIH went along with congressional wishes and appropriations because they feared that if they did not, Congress would start a competing agency. This in fact was one of the major contentions of the 1971 Cancer Act.

The interest by Congress in medical research did not stop with providing excess research support. Congress also directed the research institutes on which diseases were to be investigated. For the public to appreciate what it was doing on their behalf, Congress wanted research conducted on specific diseases and not for basic medical research.[17] Congress consequently created additional research institutes, each named for a specific disease. For example, in 1955 the Microbiology Institute became known as the National Institute of Allergy and Infectious Diseases. After all, as one congressman commented, "Whoever died of microbiology?"[18]

Increased funding for medical research also served the economic interests of medical schools. In the late 1940s, medical schools claimed that they were in financial difficulty and needed federal support. The AMA was concerned that if the federal government provided institutional support as the medical schools requested, the government would then require that medical schools increase their enrollment. (At this time there were claims of a physician shortage.) Therefore, the AMA opposed federal support.

The tremendous increase in federal support for medical research served as a substitute for direct federal support of medical education. In 1960, approximately 200 universities and medical schools received 90 percent of all federal research funds from NIH.[19] The proportion of medical schools' operating budgets that was supported by federal medical research and research training reached 45 percent in 1965. In the 15-year period from 1951 to 1966, the number of full-time medical school faculty increased from approximately 3,500 to more than 17,000.[20] This increase was largely the result of federal medical research and training expenditures. (During this same period the rate of increase in U.S. medical graduates was virtually unchanged.)[21]

A new and powerful lobby group, the Association of American Medical Colleges, now had a vested interest in ensuring that federal support to medical schools be continued. In the debate over a new cancer agency in 1971, the Association of American Medical Colleges opposed the creation of a new agency because it feared ". . . that the medical colleges it represents—which perform 30 percent of the basic cancer research funded by NIH—would suffer a loss of funds as the federal government adopts a more narrowly targeted approach to attacking disease."[22]

The dramatic increases in federal support for medical research began to level off in the mid-1960s. Competing budgetary demands for other federal programs made it difficult to fund medical research at the previous rate. Expenditures for the space program were increasing. The Vietnam

War was beginning to escalate, and President Johnson did not want to seek a tax increase for these competing demands. Medicare and Medicaid were finally approved in 1965, and expenditures under these programs rapidly exceeded their initial projections.

Overcoming the AMA's opposition to Medicare, Congress was now able to show its compassion for health by supporting other health programs (whose constituencies, including unions, the aged, and the middle class, offered greater political support than did the AMA). Congress also passed (in opposition to the AMA) the Health Professions Educational Assistance Act in 1963, which provided institutional support for medical schools to enable more middle-class children to have access to a medical education. As Congress was able to receive political support from these other groups, it began providing financing for different types of personal health service programs.

Legislators faced a budget constraint. The administration was reluctant to seek an increase in taxes, which would have cost it political support. Legislators therefore had to make choices among different health programs. As a result, medical research funding suffered; although the funds continued to increase, their growth rate declined.

Medical research was a bipartisan issue. With visible public support and no opposition, Congress recognized a good political issue. The only competition was over who would be viewed as the most compassionate legislator in seeking funding to cure diseases the public feared. Even the AMA did not oppose federal support for medical research; in fact, new discoveries would increase physicians' productivity. Physicians could now do more for their patients.

In their support for medical research, Congress was responding to the public's fears and their belief in science. This is entirely appropriate. However, Congress went too far. In catering to the public, Congress provided more funds than could reasonably be used; it appropriated more funds than requested by the research institutes, and the institutes returned funds to the Treasury at the end of the fiscal year, a rare action. Congress also directed research strategy. Many scientists favored increased funding for basic research. However, Congress required that the funds be spent on disease-specific programs (such programs were more "saleable") so that the public could better understand what their legislators were doing for them. Further, Congress was often too directive, providing research guidelines for the scientists to follow.

When government subsidizes positive externalities based on the amount of political support for such programs, then it is unlikely that the optimal funding for these programs will be forthcoming over a sustained period. As explained previously, it is an appropriate function of government to calculate the size of external benefits received by the population and provide sufficient funding so that an efficient allocation of resources to medical research occurs. Instead, the participants in the decision-making process, namely Congress and the producers of medical research (primarily the medical schools), use a different set of costs and benefits for determining medical research appropriations. Congress views the benefits in terms of the immediate political support they might receive from the interested voting public. There are no costs involved in Congress' decision as it is unlikely that they would lose political support by appropriating too much. The outcome, therefore, is excessive funding in the short run. Those seeking research funds place a greater weight than would others on the benefits of medical research. Although researchers' perspectives have a longer time horizon than does Congress,' they too are unlikely to consider the costs of such programs, because they do not bear them. (The real costs of medical research are the other uses to which the funds could be applied.)

Public Crises as a Cause for Government Intervention

Crises have been an important stimulant to the passage of health legislation. Media attention is focused on the event. And the public wants leadership from its elected representatives. Legislators or a president portrayed by the media as being the public's protector can expect to be rewarded with favorable publicity and reelection. The following examples illustrate the importance of health crises to the passage of health legislation; each case involves the issue of externalities.

Drug Legislation

The first drug legislation was part of the Pure Food Act of 1906.[23] The supporters of this act were more concerned with the quality of food than with drugs. Pure food acts had been submitted to Congress at least ten years before one was finally enacted. A great deal of publicity was generated by newspapers, magazine articles, and Upton Sinclair's *The Jungle*, with its graphic descriptions of what was being included in the foods the public was eating. The result was public outrage, to which Congress responded by passing the Pure Food Act.[24]

The act also required drug companies to provide accurate labeling information, including whether the drug was addictive. Further, if a drug was labeled (the manufacturer did not have to do so), then the manufacturer had to disclose its ingredients. The government could then verify the accuracy of the drug's contents. The drug-related portion of the act was quite limited and was modeled by the public's concern with the contents of food.

In the 1930s, the modern drug era began. As drugs were introduced, a tragedy occurred providing the impetus for new legislation. A company seeking to make a liquid form of sulfanilamide for children dissolved it in ethylene glycol (antifreeze). The company was unaware of the toxic effects, and as a result, more than 100 children died.[25] Responding to the public outcry, Congress enacted the Food, Drug, and Cosmetic Act in 1938. The 1938 law was intended to protect the public from unsafe and potentially harmful drugs. A company had to seek approval from the U.S. Food and Drug Administration (FDA) before it could market a new drug. It was left up to the drug company to determine the necessary amount and type of premarket testing before stating that the drug was safe for its intended use. The requirements for testing drugs were not changed until the thalidomide crisis.

In 1959 Senator Estes Kefauver held hearings on the drug industry. (He was running for the 1960 Democratic nomination for president at that time.) He was concerned that drug prices were too high and that drug companies undertook unnecessary and wasteful advertising expenditures.[26] The Congressional hearings were soon to take an unexpected turn.

After thalidomide was introduced in Europe, a U.S. drug company introduced it to the United States on an experimental basis. The 1938 FDA amendments permitted such limited distribution to qualified experts as long as the drug was labeled as being under investigation. As soon as reports began to appear in Europe that deformed babies were born to mothers who had taken the drug during pregnancy, the U.S. company withdrew the drug.

Congress responded to the public's fears over drug safety and passed the controversial 1962 drug act amendments. The FDA now requires a great deal more information from the pharmaceutical firm before a prescription drug is given approval. The legislation specifies the type of premarket testing, which is extensive, that the pharmaceutical firm must undertake These amendments were enacted in spite of the fact that the 1938 legislation was effective in keeping thalidomide off the market. Further, had the new amendments been in effect at the time of thalidomide, they "would not have prevented a thalidomide-type tragedy."[27]

The consequence of the new amendments was that the cost and time required to introduce new drugs was greatly increased. (In 2003, the cost of developing a new drug was estimated to be as high as $802 million.)[28] With higher development costs, the profitability of new drug research decreased and there was a decline in the number of new drugs. Further, a large time lag developed between when drugs were available for use in other countries and when they could be used in the United States. For example, drugs proven effective for treating heart disease and hypertension were used in Great Britain as early as 1965, but it was 1976 before they were fully approved for use in the United States.[29]

One analyst examining the new amendments concluded that they made the public worse off.[30] Sam Peltzman attempted to quantify the benefits of the new amendments by weighing the estimated effect of the new regulations on keeping ineffective and dangerous drugs off the market (of which there were very few before 1962) against the lost benefits of having fewer new drugs, higher prices for existing drugs (because there is less competition from new drugs), and a reduced availability of drugs because of the time lag. The decline in the development of new drugs was the greatest disadvantage of the amendments, and according to Peltzman, this factor alone made the costs of the new amendments greatly exceed the potential benefits.

The legislators' response to the drug crisis resulted in a much greater emphasis on the short-term effects of a drug's action, which are more visible to the media and to the public, than to the longer-term consequences. The media publicizes the effects of a drug that has unfortunate side effects. Victims' names are given and photographs printed. The media do not publicize all the nameless people who may have died because a new drug was not allowed to develop or was slow in receiving approval. For example, the higher cost of developing new drugs has made it unprofitable for "orphan" drugs, that is, drugs that would benefit small population groups, to be developed. (Special legislation had to be enacted to provide drug companies with a financial incentive to develop drugs for small population groups.) The benefits to legislators (and to the FDA) of protecting the public by favoring more stringent safety requirements are obvious. Less obvious and also very important are the enormous costs of decreased availability of new drugs to relieve pain and suffering.[31]

The Swine Flu Epidemic (That Never Arrived)

An example of the government's response to a possible public health crisis is found in the anticipated swine flu epidemic of 1976. The administrative and congressional actions were typical responses to public health problems, such as epidemics.

In February 1976 an army recruit stationed at Fort Dix, New Jersey, died from pneumonia of possible influenza origin. A number of other army recruits also became ill from influenza. The influenza specimens were sent to the New Jersey Public Health Laboratory for analysis. Most of the influenza strains were determined to be a common variety. Several strains, however, could not be identified. They were then sent to the federal laboratory at the Centers for Disease Control and Prevention (CDC) in Atlanta for further analysis.[32]

Additional tests revealed that the unidentified strains were similar to the swine flu virus that was believed to have been responsible for the great flu epidemic in 1918–19. This virus had not been seen for 50 years. The CDC, which is responsible for administering a variety of federal programs in preventive medicine and disease control in collaboration with state and local health officials, was alarmed. The 1918–19 epidemic caused the deaths of 450,000 people, or 400 out of every 100,000 Americans. In contrast, in an average year, influenza causes about 17,000 deaths, or 9 per 100,000 people. The population groups most susceptible to swine flu would be those under 50 years old. If a swine flu epidemic were to occur in late 1976, approximately one million Americans could die.

Unfortunately, the scientists at CDC did not know how likely it would be that such an epidemic would actually occur, given the discovery of these swine flu strains. They were by no means certain that these new strains foretold the start of a new epidemic. But given the magnitude of the tragedy that had occurred in 1918–19, the CDC proposed that a government immunization program be initiated before the next flu season. CDC stated, "[It is] better to have an immunization program without an epidemic, than an epidemic without an immunization program."[33]

Vaccinating two hundred million Americans by the fall of 1976 would have been a vast undertaking. Government funds would have to be appropriated, private drug companies would have to develop a sufficient quantity of the new vaccines, and states and localities would have to be mobilized. It would be the first time this country undertook such a large program in such a short period of time.

Once the information about the swine flu strain was released, there was a great deal of publicity. The horrors of the 1918–19 epidemic were reviewed. The media interest and the public concern necessitated a response by our country's representatives.

President Ford was provided with a set of options on how to respond to the public's fears about a possible repeat of the 1918–19 epidemic. The following choices were available to the president. If the president took no action and the feared epidemic did not occur, then the government would save $134 million, the cost of the vaccination program. However, the media, Congress, and the American people expected some kind of leadership. President Ford's advisers believed the public would prefer to have the money wasted than not have the vaccine if truly needed. Further, if the president— a Republican—did not act, then the Democratic Congress would step forward as the party concerned about the nation's health and pass a mass vaccination program.

Any legislator knows that in choosing between spending money or risking American lives the public would prefer that the money be spent. A politician cannot go to the electorate later and say that he was just trying to save money because the epidemic had such a small probability of occurring. If he was wrong, the electorate would never forgive him.

In addition, 1976 was an election year. President Ford was having a difficult time against Ronald Reagan in the primaries, and the Democrats continually characterized him as being weak and indecisive. What would happen to his reelection prospects if he appeared to be more interested in balancing the budget when the epidemic arrived in the fall, at the time of the election? President Ford consulted with a large number of prominent scientists, received their unanimous approval, and decided to go ahead with the mass vaccination campaign.

The Democrats in Congress were upstaged by a conservative president on an issue—health—they believed belonged to them. Congress, however, had to respond positively to the president's request for an additional appropriation for the vaccination campaign, because "a Presidential charge of congressional irresponsibility in the face of a health emergency would be politically unbearable."[34] However, Congress also saw the immediacy of the president's request as an opportunity to do something for its members. After attaching additional funds for temporary jobs ($1.2 billion), water pollution control ($300 million), comprehensive human resources assistance ($528 million), and community service for older Americans ($55.9 million), Congress passed President Ford's emergency appropriation of $135 million. Congress was sure the president would not veto his own program.

The swine flu program ran into a number of obstacles, however. One drug company produced the wrong vaccine, thereby setting back the date at which immunizations could start. The drug companies had early warned that unless Congress relieved them of the insurance liability of people potentially becoming ill from the vaccine, they would not proceed with production. Congress delayed enacting such relief. Then doubt began to spread in the media that there would be an epidemic in the fall. All of a sudden a new fearful disease, Legionnaires' disease, broke out in Pennsylvania. At first it was believed to be connected to swine flu. Once again, the media attention and the became concerned about the possibility of an epidemic. President Ford used his office to castigate Congress for not moving on legislation to waive immunity for the drug companies.

"This was greater heat than the members of Congress could bear. Here was President Ford, apparently willing to go before the Republican convention and into the Presidential campaign with accusations that the opposition party cared so little for the health and safety of the American people that they would let this important immunization program die. This would be unbearable during a normal year, but doubly so during an election year.[35]

Once the vaccination program finally began, it was discovered that vaccinated people were at higher risk of contracting a rare disease, Guillain-Barre syndrome. This finding finally ended the ill-fated vaccination program. By then the election was over and no epidemic had appeared. The vaccination program was not renewed. Much has been written on the swine flu affair.[36] With the media coverage of the swine flu situation gone, Congress lost interest in immunization programs.

As this country grapples with the possibility of new types of epidemics, such as the threat of avian (bird) flu that emerged in 2005, it is not clear that the country is any more able to deal with the threat of another killer epidemic. The federal bureaucracy, the CDC, is unlikely to favor saving a very small amount of government funds only to be blamed if an epidemic occurs and people die. Similarly, it is unlikely that any president would want to be accused of sacrificing lives for dollars. Given the media attention concerning a possible epidemic, the opposing political party would seek a leading role on the issue if the president hesitated. The political costs and benefits have not changed, and Congress has not completely resolved the issue of insurance liability for vaccine producers if an emergency situation were to arise.

AIDS

It is instructive to contrast the political response to the swine flu epidemic with that of a different contagious disease, AIDS. Although the first AIDS cases were reported in March 1981, the Reagan administration did not acknowledge a need for funds to combat this disease until May 1983.[37] After being relatively unresponsive, the government increased AIDS funding.

The reason behind the initial and subsequent government response was a perceived change in political support. The swine flu epidemic was expected to affect everyone. The media had made the public fearful of the recurrence of such an epidemic. The public demanded action, and legislators and the members of the administration competed with one another over who would be perceived as being more responsive.

The AIDS epidemic differed from swine flu in three important respects. First, there is no known cure for the disease. Second, a vaccine was not available and, therefore, other, more complex, policies had to be pursued. Third, and most important, AIDS differed from other contagious diseases with regard to the methods of transmission and the population groups affected. The first AIDs cases in the United States appeared about 1981; however, it was not reported in the mainstream media until about two years later.

The early victims of AIDS and those at high risk were believed to be homosexuals with multiple sexual partners and intravenous drug users, two groups considered by many as not deserving of sympathy and compassion. In fact, one political spokesperson suggested that AIDS was nature's revenge on homosexuality.[38] Members of the religious right, who were politically influential, were opposed to homosexuality and not inclined to offer political support for homosexuals' concerns. Those at high risk for the disease were unable to offer much political support of their own to legislators. It was only in those communities where high-risk groups were politically influential that treatment programs for AIDS victims were developed. In the early years the political appeal of legislating increased funding for AIDS patients was further limited by congress' calculation that few geographic areas would benefit, basically San Francisco and New York.

Three types of public policies are appropriate with regard to AIDS: funding for research to discover a cure and a vaccine against the disease, public education on methods to prevent the spread of the disease, and expenditures to pay for the care required by its generally impoverished victims. The publicity over AIDS occurred at a time when the federal government was attempting to reduce the budget deficit. The administration was reluctant to increase expenditures for a population group that offered little political support. Different constituencies were competing for portions of the federal budget; initial funding for AIDS, when it came, was achieved by reducing the allocations of other programs rather than by appropriating new dollars.

Public education to prevent the spread of the disease required public information on "safe" sex. Fundamentalist religious groups and social conservatives opposed government programs, such as the distribution of condoms and needle exchange programs (to intravenous drug users) on the grounds that such programs might seem to condon behavior that such groups opposed. Because of this political opposition, funding for such programs was limited.

The victims of AIDS often become impoverished once they contract the disease; the debilitating effects require them to give up their jobs, lose their work-related health insurance, use up their savings, and rely on Medicaid. Insurers attempted to limit their financial risk by requiring an AIDS test before selling health insurance to individuals and the self-employed. The financial burden of caring for AIDS victims has fallen on Medicaid and on hospitals providing uncompensated care.[39] These hospitals became advocates for increased funding for AIDS treatment.

Early public indifference to the plight of AIDs victims led gay activists to organize community efforts to assist AIDs victims and to mobilize broader public support for increased funding. One such group, the AIDS Coalition to Unleash Power (ACT UP) eventually became actively involved in formulating and changing many of the policy issues associated with AIDS, such as prevention and education programs, needle exchanges, treatment programs, government funding for research, and even the pricing of drugs for AIDS patients.[40]

The 1985 announcement by film star Rock Hudson that he contracted AIDs (and his subsequent death) increased public awareness of the disease. Adding to the change in the public's perception of AIDS was the story of a boy from Indiana, Ryan White, who had contracted AIDS via a blood transfusion and endured discrimination because of it. The publicity surrounding this case led to the Ryan White Act in 1990, which made treatment funds available, exceeding $2 billion in 2004. These new funds were designed to relieve the pressures placed on state Medicaid programs for their increased expenditures on HIV-related patients, although state Medicaid programs still account for the majority of funds spent on AIDS.[41]

It was only when people believed the disease would spread to the heterosexual middle class and all congressional districts would be affected that federal expenditures increased. For example, as the media increased its attention to the disease, public anxiety about the risk of acquiring it grew; there were unfounded fears about how AIDS was transmitted. Many believed sharing a drinking glass could transmit the disease. The general public became concerned for themselves. The result was special treatment for AIDS-related programs. Even though the death rate from AIDS is very small (4.9 per 100,000 population in 2002) relative to heart disease (241.7 per 100,000 population) and cancer (193.2 per 100,000 population), federal appropriations for AIDS research have grown much more rapidly.[42] New drugs for AIDS patients also receive an exception to the FDA's lengthy approval process, unlike comparable life-saving drugs for heart disease and cancer patients.

From its initial slow start, political support for AIDS programs and government expenditures has grown very rapidly. In addition to direct public expenditures for AIDS patients (Ryan White Act), indirect government expenditures on HIV-related care, such as Medicaid and Medicare expenditures on behalf of persons eligible for these programs, are substantial and outweigh direct expenditures. In 2004, total federal expenditures on HIV-related care exceeded $18 billion.[43]

AIDS was viewed as a social issue, not a public health problem. The early lack of legislative support reflected their constituent's concerns. The response would have been different if a broad constituency (the middle class) had been affected, if the disease had affected a wider geographical area of the country, if the victims had been viewed more sympathetically, if the disease were transmitted in a different manner, and if the preventive measures were not disturbing to politically influential population groups.

Environmental Protection

By the late 1960s the public had became increasingly concerned about environmental problems. "As a political issue, the country seemed unequivocally behind it. Local bond issues for environmental improvement passed handily. Much attention was given to environmental matters by the press. Congress responded by producing a wealth of legislative proposals for budgeting expenditures, for administrative reorganization, and for further regulation."[44]

As important an issue as the environment was, it did not change the congressional response or approach from what one would expect, based on the economic theory of regulation.

The federal government did not become engaged in pollution control until pollution became a visible public issue. Congress (and various administrations) did not act until several pollution crises occurred and the public became concerned about the environment. Although pollution was a health issue, it first had to become a political issue before Congress would respond.

Early federal efforts at pollution control (in 1899) were concerned with the dumping of debris in navigable waterways. The intent of the law, however, was to ensure navigable waterways rather than clean water.[45] Federal policies during the 1930s and 1940s mainly involved grants to the states for constructing waste-treatment facilities. These federal programs were also public works projects and were popular pork barrel legislation.[46]

Water pollution.

It was not until the mid-1960s that more serious efforts to control water pollution began. The Water Quality Act of 1965 stressed water-quality standards to be set by the states as well as increased federal funding for waste-treatment facilities. The states, however, were reluctant to set too stringent standards for fear of losing industry. When the Johnson administration attempted to create regional agencies to be responsible for pollution control, Congress was more "enthusiastic" about public works programs and "suspicious of regional approaches which might undermine the political base of senators and representatives . . . [and] was also reluctant to tamper with the state allocation formula contained in the existing act."[47]

The 1966 act contained a provision, inserted by a representative from the oil-producing state of Texas, which precluded any enforcement against oil pollution.[48] It was not until the oil tanker Torrey Canyon sank off the coast of England, which resulted in extensive oil pollution and media publicity, that Congress passed stronger oil pollution legislation. Further legislative refinements against oil polluters occurred as additional oil disasters received widespread media attention. In 1969, an oil rig off the coast of Santa Barbara suffered a "blowout," sending hundreds of thousands of gallons of oil onto the California beaches. The media attention lasted weeks, as did the oil spill. Congress was "forced" to act.

During this period, Rachel Carson's *Silent Spring* was published. The book pointed out the dangers of pesticides, raised the public's consciousness about pollution in the environment, and increased the public's desire to have Congress do something about the issue.

By 1970, pollution was so politically visible that President Nixon sent a special message on the environment to Congress, thereby raising the political stakes of environmental issues. In the 1972 presidential election, Senator Edmund Muskie, who was known for his environmental initiatives, was viewed as the front runner for the Democratic nomination. In April 1970, the first annual Earth Day was held, an indication of the public's interest and awareness of environmental issues. Further, studies began to be published that were critical of federal pollution control efforts. The pork barrel nature of water pollution control programs was criticized. The Nader group issued a report that was very critical of Senator Muskie's efforts. In response, Senator Muskie attempted to regain the initiative as the protector of the environment.[49]

When Congress finally passed a new water pollution bill in 1972, instead of embracing it, President Nixon vetoed it. Congress had appropriated federal expenditures greatly in excess of what the president had requested. Responding to the perceived support by their constituencies in an election year, Congress overrode the veto.[50] The main aspects of the 1972 Clean Water Act were the creation of standards in granting permits to individual dischargers and a greatly enlarged public works program to build municipal treatment plants.

The 1972 act, and subsequent amendments to that act, set unrealistic deadlines and guidelines. The EPA criticized the "ineffectiveness and unenforceability of its regulations."[51] Deadlines and goals came and went. Although the specification of too stringent standards and unrealistic deadlines may have demonstrated to the public that Congress was against pollution, they took an unrealistic approach. Given the complexity of the problem, pollution control has to be a continuing effort, unlikely to result in the total elimination of pollution in the short term. "In fact, the principal lessons to be learned from the experience of the 1970s are that the problems are far more difficult, will be with us far longer, and will require far more patience and continuous management than the [Congress] imagined."[52]

In addition to setting unworkable, rigid standards and deadlines, Congress also favored funding for waste-treatment plants. These expenditures have grown over time, and analysts consider them to be politically popular pork barrel programs for congressional districts all over the country. However, because municipal governments are the cause of approximately two-thirds of all water pollution, such large federal programs should have had some positive environmental effects. (Yet it is not clear that it is appropriate for the federal government to fund projects where the benefits and costs are so localized.)

As part of the 1972 Clean Water Act, states were required to establish water-quality standards and to conduct regular testing to see if the waterways met those standards. When waterways do not meet those standards, the states must determine how much pollution could be discharged and then implement policies designed to improve water quality. The approach the EPA currently uses for improving water quality is to award pollution permits to point sources, such as municipal and industrial dischargers. (Neither the states nor the EPA are required to control nonpoint sources of pollution.) The main approach for controlling pollution discharges is for the discharger to use EPA-prescribed technology. A 1997 Government Accounting Office report confirmed that EPA's technology-oriented approach discouraged dischargers from developing innovative approaches to achieve their pollution limits.[53]

An alternative approach to achieving specified water-quality standards would be for the EPA and the states to rely on a trading system for rights to pollute. Dischargers would be allowed to buy and sell pollution rights, and the total amount of pollution permitted would be set by the EPA and the states. Dischargers would then have the incentive to seek out and implement pollution-control mechanisms that are less costly than those mandated by the EPA. Further, dischargers would have an incentive to reduce their pollution below their permitted levels so they could sell their pollution rights. Under a pollution rights trading system, regulators would not have to be concerned with identifying and requiring specified technology but instead would concentrate on establishing water-quality standards and monitoring compliance.[54]

Air pollution.

Most pre–World War II legislation dealing with air pollution consisted of local laws against smoke. Enforcement of these laws varied greatly. The first real effort to control air pollution began in the late 1940s in Los Angeles when the public objected to odors from wartime plants and to eye-irritating smog. Then in 1951, automobile emissions were pinpointed as the major contributor to air pollution in Los Angeles. Other events increased the public's awareness of the dangers of air pollution. In 1948, for example, 6,000 people became ill from industrial smog in Domora, Pennsylvania. Fears about radioactivity arose from publicity on nuclear testing.[55]

Early federal legislation on air pollution (1955), called for a temporary program of research, training, and demonstrations.[56] Subsequent legislation was strengthened as little was done to control air pollution. Until the mid-1960s, these acts were generally believed to be "seriously defective."[57] Increased pressure was placed on Congress to act when in 1966 an air pollution problem in New York City "was estimated to have caused the death of eighty persons."[58] In the late 1960s and early 1970s, federal pollution legislation mandated deadlines to meet certain controls on automobile emissions. (The automobile industry, although against emission standards, was not strongly opposed to this federal legislation; the companies were concerned that it would be more costly to them if each state imposed its own standards on emissions. A federal standard was preferable to 50 different state standards.)[59]

Much credit is given to Senator Edmund Muskie for the stringent air pollution standards established in the 1970 legislation. These same sources, however, emphasize his presidential ambitions at that time and point out that he was sharply criticized for his performance in protecting the environment by a Ralph Nader organization.[60]

Again, the tough standards and deadlines established in the 1970 legislation were not met. The automobile industry and its union, the UAW, successfully lobbied Congress to weaken and delay the emissions standards.[61] The oil crisis in the early 1970s (when the oil-producing countries formed a cartel and sharply raised the price of oil) was an opportunity for industry groups to lobby for relaxation of the standards so as to conserve costly fuel oil. And in many cases, EPA did not have the staff or resources to monitor all the sources of air pollution. When large firms, such as the steel industry, were found not to be in compliance with air-quality standards, officials "were reluctant to force large industries with marginal profits to invest large sums in pollution control."[62]

Industrial self-interest.

Environmental regulation became an arena where firms and industries found it in their self-interest to form a coalition with "public interest" organizations to increase the industry's profits.[63] The following examples illustrate how firms have favored environmental regulations to increase their profits.

In 1988, Dupont, the world's largest producer of chlorofluorocarbons (CFCs), called for a complete global phase out of CFCs as an environmental threat. (CFCs were once the most widely used class of refrigerants, used in car air conditioners, refrigerators, aerosol can propellants, cleaning agents, and so on.) In the 1970s scientists determined that CFCs were contributing to a thinning of the earth's stratospheric ozone layer. In response to this concern, Congress banned the use of CFCs in aerosol cans in 1978, and the United Nations sponsored negotiations with the intention of banning CFCs to protect the ozone layer. As concern about CFCs increased, Dupont increased its research on possible substitutes. At the same time, foreign CFC producers were beginning to erode Dupont's market share. However, if there were a global phaseout of CFCs, consumers would have no alternative but to replace CFCs and CFC-reliant equipment with substitutes designed and patented by Dupont and other U.S. producers. Thus, the American CFC industry changed from an opponent of CFC phaseout when it was first proposed to a prime proponent of international limits on CFCs.[64]

When corporate average fuel economy (CAFE) standards were first enacted in the 1970s, they were designed so as to provide U.S. auto companies with a competitive advantage over foreign manufacturers. By basing the standards on the average fuel consumption of all of the cars produced by a manufacturer, the CAFE standards disadvantaged high-end foreign manufacturers, such as Mercedes-Benz, BMW, and Volvo. These manufacturers did not make many smaller cars with high fuel economy ratings, as did U.S. auto companies with their wide product lines. Congress explicitly rejected alternative approaches for reducing automobile fuel consumption that would not have restricted foreign auto imports.[65]

In the early 1990s, after a series of court decisions and regulatory actions to protect the Northern spotted owl, millions of federal acres of forest land and owl habitat in the Pacific Northwest were placed off limits to timber cutting. Weyerhaeuser Corporation employed wildlife biologists to search for owl habitat, but not on Weyerhaeuser's timberland. Although Weyerhaeuser was required to restrict logging on 320,000 acres to comply with federal regulations, a total of 5 million acres of timberland were taken off the market. The effect of such a large decrease in supply was that lumber prices soared and Weyerhaeuser's profits increased 80 percent over the previous year. Both the environmentalists and Weyerhaeuser were pleased with the efforts to protect the spotted owl.[66]

Clean Air Act.

The government has three alternative policy instruments to deal with air pollution. First, the government can require processes or standards that must be adopted to control pollution. Second, pollution taxes can be imposed on the polluters, and the funds collected can be used to clean up the pollution. Or third, the amount of pollution can be limited by awarding permits to pollute equal to the total amount of pollution permitted (and permit the sale and trade of these marketable permits).[67] Each of these approaches has redistributive effects—there are winners and losers.

A tradable emissions-permit system would work as follows: the government would establish an overall limit or quantity of pollution for each geographic area. The total amount of pollution defines the total number of emission permits to be issued and these emission permits may be traded within these geographic markets. A very important decision is determining how the permits will be distributed. Should they be awarded to the existing producers of pollution? Should they be awarded free or for payment? Should the government auction the permits to anyone (existing polluters, new firms, or even environmentalists can bid for them) and use the funds to clean up the pollution? And for how long should the permits be good? One year? five years? Longer? Each of these choices for allocating tradable permits will result in wealth transfers.

Both taxes and marketable permits offer incentives to reduce pollution, as the polluter can save money by reducing pollution. The polluter also has an incentive to search for the least costly method to reduce pollution. Mandating certain technology to reduce pollution offers neither of these incentives.

According to the public interest theory, the least costly policy instrument should be adopted to ensure that the (marginal) cost of decreasing pollution is equal to the (marginal) cost incurred by pollution.

According to the economic theory, the pollution-control policies adopted are unlikely to be the least costly approaches. Instead, they will reflect the political support offered by those groups having a concentrated interest in the outcome.

The 1977 Amendments to the Clean Air Act is a classic example of how interest-group politics designed air pollution policy so as to benefit polluting high-sulfur coal firms and their unionized employees, while imposing unnecessary costs on population groups in other parts of the country.

In the fall of 1973, OPEC raised the price of oil dramatically. Many electric utilities that had previously used oil switched to coal. Environmentalists were concerned that the switch to coal would increase the amount of sulfur oxides in the air and worsen air quality. The region that would suffer the most in terms of deterioration of air quality would be the Midwest, which is more industrialized and more heavily populated.[68]

Coal produced in the United States varies in sulfur content according to its origin. Western coal is low in sulfur and cheaper to mine, and is therefore a competitive threat to Eastern coal interests.

When Congress looked for an environmental policy that would reduce the amount of sulfur discharged into the air as utilities increased their use of coal, it was faced with a series of options. The simplest approach at that time would have been for Congress to set a pollution tax (or a limit) on the amount of sulfur oxide emissions produced by electric utilities. This requirement would have left it up to the utilities to determine how they might best meet that limit (or the cheapest method of paying the emissions tax). However, the approach that is most efficient and best for air quality is not necessarily good politics. And politics always takes precedence.

Faced with a limit on the amount of sulfur emissions, utilities would be expected to achieve that limit in the least costly manner. Given the lower cost and lower sulfur content of western coal, Midwestern and Eastern utilities would find it profitable to pay higher transportation charges and increase their purchases of Western coal. Such a market response would have had adverse consequences on the owners and employees of Midwestern and Eastern coal mines. Eastern coal mines are heavily unionized by the United Mine Workers, while Western mines are not. It was estimated that between 10,000 and 20,000 jobs would have been lost. Joining with the coal producers, the United Mine Workers lobbied the Carter administration to use a different approach for reducing sulfur emissions. The Carter administration was also interested in saving jobs in the Midwest and in Appalachia (Robert Byrd, the Senate Majority Leader was from West Virginia).[69]

The approach Congress selected was to emphasize the process of meeting the air-quality goal rather than the desired outcome. Congress mandated specific technology be used. Only newly constructed coal-fired electric plants, whether or not the plant burned dirty coal, had to install and use expensive "scrubbers." As long as the mandated technology was used, any type of coal could be burned.

The effect of mandating scrubbers was to decrease the incentive to use low-sulfur Western coal. Why should a utility pay higher transport cost for low-sulfur coal when they would have to install scrubbers anyway? The utility's incentive is to seek out the cheapest coal, even though it may have the highest sulfur content.

The effect of the congressional approach toward improving air quality likely had the opposite effect.

> EPA accepted evidence that scrubbers can remove as much as 90 percent of (Sulfur Oxides) from stack gases when operating efficiently, but it ignored the fact that it has neither the technology nor the resources to assure compliance with the (Sulfur Oxides) emissions limits. . . . Stack-gas scrubbers require enormous amounts of maintenance, which utilities are unlikely to provide in a diligent manner if environmental authorities do not monitor their results carefully. . . . [A] scrubber failure can lead to enormous increases in emissions. The burning of low-sulfur coal carries no such risks. Therefore, it is possible that full . . . scrubbing increases cost and emissions concurrently—hardly the result an environmental policy maker would wish.[70]

Earlier, in 1971, different air-quality standards had been set for existing and new sources of air pollution. If existing sources of air pollution, primarily electric utilities, had had to meet tighter air-quality standards, they would have passed on these higher costs to the public in the form of higher utility rates. Legislators from the heavily industrialized Midwest, whose utilities emit much of the pollution that returns to earth as acid rain, were concerned that their utilities would bear the economic burden of reducing air pollution. The utility customers would then have become upset with Congress over their higher utility bills. Further, the environmentalists' concern was to ensure that air quality did not deteriorate. To resolve both of these concerns, Congress exempted existing sources of air pollution and imposed the technology requirements *only* on new sources of air pollution.

The policy of applying more stringent requirements on new sources and mandating the use of scrubbers was harder on the Western and Southwestern regions of the country. Because population was growing more rapidly in these regions, these regions were more likely to be required to use scrubbers. Further, even though these regions had vast amounts of low-sulfur coal, and they could meet the air-quality standard in a less costly manner, all new sources of pollution had to use scrubbers.

Had flexibility in reducing pollution from acid rain been incorporated into the 1977 Clean Air Act, less costly methods would have been adopted. However, by forcing the use of scrubbers, absurd situations occurred. In the West where low-sulfur coal is used, engineers had to actually add sulfur to the scrubber to make it work.[71]

A flexible approach to reducing air pollution was, however unlikely, ". . . because the congressional committee that dominates the EPA's acid rain agenda is dominated by coal, the EPA's own acid rain approach tends to be dominated by coal. . . ."[72]

Higher utility bills and loss of jobs in the coal industry determined the approach used for reducing air pollution from high-sulfur coal.

Applying the more expensive technology only to new pollution sources also provided utilities with an incentive to postpone replacing their high-pollution plants. "In short, the new rule does very little to improve air quality in those areas that have the biggest problems while imposing very large emissions-reduction burdens upon the growing Western and Southwestern portions of the country."[73]

In 1990, Congress amended the Clean Air Act. By the late 1980s the political conditions for more stringent clean air legislation had improved. Acid rain was a greater environmental and political issue because of growing pressure from environmental groups, Northeastern states, and Canada, whose lakes, trees, and property was also being adversely affected. Further, by the end of the1980s it was determined that two-thirds of the pollution causing acid rain emitted by power plants was emitted by power plants constructed before 1970.[74]

During the 1980s, the utility and mining interests in the Midwestern and Appalachian states that produce high-sulfur coal successfully blocked any new meaningful environmental controls on acid rain. These concentrated interests were supported by two key legislative allies: Representative John Dingell (D-MI), who was chairman of the House Energy and Commerce committee, was protective of the automobile industry and concerned that any new legislation would tighten auto emission standards; Senator Robert Byrd (D-WV), the majority leader in the Senate, represented a state that produced a high amount of sulfur dioxide and would have been a big loser under any tighter air pollution standards. Western and Northeastern states opposed more stringent scrubber requirements. Thus, there was an impasse over new air pollution laws.

By the late 1980s conditions for clean air legislation changed. The environmental movement grew stronger politically, President Bush was elected and, in contrast to President Reagan, was a strong proponent of improvements in the Clean Air Act. More importantly, control over key congressional leadership positions changed as George Mitchell (D-Maine), who was a strong proponent of more stringent controls on acid rain, became the Senate majority leader. The states favoring clean air, and their representatives, were able to break the legislative impasse.

The 1990 Clean Air Act amendments included an innovative market-based approach, in which tradable permits for sulfur dioxide emissions were provided to electric utilities to reduce acid rain. The act also placed new controls on auto emissions and mandated that the use of an alternative fuel, ethanol, be increased. Ethanol, which is made from corn, is a more costly fuel than gasoline. However, if the EPA forces refineries to produce ethanol, farmers and distillers benefit, even though it increases the price of gasoline by 20 cents a gallon. The ethanol proponents (supported by Senator Robert Dole, the Senate's minority leader at the time) were the Archer Daniels Midland Co. (the largest domestic producer of ethanol), the National Corn Growers Association, environmentalists, and other alternative fuel interests. Although the legislation was opposed by the oil and auto industries, the EPA created a vast new market for ethanol.[75]

To understand these regulatory strategies for reducing air pollution, one must know which groups have a concentrated interest in the outcome rather than simply assuming that the most cost-effective approach for reducing air pollution will be adopted (the public interest theory). Given the great deal of money at stake in reducing air pollution, the EPA became a focal point for lobbyists; each interest group attempted to minimize its costs while penalizing its competitors. Existing firms in an industry seek to increase their competitor's costs, thereby gaining a competitive advantage; similarly, they try to have legislators impose pollution standards that are advantageous to old sources of production and thereby inhibit entry by new competitors.

In designing environmental regulations, congressional environmental politics tries to maximize political support by benefiting an entire industry or a subset of firms within the industry as well as environmentalists. For this reason, environmental policy is achieved by less efficient means, such as technology mandates, rather than by providing incentives for the private sector to improve the environment. Environmental policy is designed to transfer wealth to those industry segments that can provide political support.[76]

Concluding Comments

When externalities exist, such as in the case of medical research, epidemics, and pollution, it is an appropriate function of government to implement policy to match the costs and benefits in each of these areas. The public interest is served when external costs and benefits are included in the private decision-making process that determines the level of production. Not all externalities must necessarily be undertaken by the federal government. The geographic scope of the problem should determine the level of jurisdiction. Municipalities should be responsible for local pollution problems. When problems cross state boundaries, regional agencies, established by state coordination, may be the appropriate agency. Other types of problems require federal intervention.

The brief description provided of federal intervention in the issues discussed above suggests the following: Congress, when considering the benefits and costs of its actions, may at times find it in its self-interest to act in the public interest. However, Congress is unlikely to act in the public interest when there are no net gains from doing so. (Legislators could be spending their time on other activities or legislation that would provide them with greater political support.) Congress will act only when an issue gains high visibility, and the public is perceived as wanting Congress to act. The type of action, however, will depend on the strength of the opposition by concentrated interests to Congress' actions.

In the case of funding medical research, there was no opposition. Congress could not spend enough on this popular issue. (Congress bore no costs and saw large potential benefits to itself.) In doing so, Congress became very directive on how those funds were to be spent, so as to maximize public awareness of their actions. Congress also appropriated too much, more than could have been well spent, as evidenced by an agency's return of research funds to the Treasury.

With respect to a possible swine flu epidemic, no political leader would have chosen to save money at the possible expense of losing lives, no matter how remote that possibility might be. This strategy makes sense in terms of a legislator's costs and benefits. The cost is the government's money, and the benefit is the legislator's political future.

The lack of an initial federal response to the AIDS epidemic was a result of the lack of political support by those at greatest risk for contracting the disease. Once the middle class became concerned that they were also at risk, and the geographic areas affected expanded beyond New York and San Francisco, the political support materialized for legislators and the administration to take greater action. The preferences of politically important population groups, however, affected the types of prevention and educational programs. Government support for AIDS programs, such as AIDS research and treatment expenditures and fast-tracking AIDS-related drugs for FDA approval, has increased sharply. A well-organized AIDS lobby group has been very politically effective.

Eliminating pollution is politically attractive. Public awareness is very high and opinion polls indicate that public concern is also very high. Initially, environmental groups were established to lobby the federal government to protect and enlarge wilderness areas and parks. The constituency of environmental groups—largely middle class—grew during the 1960s and 1970s when concern over air and water pollution increased. By placing restrictions on "growth," however, environmental groups favored the status quo; limits on industrial growth favor the "haves" over the "have-nots." Labor unions, therefore, have been major opponents of environmental restrictions on industry. Racial minorities considered environmental issues a luxury and not relevant to their constituency.[77] By regulating growth, environmentalists preserve their quality of life as well as their relative wealth.

The political influence of environmental groups is also indicated by the large number of interest groups (approximately 5,000) that are concerned with protecting the environment in their local areas. These groups are active in lobbying for a cleaner environment, bringing lawsuits against the EPA to ensure that it enforces strict compliance standards, publicizing legislators' votes on environmental issues, and endorsing candidates at election time. Politicians compete with one another to show the public who is most concerned over the environment.

The most popular response by Congress to these issues has been to appropriate funds for municipal waste-treatment plants. Legislators can thereby be pro-environment, as well as provide projects for their home districts. There is no opposition to this approach. In fact, various associations of mayors, cities, and counties actively lobby for such funds. This is the ideal environmental policy for legislators.

When it comes to air pollution, however, it is difficult for Congress to find a comparable response. Costs must be imposed on business, and ultimately on consumers, if air pollution is to be reduced. Congress is thus forced to make choices. One person's pollution is another person's job. Initially, Congress preferred to delay or even pass symbolic legislation, which is effective when the public has little information. With a pollution crisis, there is a great deal of media attention, and Congress cannot delay any longer. To demonstrate concern for the public and because of pressure by environmental groups, Congress establishes strict and unrealistic deadlines to achieve environmental goals. The short-term political benefits to Congress of this aggressive action in time of crisis are high. Once the crisis and media attention have passed, Congress can gain greater political support from companies and unions by delaying deadlines and requirements that may adversely affect company profits and jobs.

A large industry with many employees will often use the excuse of loss of jobs in an area if the EPA, the governmental agency responsible for carrying out congressional environmental mandates, forces them to undertake heavy expenditures. This occurred with the steel and automobile industries. Compromises are then worked out between the industry and the EPA. Often the penalties for noncompliance are so severe they cannot be imposed, for example, stopping Chrysler Corporation's auto production.[78]

The experience of one EPA administrator, Anne Burford, and one of her deputies, Rita Lavelle, administrator of the Superfund (to clean up toxic wastes), is instructive. The large degree of discretion permitted by the EPA in administering environmental guidelines led to a public scandal. The EPA was more concerned with minimizing the consequences of its guidelines on industry than in carrying out its mandate. Protection of the environment was an important value held by the public. The loss of public support on a popular issue became too great a political liability for the Reagan administration to bear. The two administrators were fired.

Economists focus on the use of taxes, emission fees, and marketable pollution credits to limit air pollution. Legislators and regulators have generally favored process measures, such as mandating the use of specific technology and differential standards for new and old firms. The reason for these inefficient approaches and differential treatment is to benefit existing firms over new competitors. Restrictions on the total amount of pollution inhibit entry by new firms and prevent increases in output by existing firms, thereby enabling firms to raise their prices; the consequence is the same as when firms form cartels. Industry also favors environmental regulations that require its competitors to meet more costly standards. The use of catalytic converters to control auto emissions, the method chosen by U.S. automobile companies, is a high-cost method that reduces gas mileage and adds equipment to the car. Converters can be, and are, easily tampered with. These pollution-control requirements were more costly for foreign-made cars thereby provided a competitive cost advantage to U.S. automakers.[79] In another example, requiring scrubbers, rather than direct limits on sulfur oxide emissions, imposed large costs on Western utilities, while protecting Midwestern and Eastern coal mines and workers from their competitors—low-sulfur Western coal producers. New sources of pollution are subject to greater pollution costs than existing sources, thereby providing a competitive cost advantage to existing firms.

Some legislators, such as Senator Muskie in the 1960s, were able to anticipate the public's interest in the environment. However, little meaningful legislation was able to pass Congress at that time. Only when the public's awareness was heightened by a series of crises and by media attention did Congress respond. The initial response was to spend federal dollars. There is no reason, other than political, why municipalities should not have been required to spend their own funds to clean up their own wastes. However, members of Congress were able to provide a benefit to their districts without having to be accountable for the costs.

Although environmentalists are interested in the broader principle of improved air quality, it is with respect to the details of the regulations that the affected industry uses to provide itself with a competitive advantage. When Congress perceived political support from the public by imposing more stringent pollution standards, it chose inefficient methods (specifying equipment), rather than establishing effluent charges. By lessening the impact on existing firms, and even exempting these firms from the regulations, Congress was able to satisfy the environmentalists while providing benefits to a politically important industry.

The benefits of improvements in air quality could be achieved at lower cost if greater flexibility were permitted in achieving specified targets. However, public policy to resolve problems concerning externalities is unlikely to adopt the most efficient solution as long as the costs and benefits of the decision makers are different from the costs and benefits required for an efficient solution.

Study Questions

1. Explain why an "externality" can be used to justify government intervention in the marketplace.

2. Explain how congressional funding for medical research accommo-dated both producer interests and the public's political support for such funding.

3. Contrast the political response to the swine flu epidemic with the response to the AIDS epidemic.

4. Using the public interest and economic theory, provide separate explanations for the congressional approach of mandating "scrub-bers" to reduce air pollution.

5. Explain why legislation promotes the use of "process" measures to reduce air pollution rather than more efficient mechanisms, such as the use of emission taxes or marketable pollution credits, which allow industry to have greater flexibility in achieving pollution goals.

Notes

1. Taxes and subsidies are not the only approach that can be used to deal with externalities. For example, the government may sell rights to produce pollution once the appropriate level of pollution is determined. Government regulations that every child attending school be vaccinated do not require taxes or subsidies to achieve the efficient number of vaccinations.

2. Richard H. Shryock, *American Medical Research* (New York: Commonwealth Fund, 1947), 99.

3. Ibid., 111.

4. Ibid., 111.

5. Ibid., 44.

6. Edward J. Burger, Jr., *Science at the White House* (Baltimore, MD: The Johns Hopkins University Press, 1980), 21.

7. Stephen P. Strickland, *Politics, Science, and Dread Disease* (Cambridge, MA: Harvard University Press, 1972), 34.

8. Ibid., 54.

9. Senator Hill also coauthored the Hill-Burton Act. This popular leg-islation provided federal support for hospital construction based on a formula that gave each state a share of the funds. Thus, this legis-lation had all the ingredients of a successful bill; senators and repre-sentatives could all show what they did for their constituents.

10. Ibid., 79.

11. Congressional subcommittees were the main determinant of legisla-tion and the level of appropriations. When there was unanimity among subcommittee members, the subcommittee's recommenda-tions were generally accepted by the full committee and subse-quently by the House itself. The bipartisan approach to medical

research led to unanimous recommendations by the subcommittee; thus, these subcommittees had a great deal of power.

12. Stephen P. Strickland, "Medical Research: Public Policy and Power Politics," in *Politics of Health*, eds. Douglass Cater and Philip R. Lee (New York: MEDCOM Press, 1972), 75.

13. Stephen P. Strickland, *Research and the Health of Americans* (Lexington, MA: Lexington Books, 1978), 17.

14. Ibid.

15. Strickland, "Medical Research," 126.

16. Ibid., 127.

17. Under the able leadership of Dr. Shannon, the NIH continued its basic research while following the guidelines set down by the congressional subcommittees.

18. Strickland, "Medical Research," 192.

19. Ibid., 170.

20. Ibid., 249.

21. Paul J. Feldstein, *Health Care Economics*, 6th ed. (Albany, NY: Delmar Publishers Inc., 2004), 345.

22. Strickland, "Medical Research," 95.

23. Peter Temin, *Taking Your Medicine: Drug Regulation in the United States* (Cambridge, MA: Harvard University Press, 1980), 27–31.

24. The Pure Food Act also presented an opportunity for firms to use it to gain a competitive advantage over their rivals. For example, the dairy industry was able to restrict the sale of oleomargarine. Ibid., 30.

25. William M. Wardell, "The History of Drug Discovery, Development, and Regulation," in *Issues in Pharmaceutical Economics*, ed. Robert Chien, (Lexington, MA: Lexington Books, 1979), 8.

26. A history of the 1962 FDA amendments is found in Richard Harris, *The Real Voice* (New York: Macmillan Company, 1964).

27. William M. Wardell and Louis Lasagna, *Regulation and Drug Development* (Washington, DC: American Enterprise Institute, 1975), 1.

28. Joseph A. DiMasi, Ronald Hansen, and Henry Grabowski, "The Price of Innovation: New Estimates of Drug Development Costs," *Journal of Health Economics* 22, no. 2 (2003): 151–85.

29. William M. Wardell, "The Impact of Regulation on New Drug Development," in *Issues in Pharmaceutical Economics*, ed. Chien, 147.

30. Sam Peltzman, *Regulation of Pharmaceutical Innovation* (Washington, DC: American Enterprise Institute, 1974).

31. For additional discussion on the FDA's approval process, its consequences, and drug firm profitability, see Paul J. Feldstein, *Health*

Policy Issues: An Economic Perspective (Chicago: Health Administration Press, 2003), chapter 24.

32. The following account of the 1976 swine flu episode is based on Arthur M. Silverstein, *Pure Politics and Impure Science* (Baltimore, MD: The Johns Hopkins University Press, 1981). The author is a professor of Ophthalmic Immunology at The Johns Hopkins University School of Medicine. The book was based on the author's year as a congressional science fellow on the staff of Senator Kennedy's Senate Health Subcommittee at the time of the swine flu episode. In the preface to his book, the author states, "I was quickly disabused of the notion that this was a question [swine flu] on which Science would triumph. As the months passed and Congress dealt with the swine flu issue in its various forms, it soon became apparent that the course of events was being decided more by political and occasionally economic considerations than by scientific ones. For the first time, I witnessed in great detail the sometimes subtle, sometimes not so subtle, influences that affect the course of events in government. The swine flu issue brought into play the frictions that exist between a Republican presidency and a Democratic Congress, the frictions and differences of style between the Senate and the House of Representatives, and the frictions between congressional committees vying to protect their own jurisdictional rights. Finally and not least, there were the political consequences of all of this happening in a Presidential election year."

33. Arthur J. Viseltear, "A Short Political History of the 1976 Swine Influenza Legislation," in *Influenza in America 1918–1976*, ed. June E. Osborn (New York: PRODIST, 1977), 49.

34. Silverstein, *Pure Politics and Impure Science*, 67.

35. Ibid., 102.

36. After President Carter took office, Health, Education, and Welfare Secretary Califano asked two distinguished scholars to conduct a study to determine what went wrong. Richard E. Neustadt and Harvey Fineberg, *The Epidemic That Never Was* (New York: Vintage Books, 1983).

37. Randy Shilts, *And the Band Played On: Politics, People, and the AIDs Epidemic*, (New York: St. Martin's Press, 1987).

38. Patrick Buchanan, "AIDS Disease: It's Nature Striking Back," *New York Post*, May 24, 1983.

39. John K. Iglehart, "Financing the Struggle Against AIDS," *New England Journal of Medicine* 317 (1987): 183.

40. Patricia D. Siplon, *AIDS and the Policy Struggle in the United States* (Washington, DC: Georgetown University Press, 2002).

41. Institute of Medicine, *Measuring What Matters: Allocation, Planning, and Quality Assessment for the Ryan White CARE Act* (Washington, DC: National Academies Press, 2004).

42. National Center for Health Statistics, 2005, http://www.cdc.gov/nchs/data/nvsr/nvsr53/nvsr53_05.pdf.

43. Marty McGeein, "Issues in HIV/AIDS Policy," Office of the Assistant Secretary for Planning and Evaluation, U.S. Department of Health and Human Services, (mimeograph), January 12, 2005. See also, Jeffrey Levi, "The Evolution of National Funding Policies for HIV Prevention and Treatment," in *Dawning Answers: How the HIV/AIDS Epidemic Has Helped Strengthen Public Health*, ed. Ronald O. Valdiserri (New York: Oxford University Press, 2003), 118–134, Table 6-1.

44. Burger, *Science at the White House*, 75.

45. J. Clarence Davies and Barbara S. Davies, *The Politics of Pollution*, 2nd ed. (Indianapolis, IN: Pegasus, 1975), 27.

46. Kenneth J. Meier, *Regulation: Politics, Bureaucracy, and Economics* (New York: St. Martin's Press, 1985), 142.

47. Davies and Davies, *The Politics of Pollution*, 35.

48. Ibid., 36.

49. Meier, *Regulation: Politics, Bureaucracy, and Economics*, 144.

50. Davies and Davies, *The Politics of Pollution*, 40–43. President Nixon proposed $1 billion for each of four years; the cost of the congressional bill was $24 billion over three years.

51. Larry E. Ruff, "Federal Environmental Regulation," in *Case Studies in Regulation: Revolution and Reform*, eds. Leonard W. Weiss and Michael W. Klass (Boston: Little, Brown and Company, 1981), 235–61.

52. Ibid., 259.

53. *Challenges Facing EPA's Efforts to Reinvent Environmental Regulations*, GAO/RCED-97-155 (Washington, DC: Government Printing Office, 1997).

54. Kurt Stephenson and Leonard Shabman, "The Trouble With Implementing TMDLs," *Regulation*, Spring 2001, 28–32.

55. Davies and Davies, *The Politics of Pollution*, 19.

56. Burger, *Science at the White House*, 86.

57. Ruff, "Federal Environmental Regulation," 240.

58. Davies and Davies, *The Politics of Pollution*, 49.

59. Ibid., 48.

60. Ibid., 54–6.

61. Meier, *Regulation: Politics, Bureaucracy, and Economics*, 149–50. When GM faced a $386 million government fine for failing to meet

federal fuel economy standards on its 1987 and 1988 model cars, GM threatened to close some plants and lay off workers if the Department of Transportation (DOT) did not ease its standards. The DOT received 12,000 letters from GM workers, dealers, and shareholders, as well as 100 letters from representatives in support of GM's position. The rules were relaxed by DOT because, as they explained, they did not want to be accused of causing the loss of tens of thousands of jobs and worsening the trade deficit as more auto production is shifted overseas. *The Wall Street Journal*, October 2, 1986, 56.

62. Meier, *Regulation: Politics, Bureaucracy, and Economics*, 153.

63. An industry's profits can be increased by regulations that restrict the output of its industry (thereby resulting in an increase in price) by causing an increase in their competitor's costs, thereby gaining a competitive advantage, and by entry-inhibiting standards that are advantageous to old sources of production.

64. Jonathan Adler, "Rent Seeking Behind the Green Curtain," *Regulation* 19, no. 4 (1996): 26–34.

65. Ibid.

66. Bruce Yandle, "Bootleggers and Baptists in Retrospect," *Regulation* 22, no. 3 (1999): 5–7.

67. Georges A. Tanguay, Paul Lanoie, and Jerome Moreau, "Environmental Policy, Public Interest, and Political Market," *Public Choice* 120 (2004): 1–27; and Gebhard Kirschgassner and Friedrich Schneider, "On the Political Economy of Environmental Policy," *Public Choice* 115 (2003): 369–96.

68. This discussion is based on Robert W. Crandall, "Air Pollution, Environmentalists, and the Coal Lobby," in *The Political Economy of Deregulation*, eds. Roger G. Noll and Bruce M. Owen (Washington, DC: American Enterprise Institute, 1983), 84–96. See also, Bruce A. Ackerman and William T. Hassler, *Clean Coal/Dirty Air: Or How the Clean Air Act Became a Multibillion-Dollar Bail-Out for High Sulfur Coal Producers and What Should Be Done About It* (New Haven, CT: Yale University Press, 1981).

69. Ibid., 87.

70. Ibid., 91–2.

71. C. Boyden Gray, *The Fettered Presidency: Legal Constraints on the Executive Branch* (Washington, DC: American Enterprise Institute, 1988).

72. Ibid, 216.

73. Crandall, "Air Pollution, Environmentalists and the Coal Lobby," 93.

74. Paul L. Joskow and Richard Schmalensee, "The Political Economy of Market-Based Environmental Policy: The U.S. Acid Rain Program," *Journal of Law and Economics* 41 (1998): 37–81.

75. Fred L. Smith, Jr., "Markets and the Environment: A Critical Reappraisal," *Contempory Economic Policy* 13, no. 1 (1995): 62–73. See also the following articles in the same issue, W. Michael Hanemann, "Improving Environmental Policy: Are Markets the Solution?", 74–9, and Robert W. Crandall, "Is There Progress in Environmental Policy?", 80–3.

76. For a discussion of using market mechanisms, such as trading pollution allowances to control acid rain, rather using than traditional command-and-control approaches to reduce sulfur dioxide emissions, see A. Denny Ellerman, Paul L. Joskow, Richard Schmalensee, Juan-Pablo Montero, and Elizabeth M. Bailey, *Markets for Clean Air: The U.S. Acid Rain Program* (Cambridge, MA: Cambridge University Press, 2000).

77. Rochelle L. Stanfield, "Environmental Focus," *National Journal*, January 31, 1987, 292. Further, through the use of zoning restrictions to "protect nature," environmental concerns were also used by the middle- and high-income groups to limit growth in their surrounding areas, thereby increasing its value.

78. Ibid., 207. "Former EPA Administrator Ruckelshaus, when he announced his decision on the 1975 auto standards, stated, 'The issue of good faith as it relates to Chrysler Corporation has been particularly troublesome for me in these proceedings. . . . If Congress provided me with some sanctions short of the nuclear deterrent of in effect closing down that major corporation, my finding on good faith may have been otherwise.' Solutions to this problem, such as a tax on emissions, are possible, but the industry is undoubtedly happier with an unrealistic 'nuclear deterrent.'"

79. Meier, *Regulation: Politics, Bureaucracy, and Economics*, 150.

REDISTRIBUTIVE PROGRAMS

After completing this chapter, the reader should be able to

- contrast the two types of broad redistributive programs using the economic theory of regulation,
- explain why "in-kind" redistributive programs are used instead of cash,
- evaluate the effectiveness of medical school subsidies for low-income students,
- describe how the "pay-as-you-go" financing method of Social Security works,
- contrast Society Security's financing by a payroll tax that is a flat percentage of earning up to a maximum wage base to one where no maximum wage base exists, and
- name reasons why the aged are considered politically powerful.

Medicare and Medicaid were broad redistributive programs. The intended beneficiaries were population groups: the aged (Medicare) and the poor (Medicaid). Although health providers also benefited from these programs, Medicare and Medicaid were clearly different from producer-type regulations (which are also redistributive). Medicare and Medicaid were "visible" forms of redistribution, the legislative debates were publicized, and the intended beneficiaries were specific population groups.

Examples of broad redistributive programs outside the health field are welfare, Social Security, food stamps, farm subsidies, and subsidized higher education. To understand the development of Medicare and Medicaid, as well as these other broad redistributive programs, it is necessary to view such programs within the context of the economic theory of legislation.

The underlying assumptions of the self-interest paradigm are that individuals and groups, as well as legislators, act according to their self-interests and that legislation is a means of transferring wealth to those with political power from those without. Such a theory is more readily understood when it is applied to producer-type legislation. The previous chapter applied the theory to explain the legislative response in the face of externalities. Another generally acknowledged function of government is an explicit redistribution of wealth, for instance, to the poor. In this chapter, the self-interest paradigm provides an explanation as to why Congress passes broad redistributive legislation and how that legislation is designed.

Chapter 9 uses the concepts developed in this chapter to explore why Medicare and Medicaid were enacted. Why were two redistributive health programs legislated rather than one? Why were these programs structured so that rapid increases in medical prices were inevitable? Why are the solutions to the current financial problems of these two programs likely to be less equitable and less efficient than need be? *In fact, why was the original Medicare program deliberately designed to be inequitable and inefficient?*

The equity of a program is defined by those who receive the benefits and those who bear the costs. In nonredistributive programs, such as city garbage collection, the government provides a service in return for a user fee. Those who receive the benefits also pay the cost. No explicit redistribution of wealth occurs, nor is it intended.[1] With explicit redistributive programs, however, beneficiaries (presumably those with lower incomes) are expected to receive benefits in excess of their costs, that is, the taxes they pay to finance those programs. The "losers" under redistribution programs are expected to be those with higher incomes; the taxes they pay to support such programs are expected to be greater than the benefits they receive. The public interest theory would predict that explicit redistribution would be from higher-income groups to lower-income groups. A self-interest analysis of such policies hypothesizes that redistribution will be toward those who are able to provide political support, regardless of their "need" for wealth transfers. In the latter case, the redistribution is likely to be inequitable; lower-income groups are likely to bear costs in excess of their benefits.

The public interest theory would also predict that the distribution of services from redistributive programs would be provided in an efficient manner. Efficiency is defined in terms of the cost for producing a given level of output or service. A more efficient program will be able to achieve a greater output for the same cost than an inefficient program. Price-competitive markets, with their incentives for both purchasers and suppliers, are the yardstick for achieving efficient market outcomes.

A Theory of Broad Redistributive Programs

Broad redistributive programs can be classified into two types: charitable and universal. Beneficiaries of charity (or welfare) programs are people with low incomes. Universal programs do not use income as a basis for determining beneficiary status. Universal programs either provide benefits to everyone or to a particular class, such as to all the aged. Because the motivations underlying these two types of programs differ, it is important to be able to distinguish between them.

Charitable redistributive programs are specifically designed to assist the poor. Program eligibility is based on income, and program financing comes from general taxes. According to these criteria, the program's benefits go to those with low incomes. The costs of these programs are borne by those with higher incomes who carry the tax burden. Charitable programs redistribute income from those with higher incomes to those with lower incomes.

Universal programs, on the other hand, do not require an income-related means test for eligibility for the program's benefits. Instead, everyone in the appropriate category is eligible, regardless of income. The financing of universal programs often, although not always, comes from excise taxes that are applied to all, regardless of income (for example, a payroll tax, which is an excise tax on labor).

Charitable Redistributive Programs

Charitable programs are based on the public's desire to help the less fortunate members of society. Although some individuals contribute to private charities (or organizations whose goals they share), taxes can also be used to provide for charity. In fact, some persons may prefer that the government be the mechanism to provide the charity because everyone would contribute (according to the taxes they pay). Otherwise, if only some persons donate to private charity, others who benefit from seeing the poor cared for do so without having to contribute. They have a "free ride." Having the government provide the charity is a way of overcoming this free rider problem.[2]

The poor are typically not able to offer a great deal of political support to legislators. Therefore, the political support for welfare programs must come from other groups, those with middle and high incomes who finance welfare programs through their tax payments. Middle- and high-income groups are also politically more powerful than the poor: they are more numerous and more likely to vote, and they provide campaign contributions and volunteer their time. Unless the middle- and high-income groups favor the welfare programs, they are unwilling to support them. They are the ones whose political demands for welfare must be listened to by Congress.[3]

If the only objective of charity programs was to improve the condition of the poor, then the most efficient way to do so would be to provide the poor with cash.[4] Instead, most of the benefits provided to the poor are for specific services (referred to as "in-kind benefits"), such as food stamps, housing, medical care, and so on. If the poor could have the cash equivalent of the in-kind benefits, they would be better off. They could spend the cash on those goods and services they believe they need most.

Welfare programs, however, are designed not just to aid the poor, but, perhaps more important, to match the preferences of the two powerful groups supporting welfare legislation. Welfare programs must accommodate both the donors' (middle- and high-income groups) and producers' desires rather than those of the poor. For this reason, welfare programs provide specific services rather than cash.

The middle class may prefer to provide in-kind subsidies because they may distrust the ability of the poor to make the "right" choices. The donors may favor subsidies to the poor only if the poor buy those services that the donors believe they need.

Welfare programs are often provided under conditions that differentiate these programs from those that the rest of society is able to purchase. It is unlikely that the middle class, particularly the lower-middle class (the working near-poor), would favor providing services to the poor that are more generous than they themselves could afford. And, if the same services are provided to the poor, then those services should be provided in a differentiated manner. After all, the recipients of charity should not fare better than the donors. For this reason, means-tested programs have, in the past, been administered using obvious and embarrassing methods. Requiring persons on welfare to work is also based on donor preferences.[5]

The second group that promotes subsidies to the poor are those industries that would benefit from an increase in demand by the poor. Producers, whether in agriculture or in medical care, have a concentrated interest in increasing the demand for their industry's output. Whether originated by the industry or by those with a redistributive motive, welfare programs are provided in accordance with producer interests. Thus, the legislature responds not only to the public's demand for charity but also serves the industries that have an interest in the services being provided.

In this way redistributive programs motivated by charity reflect the charitable desires of the middle- and upper-income groups—and the economic interests of the suppliers of those services—rather than the political power of the poor.[6]

Political support by the middle class for welfare programs is also high when the beneficiaries are viewed as being "deserving." Typically, deserving means that the beneficiaries are similar to those of the middle class but, because of unfortunate or temporary circumstances, find themselves in need of charity. Examples of deserving groups are those who are temporarily unemployed, the aged, children, and widows. Welfare programs that do not have these groups as their beneficiaries rapidly lose political support.

Universal Redistributive Programs

Universal redistributive programs do not have the same underlying motivation as charitable programs, although they are often promoted on the grounds that they will benefit the poor. Proponents of universal programs claim that by eliminating means tests for determining eligibility, the poor can be treated the same as others. The actual effect of universal programs, however, is that they are more likely to provide net benefits to groups other than the poor. Universal programs are hypothesized to have economic self-interest, rather than charity, as their prime motivation. In fact, as will be discussed, universal programs may leave the poor worse off than a means-tested (income-related) program.

Proponents of universal programs are more likely to favor expanding population eligibility than just increasing the benefits to those who are poor. However, to include a greater number of eligible persons requires a greater cost. An increased cost can be promoted only by including politically powerful groups as part of the eligible population. Consequently, the cost of the expanded program is shifted to those who are less politically powerful, generally those with low incomes.

Regardless of the initial motivation for universal programs, whether it is based on a sincere desire by some to abolish means-tested programs for the poor, or a desire by some to expand the opportunities of the program to everyone (including themselves), the analysis of such programs can best be explained within the framework of self-interest. Although it is difficult to know what someone's intentions really are, inferring a selfish interest on the part of the group that benefits provides a fairly good explanation of the effects of universal programs.

Universal redistributive programs are designed to benefit persons belonging to certain income or age groups, which are categories related to tax and expenditure policies of government. Income and age groups, therefore, provide a basis for the formation of political interests and voting coalitions. When universal programs are instituted regardless of income, then the prime beneficiaries will be the middle-income groups. The losers will be those in either the lowest- or the highest-income groups, most likely the lower, as more money can be raised from a diffuse, regressive, tax than from a highly visible increase in income taxes. When universal programs are designed according to age groupings, then the beneficiaries will be the aged, that is, those aged 65 years and older, who also have the political support of the near-aged and their children. The costs of universal programs based on age will be borne by the young.

Universal programs that subsidize particular services will, as in the case of welfare programs, be designed according to producer preferences.

Income groups in society may be classified into any number of categories; for example, the nonworking poor, the working near-poor, middle-income groups, upper middle-income, and so on. For simplicity, three income groups are used: the poor or low income, the middle class, and the rich.

Each of these income groups may be viewed as a special-interest group; through their votes and political power they would like to use the government to transfer wealth to themselves by imposing the cost on another group. Different voting coalitions are possible among these three groups. All that is required is for a particular group to be part of the winning coalition, which can then impose its will on the minority.

Generally, the middle class is likely to be able to form a coalition with either the rich or poor against the other. After all, the median voters are the middle class; under majority voting the median voter and the median political view receive a disproportionate share of influence. To be reelected, and hence receive a majority of the votes, a legislator moves to the position favored by the median voter. Political competition enhances the political influence of the median voter. The median voter holds the key to the formation of majorities, hence political power.[7] Further, because the middle class is the determining factor in any majority coalition, the middle class is able to extract a higher price than their coalition partners and to be favored by any explicit redistributive programs.

Gordon Tullock claims that majority voting coalitions between the rich and the poor have been unsuccessful largely because of the miscalculations of the poor. A redistributive program based on a means test would transfer funds from high-income to low-income groups. By excluding transfers to the middle class, the poor could receive more than if they were in a coalition with the middle class. The wealthy would benefit because such a redistribution would cost them less than if they also had to subsidize the middle class. Tullock believes, "The poor realize that the interests of the wealthy are clearly not congruent with their interests, but they do not realize that the interests of people between the 20th and the 51st percentile of the income distribution are also not identical with theirs. They therefore tend to favour a coalition with the second group (the middle class) rather than the former (the wealthy)."[8]

Previously, various majority voting coalitions, by income level, have been formed to receive economic benefits by imposing the costs on low-income groups. A coalition between the middle class and the rich against the poor would require only that a small diffuse tax be imposed on those with low incomes. A coalition against those with high incomes would require very large taxes on the wealthy as there are fewer persons with high incomes and a great many persons with middle and low incomes. Faced with a large, more obvious tax, the rich would be expected to offer greater opposition than would the poor; the voting participation rates of the rich are higher and they can provide more funds to legislators than can the poor.[9]

Given that the middle class is likely to hold the majority of power in any coalition, the objective of universal redistributive programs is assumed to be to provide the middle class with benefits in excess of their costs.

Examples of Charitable Redistributive Programs

The major means-tested programs are those providing subsidies for housing, food, medical care, and cash payments under the category of AFDC. Medical care for the medically indigent (Medicaid) will be discussed along with Medicare in the next chapter. The following examples illustrate the application of the self-interest paradigm to welfare redistribution programs.

Food Subsidies

In 1946 the National School Lunch Act was enacted. The objective of the program was to help states establish, maintain, operate, and expand school lunch programs.[10] In 1954 a school milk program was passed, and in 1965 Congress added a breakfast program to schools located in poor areas. Although the legislation received widespread support from educators, women's groups, and labor unions, the legislation was originated in the House Agriculture Committee, whose primary purpose was to benefit farmers. In its report, the House Committee on Agriculture stated:

> The Federal Government has always had an active interest in providing markets for agricultural production and for maintaining agricultural production at a high level. Any measure that will expand the domestic production of agricultural products, both immediately and in the future, and assume a larger share of the national income to farmers, should receive support. With an established school lunch program, a means of disposal of surplus products is likewise available. It has been demonstrated time and time again that price-destroying surpluses, even though of relatively small amount compared with the total production, must be disposed of if a fair price is to be maintained by the farmer.[11]

The origin of the 1954 school milk program was "an Act to provide for greater stability in agriculture . . . and for other purposes." Further, "it is the policy of Congress to assure a stabilized annual production of adequate supplies of milk and dairy products."[12]

By 1965, food product surpluses were smaller, and the Johnson administration wanted to reduce its expenditures for farm subsidies. The administration therefore proposed that the lunch and milk programs be reduced by redirecting them from areas that could afford to pay for these programs to poor school districts. Congress rejected that proposal and instead authorized a new program to provide breakfasts to schools located in poor areas, while retaining the earlier school lunch and milk programs.[13] Congress gave the U.S. Department of Agriculture (USDA) the authority to oversee the school lunch, milk, and breakfast programs.

These programs were primarily enacted because Congress wanted to serve a powerful constituency, the farmers. The legislation did not visibly impose costs on the public (although they paid for the programs through increased taxes and higher food prices). Congress could thereby do good while serving their farm constituents.

The original intent of the legislation became clearer when subsequent legislation was proposed to achieve its more "public" goals directly. It was suggested that the milk program be incorporated as part of the school lunch program and as part of child nutrition programs. Senator William Proxmire, from the dairy state of Wisconsin, objected on grounds that "it would be far easier to sharply slash school milk programs that were an unidentified part of a general nutrition effort."[14] The school milk program was not incorporated into these other programs, even though a study had shown that it was not directed to the needs of the poor. Only $7 million of the $104 million went to needy children.[15]

Food stamps to low-income persons help remove agricultural surpluses from the market. The food stamp program replaced an earlier food distribution program, under which the federal government gave surplus food to the states to distribute to their needy. Under the food stamp program, the recipients would have to buy the food stamps (a requirement since dropped), which could then be used to purchase food at a retail store. Imported food products could not be purchased with food stamps. When the permanent food stamp legislation was signed by President Johnson in 1964, he stated that it was "one of our most valuable weapons for the war on poverty . . . [and a step toward] the fuller and wiser use of our agricultural abundance."[16]

Housing Programs to Benefit the Poor

Federal involvement in housing construction started during World War I, when it was feared that there was insufficient housing for shipyard and defense industry workers.[17] But it was not until the New Deal that a major federal commitment to housing was initiated. It would be a mistake to believe the Wagner-Steagall Act of 1937 was solely concerned with helping the poor. There were two main reasons for a new housing initiative. One was the large number of unemployed, the new poor, those who had lost their jobs because of the depression. These people were considered the deserving poor. The other reason was the government's desire to create jobs.

Private housing construction had fallen from 900,000 units in 1925 to 60,000 units in 1934. Yet, with the decrease in new construction, there was no housing shortage: rents were low, there were vacancies, and many people lived in "Hoovervilles" and shanties. A federal program to increase the supply of housing could, however, have adverse effects on the private housing market. To address this, federal housing legislation required that existing dwellings be destroyed in number equal to the number of new units being built. This policy eliminated potential opposition from landlords and the housing industry. At the same time, the policy was appealing to those who favored eliminating slums for the submerged middle class, the new poor, and to those who favored increased jobs. Building trades unions lobbied vigorously for the public housing act. The original public housing projects were row houses built mostly in the suburbs.

At the end of World War II, there was a large demand for housing by returning veterans and the rising middle class. Federal housing policy provided tax breaks and mortgage insurance for veterans and had the effect of stimulating the construction industry. At the same time, the government was concerned that the country not return to the depression. Public housing lost its initial clientele as the middle class moved out and suburban sites were taken over for veterans' subdivisions. Public housing became confined to the inner city. The new middle class did not want the poor, no longer the submerged middle class, in their neighborhoods. And as land for public housing in the city became expensive, the size of the buildings increased. As the inhabitants of public housing began to change, fewer from a middle-class background and a greater proportion of blacks, the political support for public housing declined.

By the 1960s, public housing was in disrepute with the exception of public housing for the elderly, which still has a political constituency even now. Communities that have traditionally been hostile to public housing have welcomed housing for the elderly, who are predominantly middle class and white and who tend not to be vandals. Subsidized housing for the elderly also helps the middle class find a place for their parents to live.

Other federal housing programs were also enacted, such as urban renewal.[18] Rather than benefiting them, however, the urban poor were, on net, displaced. Urban renewal destroyed more units than were built, thereby decreasing the available supply of housing. According to the 1949 act, federal funds were available if slums were torn down. However, the slums could be, and were, replaced by nonresidential projects.[19] Urban renewal was used to revitalize cities by eliminating urban slums, but there was little concern for the displaced urban poor. Cities built coliseums and civic centers. The beneficiaries were downtown businesspeople, construction workers and firms, and those who wanted a revitalized city. Middle- and high-income groups were attracted back to the city to live in newly constructed housing.

Two other federal housing programs of interest are the rent-supplement and leased-housing programs. In 1965, a rent-supplement provision was added to the Housing and Urban Development Act. By providing supplements to low-income people, the government would avoid owning public housing. Initially, the rent supplement was to be used in new projects or in projects requiring major rehabilitation, thereby assisting the building unions. A number of the groups that took advantage of this program were churches and nonprofit organizations. (The landlords were able to select their tenants.) Thus, these organizations could serve the housing needs of their needy members.[20]

The leased-housing program (1965) authorized local authorities to lease private apartments and homes (with the landlord's approval). This program was welcomed by landlords, because it helped eliminate vacancies in areas with high vacancy rates and guaranteed government rent payments. The leasing program was to "take full advantage of vacancies or potential vacancies in the private housing market."[21] There were also incentives for buildings to be rehabilitated. To avoid increasing rents to the middle class, the lease program could not leave the area with too few vacancies.[22]

Both the rent-supplement and leased-housing programs benefited landlords, the elderly (who were often the recipients), and others from the submerged middle class.

Aid to Families with Dependent Children

The AFDC program differs from all other welfare programs in that it provides cash to the recipient, rather than in-kind services, such as food, housing, and medical care. Therefore it is of interest to determine why a cash subsidy, which does not benefit any specific producer group, is provided. Subsequently, a producer group was created—welfare employees to administer the program, who developed a concentrated interest in its continuance.

The AFDC program had its roots in the "mothers' pension" movement. In the early 1900s, there was concern that children not be denied the benefits of a home life because of poverty.[23] If a mother became a widow, her children might have to be cared for in an institution. The social reformers of the day wanted to establish a program that would provide financial assistance to children in their own homes.

The states started their own programs to aid needy children; however, they were not meant to aid all needy children. The rules the states promulgated were quite explicit on who the beneficiaries should be. The children had to have parents of "worthy" character, that is, parents who had suffered from temporary misfortune. Further, the mother had to be able to provide a "suitable" home.

To determine "fit" mothers, the state focused attention on two issues. The first was the father's status. Was the father dead or was he imprisoned, divorced, or unmarried? The second criterion was the mother's fitness to have children. The local determining agencies established the criteria known as "gilt-edged widows." Typically, in familys that qualified for aid the father was dead, the mother was white, and both came from a middle-class background. Blacks and unmarried mothers were excluded. Caseworkers were also encouraged to visit the mothers after their grants had been approved to ensure that a suitable home continued to be maintained.

Thus, the AFDC program was not meant to provide for all the poor. Instead, it was meant to aid those who were from the same middle-class background as the donors. During the depression, many states' funds became depleted as more workers were temporarily unemployed. Additional funding was required to assist the states. After the passage of the Social Security Act in 1935, both the federal and state governments became involved in financing the AFDC program. Basic control over the program, however, was asserted by the states, and states varied greatly in their eligibility determinations. Blacks were widely discriminated against.

During the 1950s and 1960s, the program changed because of demographics and economics. As more of the recipients were black mothers, public support for the program began to fade. Instances of welfare fraud occurred, and the program was blamed for causing an increase in illegitimate births. The AFDC program came under permanent attack. The middle-class constituency that had initially favored the program now withdrew its support. The desire to impose conditions, such as "workfare," is an indication of this change. Another indication of the lack of public political support is the fact that Congress had never tied AFDC benefits to the consumer price index, as had been done for many middle-class entitlement programs.

The Nixon and Carter administrations tried to change the welfare system. Both administrations failed. The objective of these welfare reform proposals was to eliminate the various in-kind subsidies currently being provided to the poor and instead provide them with cash. However, the political constituencies favoring continuance of the multiple program approach were too powerful. They argued that the special needs of the poor could best be met by in-kind subsidies—which incidentally benefit powerful producer groups—rather than a single, simple, integrated cash system. Obviously, the poor would prefer cash, but the poor do not have a strong political constituency.

> Welfare reform has no natural political constituency. Although the poor can play on the national conscience successfully at times, they do not organize themselves or vote to the extent that other groups do; in any event, there aren't enough of them to wield a lot of political power.[24]

One might think that welfare workers would represent the interests of the poor. Unfortunately, that is not necessarily the case. By 1970, more than 100,000 employees were involved in the administration of various welfare programs. These state bureaucracies have themselves become an important political constituency.[25]

> It was . . . instructive . . . to observe the opposition of social workers to the family assistance program [President Nixon's welfare reform proposal] under which federal dollars would have been channeled directly to the poor to permit each poor family to decide for itself how best to spend its allotment. We should not be surprised that many social workers supported the retention of the existing system, under which a large portion of those dollars go to social workers, a middle-income group, in return for supervising the allocation of in-kind benefits and the expenditure of funds by the poor.[26]

In his discussion of why President Nixon's Family Assistance Program was not enacted, Daniel Moynihan spoke harshly of the role played by the leadership of middle-class welfare professionals, who wanted to ensure that welfare workers would benefit (or at least not be harmed) by any new poverty program: "The de facto strategy of social-welfare groups was to seek to kill the program, . . . by insisting on benefit levels that no Congress would pass and no president would approve."[27] Moynihan added, "A proposal to put an end to poverty, or the largest share thereof, through direct cash payments was by definition a threat to an agency proceeding at the same task by indirect means."[28] Instead of the Family Assistance Program, community action agency directors (whose agencies were funded by the federal government) wanted a program of block grants to their own agencies. They wanted to ensure that their own federally paid antipoverty workers would participate in the funding.[29] Jerry Wurf, head of the American Federation of State, County, and Municipal Employees, the largest public employee union in the United States (approximately 30,000 members), testified about his opposition to the Family Assistance Program before the Senate Finance Committee: "This legislation threatens to eliminate the jobs of our people."[30]

Examples of Universal Redistributive Programs

Universal redistributive programs do not use a means test to determine beneficiaries. The users or beneficiaries of the service receive the same subsidy regardless of income level. Such programs appear to be egalitarian. However, the effect of universal redistributive programs, as will be shown by the following examples, is that the middle-class and even high-income groups receive most of the subsidies. The methods by which the subsidies are provided are according to the producer's preferences.

Higher Education

State and federal subsidies are provided to institutions of higher learning. Higher education, including undergraduate, graduate, and professional schools (such as medical schools), are all examples of places where the majority of the benefits are received by students from the middle- and upper-income groups. Typical of state-supported educational institutions is the California system of higher education. Hansen and Weisbrod found that family incomes of students who attended the state-supported universities were on average higher than families whose children did not attend the state university system.[31] Further, the annual amount of state subsidy (the difference between tuition and cost of education) per student who attended the state university system exceeded, on average, their family's yearly payment of state taxes. Thus, families who sent their children to the state universities, predominantly the middle- and upper-income groups, received a net subsidy from the state. Even after considering the additional state taxes the students paid once they started working (assuming they remained in California), the state subsidy still exceeded the additional taxes paid, on a present value basis. Because the annual state subsidy exceeded the annual amount of state taxes paid by families with children in the state system, the subsidies for the state university system had to be paid by those families whose children did not attend the university and whose incomes were on average lower. This system of providing subsidies to middle- and upper-income families for their children's higher education exists in all states that have publicly supported state universities.

The reason often stated for such education subsidies is that without them students from low-income families would not have the opportunity to attend college. Although this would appear to be a charitable motivation, why is it necessary to subsidize in an equal manner all students who attend state universities, particularly those from the highest-income groups? The true motivation for such programs can again be questioned when it is realized that most of the students are not from low-income families, but from middle- and upper-income families. Thus, one important characteristic of universal programs is that the subsidized services are used predominantly by those with middle and higher incomes.

A second characteristic of universal redistribution programs is that the subsidies are provided in a manner in accordance with the producers' preferences. State subsidies for college education could be provided to state universities, as they are now, or they could be provided to students to be used at the college of their choice. If the state provided students with a "voucher," that is, a fixed-dollar subsidy for education (to be mailed to the university selected by the student), then the state university would have to compete with other universities for that subsidy. It is more in the state university's interest that the subsidy be given directly to the state university. Thus, a student who wished to be subsidized would have to go to the state university. The state university receives a competitive advantage over other, nonstate-supported universities; its price of education is lowered.

It is not surprising, therefore, that state universities are the major lobbyists for state subsidies to higher education. After all, the members of the university community have a concentrated interest in the size and method of distributing those subsidies.

Medical Education

A more obvious case in which the net benefits accrue primarily to those in the middle- and higher-income groups is that of medical education. (The same analysis would apply to all professional education except that the size of the subsidies per student is so much greater for medical education.) Public medical schools are primarily subsidized by the state, although in the past the federal government has also provided large subsidies. In 2001, the average annual government subsidy for four years of medical education was more than $500,000 per student.[32] These subsidies are in addition to those received during the student's four years of undergraduate education.

How are these medical education subsidies distributed with regard to family incomes? In 1967, only 12 percent of families in the population had incomes greater than $15,000, whereas 42 percent of the families of medical students had incomes greater than $15,000. In 1975, three times as many families of medical students had incomes greater than $25,000 than did families in the population at large. In 2001, more than five times as many families of medical students had incomes greater than $250,000 than did families in the population at large.[33] And once these medical students graduate, they enter the top 10 percent of the income distribution in society.

A charitable motivation is again used as the justification for extensive medical education subsidies; without subsidies, low-income and minority students would be unable to afford a medical education. Only the children of the rich would be able to become physicians. However, if the motivation were truly to aid low-income persons, then it would be more efficient to provide the subsidies according to the family incomes of the medical students. A smaller state subsidy would be required if only low-income students qualified (or if the subsidy was graduated according to family income). A medical education subsidy is a universal redistribution program: all students, regardless of family income, receive the benefits. Because the large majority of medical students come from the middle- and upper-income groups, the subsidies go predominantly to these groups. Low-income groups pay state taxes, which are used for such subsidies; the benefits they receive from these programs are less than their costs.

The method by which these subsidies are provided is again based on producers' (the medical schools) preferences. The subsidies go to the schools, which enable them to lower tuition rates. In this way, students are subsidized only if they attend a state medical school. Given the higher tuition at private medical schools, state-subsidized medical schools have a large price advantage when competing in the market for medical students.

Based on the distribution of education benefits, both undergraduate and professional, particularly for medical education, the most likely reason for such subsidies is not altruism but the economic self-interest of the middle- and upper-income groups as well as the subsidized medical schools. These beneficiaries are aware of the program's economic benefits and are likely to oppose any attempts to make the program more efficient or more equitable.[34]

Farm Policy

Another example of a large universal redistributive program has been this country's farm policy. In 1929, the Federal Farm Board was established with the mission of "stabilizing" (raising) prices for farmers' crops. President Hoover and then President Roosevelt (and succeeding presidents) also urged "plowing under crops" as a means of reducing supply and raising prices. The stated intent of these programs was to assist the family farmer. However, rather than being a means-tested program, which would supplement family farmers' incomes, the farm program treats all farmers alike. The approach used to subsidize farmers is to raise the price of their crops above what they would be otherwise. The methods used to raise farm prices above market level have varied over time, from guaranteed farm prices to restrictions of farmers' output.

Neither Congress nor the USDA have adequately explained why some crops are subsidized and many other crops are not. Corn, wheat, cotton, soybeans, and rice receive more than 90 percent of all farm subsidies; the growers of nearly 400 other domestic crops receive virtually no subsidies.

The main beneficiaries of this universal subsidy program have been the larger, well-to-do farmers. In 2002, 1.4 percent of the farms received 47.5 percent of total farm income, and 71 percent of the farms earned less than $25,000. (Less than 4 percent of U.S. landowners own more than 50 percent of farm land, and the bottom 70 percent own just 11 percent.)[35]

When the price of farm products is artificially increased, those who benefit the most are those who are the most productive. Thus, most of the subsidies do not go to the small farmers who most need assistance. Family farmers with small acreage receive little, if any, subsidies. Large farms and agribusinesses receive the largest subsidies because they have the most land, use the latest technology, and are the most productive; they are able to take advantage of economies of scale. Since 1991, subsidies for large farms have nearly tripled, while subsidies for small farms have not increased.[36] These large farms, with the aid of farm subsidies, are buying out small farms and consolidating the industry. By buying smaller farms, these large farms are able to benefit from their economies of scale, increase the productivity of their land, increase their federal subsidies, and buy out additional small farms. The number of farms decreased from 7 million in 1935 to 2 million in 2002 (only 400,000 of which are full-time farms).[37]

Large numbers of small family farmers are still being forced into bankruptcy. Despite their worsening financial condition, farmers who own the small- and medium-sized farms receive a small percentage of federal subsidies. In 2002, the top 10 percent of farm subsidy recipients received 71 percent of all farm subsidies. The bottom 80 percent, including most family farmers, received just 19 percent of all farm subsidies, or on average $846 per year.[38]

Wealthy farmers and agribusinesses are a powerful political lobby; they contributed more than $11 million in campaign contributions in the 2002 elections.[39]

In previous years, to prevent large corporations from receiving millions of dollars in farm subsidies, Congress placed a total limit of $350,000 in subsidies per farm. However, loopholes in the law, such as by (theoretically) dividing the farm into smaller farms each owned by a relative, and lack of enforcement of the limit by the USDA, has enabled large farms to continue receiving huge subsidies.[40]

The cost of the farm program is borne by the public in two ways: as consumers of farm products they have to pay a higher price; as taxpayers they must pay to enable the government to purchase and store the farm produce that cannot be sold at the higher prices. The higher price to consumers is similar to an excise tax, which is a regressive tax; all consumers of food pay higher prices regardless of differences in their incomes. Thus, those with low incomes pay a greater proportion of their incomes for higher-priced farm products.

Every several years new farm legislation is enacted. For example, in 1985 it was estimated that the three-year farm bill would cost in total between $50 to $75 billion. Yet this farm bill did not include any new aid for the nation's most troubled farmers. In fact, it was estimated that the losers under this farm legislation, the most costly ever, were those farmers who were the most distressed. The taxpayers were also considered to be the losers, as they pay for these huge subsidies.[41]

In 1995, congressional Republicans promised to reduce the federal deficit and balance the federal budget in 7 years without increasing taxes. The Republican leadership in congress believed failure to keep this promise would cost them a great deal of political support among voters. However, keeping this promise required the Republicans to make reductions in many programs previously considered sacrosanct to various interest groups. The overriding concern with reducing the federal budget deficit resulted in changes in the farm program that would not otherwise have occurred.

The Freedom to Farm Act of 1996 was portrayed as a radical departure from the farm policies of the past 60 years. Proponents of the reform hoped it would provide a transition away from the price-support programs that had been in place since the 1930s and would eliminate commodity support programs and acreage limitations after 2002. The act provided for $43 billion over 7 years to phase out farm subsidies over that same period.[42]

As early as 1998, Congress changed its mind and started providing annual "emergency" subsidies to farmers. A presidential election in 2000 and the necessity to court the farm vote in several swing states led to an additional $30 billion in farm subsidies in 2000. The Freedom to Farm law was abandoned before the 2002 elections, and farmers were promised $180 billion in additional subsidies over the next 10 years.[43]

An extreme example of farm subsidy programs is dairy price supports.[44] The dairy industry, however, does not consist solely of small farmers trying to eke out a living. Instead, the dairy industry is a modernized, $27 billion industry, dominated by large milk cooperatives.[45] Two such cooperatives are among this country's 50 largest diversified businesses. The reason for the success of the dairy industry in securing subsidies worth billions of dollars a year is that the industry is very well organized. The fees dairy cooperatives charge farmers include an amount for political activities. The highly focused political activity by the cooperatives is the maintenance of high milk price supports.[46]

The inequities of the farm program, that is, low-income consumers subsidizing wealthy farmers and large corporate farms, have been brought to the attention of Congress numerous times. In addition, for some time Congress has been aware of the inefficiencies of this subsidy system, that is, greater subsidies could be received by the low-income farmers if a means-tested rather than a universal program based on price supports were used. Although the stated intent of farm legislation is to help the family farmer, the subsidies primarily benefit large agribusinesses, and the number of family farmers continues to diminish. Thus, the continued existence of both the farm problem (low-income family farmers) and farm policy (universal price supports) cannot be attributed to altruism. Economic self-interest on the part of the majority of well-to-do farmers is a more accurate explanation.

Social Security

The last example of a universal program, whose underlying motivation can best be explained by economic self-interest rather than altruism or charity, is the current Social Security program. Because Medicare is more directly related to this type of universal program, a more extensive discussion of Social Security is provided.

The Social Security program currently (and since its beginning) provides benefits to the aged in excess of their contributions.[47] Congress has increased these benefits over time. The beneficiaries of this subsidy are the aged, regardless of their income. Those who bear the cost of these subsidies are the working young. Both the size of the tax and the base on which it is levied have increased over time. The Social Security system is not based on insurance principles; the benefits are not related to the amount a worker has invested in the system. Rather, it is a "pay-as-you-go" method of financing. The benefits are paid from current tax contributions made by employees and employers.

Each time Social Security benefits are increased, those who receive the greatest benefit are the oldest, as they pay less of the additional tax needed to finance the new benefits. Thus, those aged 65 years and older would be expected to favor increased Social Security benefits, because they would be the immediate beneficiary of the benefits without having had to finance them. Those at least 55 years old would also receive benefits in excess of their costs as they would not have to pay the full costs of the additional benefits. If those in older age groups receive a higher rate of return when benefits are increased, then those who have the longest to work must receive a lower rate of return on their contributions. The benefits are not proportionate to taxes paid, but are inversely related to the taxes.[48]

When the value of Social Security benefits relative to Social Security taxes paid by the typical worker is compared for workers of different age groups, studies have found a substantial drop in the expected net benefits for younger generations.[49]

Further, if the working young receive fewer Social Security benefits when they retire than do the current elderly, then their burden will be even greater. The number of persons in the different age cohorts are not equal. In 1940, the approximate ratio of workers to Social Security beneficiaries was 9 to 1. By 1960 this ratio had fallen to 5 to 1, by 2005 the ratio had declined further to 3 to 1, and by 2031, the ratio is expected to be only 2 to 1.[50] (This support ratio is important in economic terms because the working population can be thought of as supporting nonworking age groups.) Because Social Security is on a "pay-as-you-go" financing system, to provide the same set of benefits to the current working young would require future generations to pay even greater Social Security taxes. Thus, by providing additional benefits to the current aged, Congress shifts the burden of financing those benefits to those currently working and to future generations and raises doubts that future generations will receive the same benefits as the current aged.

Various comparisons have been made of the economic status of the aged and nonaged. When such comparisons are made, it is important to adjust for differences in family size, in-kind benefits received by the aged, and their different tax advantages. One of the conclusions from these studies is that the economic status of the elderly has sharply improved over time. In 1966, 28.5 percent of the aged were at or below the poverty rate, whereas the poverty rate was 10.6 percent for nonaged adults. By the late 1980s, the poverty rates for both groups were much closer: 12.4 percent for the aged and 10.8 percent for nonaged adults. In 2003, the aged had a slightly lower poverty rate than the nonaged, 10.2 percent compared with 10.8 percent for the nonaged.[51] These figures, however, mask wide differences in income among the aged. Minority aged, women, and those over 75 years old are most likely to be impoverished. It is clearly inequitable when the burden of financing increased benefits for all aged, including high-income aged, is placed on low-income workers.

Social Security is financed by a tax on earnings, not on income from all sources. The amount of an employee's earnings (the base) subject to this payroll tax, as well as the size of the payroll tax, has been increased in recent years. The tax is paid equally by both the employee and the employer. However, regardless of whether the entire tax is placed on the employee, is placed on the employer, or is shared, as is currently done, the effect of who bears the tax burden is the same. Brittain's findings indicate that the worker generally bears all the tax.[52] Although the legislation divides the tax between the employee and the employer, this appears to be more of a device for diminishing the visibility and the employee's awareness of the size of the tax than for sharing its burden. Employees are misled into believing they bear only half of their actual Social Security tax when in reality they are paying all or most of it.

The Social Security tax is a flat percentage on earnings up to a certain earnings base. Each worker who earns up to that limit pays the same dollar amount of tax. Thus, low-income workers pay a greater proportion of their earnings in Social Security taxes than higher-income workers.[53] The burden of financing the Social Security system falls on those who are younger each time benefits for the current retired are increased. Further, those who earn lower wages pay a greater portion of those wages for Social Security taxes.[54]

Despite the expansion of benefits to the Social Security system over time, many aged are still poor. For these aged persons, as well as for the blind and disabled, a separate cash assistance program, Supplemental Security Income, is provided. This federal program is financed from general tax revenues, and eligibility is based on a strict means and asset test.

Because the "pay-as-you-go" financing system, which places the greatest burden on the working poor, is not sufficient to provide a minimum income (above the poverty level) to all the aged, a separate means-tested program is required. The universal program, however, does provide higher-income aged with benefits in excess of their contributions; the burden of financing these benefits are borne by younger working populations with lower incomes. And it is unlikely that in the future their benefits will be equal to their contributions.

Social Security is an inequitable method of helping those who are less well off. The proponents of Social Security, however, have never called it a welfare program, even though it is a massive redistributive program. If the current Social Security system is not based on providing for low-income aged, then what is the motivation for continually expanding the benefits to all aged, regardless of their incomes, and placing increased burdens on future generations? The only credible explanation is one based on economic self-interest of the aged and their supporters.

The Social Security system is financially unable to provide the promised benefits to today's younger generation. The estimated shortfall in the Social Security Trust Fund is $7 trillion. Before the Social Security Trust Fund is bankrupt, Congress will have to change its benefits and its financing. Thus, another test of the public interest and economic theories is how equitable will be the changes in benefits and taxes for making the Social Security system financially solvent. It is highly likely that the aged and near-aged will not incur any reduction in benefits while the burden of reduced benefits and increased taxes will fall most heavily on the youngest workers.

Political Power of the Aged

Since the changes in the Social Security system are hypothesized to be based on economic self-interest, it is necessary to examine whether the aged have sufficient political power to achieve their economic goals. Those population groups favoring wealth transfers to the elderly at the expense of other population groups are the elderly themselves, those members of the working population who view Social Security as a substitute for the family support they themselves may have to provide their parents, and the near-aged, who are voting on behalf of themselves for when they reach old age.

At whose expense are these benefits transferred to the elderly? If the redistribution of wealth is determined by the political process, then the financial burdens must be imposed on those who have less political power. The natural groups to bear these burdens are the young and future generations.

The young and children do not vote. The young working-age population has relatively low voting-participation rates. The lowest voting-participation rates are among 18 year olds. Their voting participation rate was 13 percent in the 2002 congressional election and 39 percent in the 2004 presidential election. Those aged 19 to 23 years old had a slightly higher voting rate (about 17 percent and 40 percent, respectively). The voting participation rate then increased with age. The highest participation rates were in the 55- to 74-year-old age group: about 60 percent in the 2002 congressional election and 70 percent for the 2004 presidential elections. Typically, one-third of those voting are 55 and older.[55]

The rewards to be gained from the political process have provided the aged with the incentive to become more politically aware. The increasing political power of the elderly can be seen from examining other statistics. The elderly are the fastest-growing proportion of the population. And more of the aged can name their congressional representative than any other age group.

Policies favoring the aged also have the political support of the nonaged. The percent of households with children is decreasing (35 percent of voters live with a child).[56] Preston, studying voting patterns in an earlier election, found that the voting participation rate of households with no children under 18 years old, that is, older couples, voted at a 60 percent rate compared with households with children younger than 6 years, who voted at a 40 percent rate.[57] Couples with children, for example, a 40-year-old couple, likely have a greater number of living parents than they do children living at home.[58]

The potential financial and social burden of caring for a greater number of elderly parents exceeds the costs of caring for their declining number of children. Therefore, even couples with children have an economic self-interest in shifting concern with their parent's economic well-being away from themselves.

The above facts, however, are of interest only if people vote according to their economic interests. It is important, therefore, to determine whether this in fact occurs.

Few empirical studies enable one to distinguish between contrasting studies of voting behavior. Parsons examined welfare payments to the aged by states in two periods: in 1934, before the Social Security Act of 1935, and again in 1940. In this latter period, states were provided with federal matching funds. The purpose of Parsons' study was to determine whether "the increased voting power of the aged in states with relatively more older individuals offset[s] the effect of the increased tax burden on the working population."[59]

After controlling for other factors affecting public generosity, such as per capita incomes and the proportion of the population that is white, Parsons concluded that benefit levels in states with a disproportionate number of aged were not significantly reduced; this "would suggest that the increased welfare burden on the younger voters of more aged dependents is approximately offset by the increased voting power of the aged." The results of a study based on a period 50 years ago may not be applicable to today's situation. However, Parsons suggests that as the proportion of the elderly increases, the intensity of the debate over transfer payments to the elderly will become greater, but that aged benefit levels are unlikely to be altered.

Additional information is also instructive in this regard. A 1983 Gallup survey on attitudes toward public schools asked whether people would vote for increased school taxes. Acting according to their self-interest, the aged would be expected to oppose these increases. For those over the age of 50, opponents of increased school taxes easily defeated proponents, 62 to 28 percent.[60] With regard to the question of how the Social Security crisis can best be resolved, a 1982 survey found that the elderly were in favor of increased contributions by the working-age population and a delay in the retirement age.[61]

Still another example of the political power of the aged was Congressional passage of the Age Discrimination Act of 1975. In an analysis of that act, Peter Schuck describes the source of the aged's political power.

> A number of ingredients combined in the case of the ADA (Age Discrimination Act of 1975) to yield a formidable, indeed irresistible, political offering. It promised benefits to a visible, politically influential group that all Americans hoped someday to join;

its sponsors argued that it could confer these benefits at no additional cost; its redistributional implications were not clear, or at least were not noticed; and it was a small and inconspicuous part of a large omnibus bill that both Congress and the Administration supported. Perhaps most important, it drew strength from the moral legitimacy and rhetorical force of the civil rights movement of the 1960's and early 1970's, a provenance that is critical to understanding how Congress conceptualized and responded to the problem of age discrimination.[62]

Further,

If the elderly constituted a powerful political force simply by virtue of their numbers (and their marked propensity to register and vote), their real strength had additional sources including, among others, the absence of any consistent opposition to their agenda, their ability to form political alliances, and a strong public image of legitimacy stemming from their status and broad distribution throughout all strata of society. As Peter Drucker has observed, "[I]n sharp contrast to every other minority group, the older population has a very large constituency outside its own ranks."[63]

Schuck concludes that the results of this political power are as follows:

The elderly translated their political power into a series of formidable legislative achievements. By 1975, their successes included Medicare and Medicaid, which together pay for over two-thirds of the healthcare costs of the elderly; rapidly rising Social Security benefits indexed against inflation; the Supplementary Security Income program, which established a minimum federal income for the elderly, blind, and disabled and also is indexed against inflation; special housing programs; pension reform; the Age Discrimination in Employment Act of 1967; and preferential tax treatment. Another example of the political effectiveness of the elderly is the extraordinary growth in appropriations under the Older Americans Act of 1965. The Act, which authorizes a pastiche of grant programs for services, planning, research, and training, was implemented by appropriations that mushroomed from $7.5 million in 1966 . . . to . . . [*$2.8 billion in 2005*].[64] As one observer recently noted, "the aging have proved a difficult group for officials to ignore or 'buy off' with purely symbolic concessions."

And finally,

Although the most important effects of the ADA, as of any social reform, may well be those that cannot now be anticipated, several predictions may nevertheless be ventured. First, the ADA is likely to increase the proportion of total program resources allocated to the elderly. If Congress may be said to have had any single coherent expectations in enacting the ADA, it was that the elderly would receive a larger share of program benefits in a world free of "ageism." But if resource levels remain unchanged, increases for the elderly will be at the expense of members of every other age group.[65]

An important indication of the rewards to political activity is the allocation of the federal budget. In 1960, less than 15 percent of a $93 billion federal budget went to the elderly (in the form of cash or in-kind benefits). By the late 1980s, the elderly received more than 25 percent of a much larger federal budget. In 2004 the elderly received 34 percent of the federal budget, and it is estimated that this will increase to 44 percent by 2015.[66]

A further display of the aged's political power (and perhaps later generalizability to Medicare's problems) was the approach agreed on by Congress to solve the Social Security crisis in the early 1980s. Changes were made to Social Security in 1983 to enhance its financial viability. These changes, however, had minimal effect on current (or soon to be) beneficiaries. The age of eligibility was increased to age 67, but this was to be phased in after the year 2000. In addition, beginning in 1984, a portion of Social Security benefits would be included in taxable income. Aged couples whose adjusted gross income, including 50 percent of their Social Security benefits, is $32,000 would be subject to taxes on half of their Social Security income. The proportion of the current aged affected by this provision, however, was very small. (In 1980, only 3 percent of the elderly had cash incomes greater than $35,000.)[67] Future generations, however, will have greater private pensions and individual retirement accounts. Together with inflation-induced increases in incomes (the earnings base is not adjusted for inflation), this 1983 legislation will cause many future retirees to lose part of their Social Security payments to income taxes.

Congress then voted to increase both Social Security taxes and the earnings base on which those taxes apply. Thus, the approach used for saving the Social Security system was to impose increased taxes on the working population. The major loss to the current beneficiaries of ensuring the viability of the Social Security system was a six-month delay in their cost-of-living adjustment (COLA).

Since 1981, there have been numerous reductions in federal programs in an attempt to reduce the federal budget deficit. Examining which constituencies have had the largest program cuts once again indicates the relative political influence of the aged. A study of these budget reductions found that "elderly households face much smaller reductions in benefits than do younger households. Benefit reductions since 1981 have, in general, fallen more heavily on means-tested programs than on social insurance programs on which the elderly are more likely to rely. . . . In contrast, programs serving the non-elderly have had larger reductions. For example, . . . the child nutrition programs were cut by about 28%."[68] A conclusion of the study was that "households with elderly members have been less severely affected by benefit reductions, relative to the share of benefits they receive, than have any other population group."[69]

Before 1972, Congress continually voted for increases in Social Security benefits during election years. Fiscal conservatives were alarmed at this attempt to buy the vote of those on Social Security. To halt this practice, Social Security benefits were indexed for inflation. If inflation was below 3 percent then there would be no COLA that year. However, if the cumulative rise in inflation in the following year reached 3 percent, then the aged would receive their COLA. Thus, if a COLA is not received in one year it could be received the next; it would not be lost, merely delayed.

Because of the low rate of inflation in 1986, an election year, the aged were not due to receive their COLA increase. The statistics that determine the COLA are published two weeks before the November elections. Both Congress and the administration came out in favor of giving the aged an increase in benefits, even though inflation was less than 3 percent. As John Rother of the American Association of Retired Persons (AARP) said, "I don't think we have to do anything to preserve the COLA. It's an election year."[70]

A further example of the use of age as a basis of redistribution was the issue of the federal budget deficit. By spending in excess of revenues, the administration and Congress were able to provide benefits in excess of costs to current taxpayers. To bring the budget into balance, it would have been necessary for Congress to reduce spending or increase taxes. In either case, some groups of current taxpayers or beneficiaries would have been adversely affected. Maintaining current expenditures with a deficit, therefore, requires that the revenues that will have to be made up, i.e., increased taxes, are shifted to future generations. The effect is the same as an intergenerational transfer of resources from the young to current taxpayers. The political support for this transfer comes from those who vote, who are also the current taxpayers.

Concluding Comments

The self-interest paradigm provides a rationale for why both producer and nonproducer groups receive legislative benefits. Population groups are large and have high costs of organization. However, certain population groups, measured either by income level or age, are able to use their political support to transfer wealth to themselves by imposing the cost of programs on those unable to provide much political support. These programs are referred to as explicit redistributive programs. The motivation underlying both producer and explicit redistributive legislation is the same: economic self-interest. Producer groups and population groups attempt to use the political process to enrich themselves at the expense of those with little political influence.

An important distinction between producer legislation and explicit redistributive legislation is visibility. Producers are provided with their benefits in an indirect manner. And the public is generally unaware of the consequences of producer-type legislation. Therefore, they offer little opposition. Explicit redistributive legislation has to be very visible, otherwise the beneficiaries of such legislation would not offer their political support.[71]

When redistributive legislation provides services regardless of income level, then the prime beneficiaries are the middle class. The middle class represents the median voter. It holds the key to the formation of coalitions; it is likely to form a coalition with either the high- or low-income groups. Because high-income persons are fewer in number and more capable of political action, low-income groups are more likely to bear the burden of redistributive programs. The least obvious method of imposing a tax on those with low incomes is to finance the service through an excise tax, either on property, products, or labor, which everyone has to pay. In this manner low-income workers or consumers pay a cost greater than the benefits they receive, because their use of the benefit, such as medical education, is less than the taxes they pay for that benefit.

When age is the criterion for providing redistributive benefits, then the aged are likely to be the beneficiaries. The aged participate more in the political process than do the young, particularly those who are too young to vote. The aged also have a great many supporters—their children, who are relieved of a financial responsibility, and the near-aged.

Empirical support for the distinction between charitable and universal redistributive programs is provided in the federal budget. According to the Congressional Budget Office, $341 billion was spent on means-tested programs in 2004. (These programs included Medicaid, SCHIP, food stamps, family support, Supplemental Security Income, veteran's pensions, child nutrition, student loans, foster care, and the Earned Income tax credit.) In that same year, $1,005 billion was spent on non–means-tested programs, the largest ones being Social Security and Medicare. The non–means-tested programs are also expected to have a much larger absolute increase over time.[72]

Producer groups are often strong supporters of explicit redistributive policies. The rules and regulations implementing such policies are complex and not very visible to the public. By designing redistributive legislation so that it also serves producer interests, Congress is able to garner political support from the major participants affecting redistributive legislation.

The motivations underlying charitable redistributive programs are also in accordance with the self-interest paradigm. The legislative process is used to implement the preferences of the middle class, the median voters. Based on the examples cited, the middle class, which provides the political support for charitable redistribution, prefers to provide such charity to the "deserving" poor; that is, those who come from the middle class. This was the basis for the AFDC program (white widows who could provide a suitable home for their children) and for federal housing subsidies (the unemployed during the depression and returning veterans from World War II). Once these programs lost their middle-class recipients, the political support for them declined.

Charitable redistributive programs are based on a means test. Because the benefits to the recipients are intended to outweigh their costs, the financing for such programs is based on general tax revenues, to which the poor contribute less than other income groups.

The self-interest role of producers (and labor unions) in promoting charitable redistributive programs cannot be underestimated. Producers may often be the ones who initiate such programs (housing programs; school lunch, milk, and breakfast programs; and food stamps).[73] Their motivation is the same as for other forms of producer-type legislation. Producers are interested in legislation that increases the demand for their services when they have excess capacity. Such legislation is rarely proposed when producers are at capacity. Charitable redistribution is primarily in the form of in-kind subsidies because it benefits the producers and reflects the values of the middle class. The donors who provide the public support for such legislation want to help the recipients according to what the donors believe is necessary, not according to what recipients believe is most needed.

This self-interest view of redistribution describes the principles underlying explicit redistributive programs. These same self-interest principles form the basis of producer-type legislation. The next chapter applies these principles to the main redistributive program in the health field: Medicare.

Study Questions

1. Using the economic theory of regulation, contrast the two types of broad redistributive programs (charitable and universal) in terms of their motivations, the basis of their political support, the intended beneficiaries, and the methods of financing.

2. Economists claim that "in-kind" redistributive programs, whereby the recipient receives goods and services, such as food stamps or housing, are less efficient than providing the recipient with just cash, which enables them to purchase those goods and services they need most. Why is it unlikely, therefore, that cash will be used instead of in-kind services?

3. Evaluate subsidies to medical schools (which enable public medical schools to reduce their tuition to all students) in terms of whether this approach is the most equitable and efficient method for enabling low-income students to attend medical school.

4. Social Security is referred to as a "pay-as-you-go" financing method. Describe how this approach works. Also discuss the redistributive effects inherent in a "pay-as-you-go" system.

5. Social Security is financed by a payroll tax that is a flat percentage of earnings up to a maximum wage base. Evaluate this method of financing versus one where there is no maximum wage base. Similarly, what would be the redistributive effects of applying this flat tax to income from all sources or from just earned income?

6. Why are the aged considered to be politically powerful?

Notes

1. Actually, government programs, such as garbage collection, do involve redistribution when the service is performed by government employees. These government employees are likely to receive higher wages and benefits than if these services were provided through a competitive bid process. These higher costs are financed by the higher costs to the users of such services.

2. Once the government provides charity, determining the appropriate amount and method of providing it is not an easy task. Voters are unlikely to disclose their true preferences on the amount of government charity to be provided. Voters both favoring and opposing greater amounts of government charity will exaggerate their preferences expecting to offset their opponent's exaggerated preferences.

3. There is another hypothesis regarding why charity or welfare is provided. Piven and Cloward hypothesize that society provides welfare to achieve two objectives: to maintain civil order and to enforce

work. To forestall revolution or property losses, such as was feared would occur during the Great Depression of the 1930s or during the civil unrest of the 1960s, the welfare system was expanded. In stable periods, welfare was provided in such a manner as to ensure that those who were able to work would do so. Frances F. Piven and Richard A. Cloward, *Regulating the Poor: The Functions of Public Welfare* (New York: Vintage Books, 1993).

Whether the motives underlying charity differ, that is, altruism or to control labor, is not essential to the argument presented, as both hypotheses assume that the political power of the nonpoor decides the amount and conditions by which welfare is provided to the poor. The acceptance of higher taxes to pay for welfare, either for purposes of altruism or because of a desire to control the poor, is based on the self-interest of the nonpoor.

4. Edgar K. Browning and Mark A. Zupan, *Microeconomic Theory and Applications*, 8th ed. (Hoboken, NJ: J. Wiley, 2004). ("There is no case, however, where the recipient is better off with a subsidy to a particular good than with an equivalent cash subsidy.")

5. Rather than basing welfare spending on a charitable motivation, Overbye claims such programs are consistent with the self-interest of the median voter, based on a demand for insurance among different risk categories in the electorate. Even though the beneficiaries may, at any time, be those with low incomes, the demand for such insurance programs results from market failure and has majority backing. For example, everyone runs the risk of growing old, not having a pension, or not having the funds to pay for medical care. Unemployment can also occur to anyone during his working life. Market failures may make it too costly to purchase private insurance against such events, and those who perceive themselves to be of higher risk in these categories want to shift their insurance costs toward lower risks. Einar Overbye, "Explaining Welfare Spending," *Public Choice* 83 (1995): 313–335.

6. A prediction of the above theory could be made with respect to Secretary of Education William Bennett's proposal in the first Bush administration. At that time, the federal government was spending $3.6 billion a year for remedial aid. These funds were distributed directly to the school districts and were in addition to the large support provided by each state to its own school systems. Bennett's proposal was to take an average of $600 per student from the federal monies and, instead of giving it to the school district, give it directly to the parents of educationally disadvantaged children in the

form of a voucher, which could only be used for education. The voucher could then be used at a public school in that district or at another school outside that district. Thus, if a school in a ghetto area is not adequately serving its children, the parents could use that voucher to secure a better education for their children at another school.

The New York City Board of Education, among others opposed Bennett's proposal. A voucher system permits parents of disadvantaged children greater choice in finding a school that would best serve the children's educational needs. However, a voucher threatens the monopoly position of the schools that do a poor job in serving disadvantaged children. Producer (teacher's union) interests have prevailed over those of low-income families regarding the education of their children.

7. Anthony Downs, *An Economic Theory of Democracy* (New York: Harper & Row Publishers, 1957), 198–201; George J. Stigler, "Director's Law of Public Income Redistribution," *Journal of Law and Economics*, 13, no. 1 (April 1970): 1–10; and Gordon Tullock, *Economics of Income Redistribution* (Boston: Kluwer Academic Publishers, 1997).

The median voter model is similar to the consumer choice model in the private market for explaining demand for goods and services and the supplier response to those demands. Utility maximization by consumers and profit maximization by firms lead those firms to produce goods and services according to consumer preferences. Consumer demands are expected to vary according to relative prices and their incomes. Utility maximization by voters and legislators, and political competition among legislators, is similarly expected to result in policies that reflect the interests of the median voters, who are assumed to be those families with median income. Comparable to the outcomes expected in the private sector, the output of the public sector, namely tax and expenditure policies, is expected to be consistent with the demands of the median voter. The use of a "taxpayer choice" model suggests that governments are hypothesized to act as if they were attempting to maximize the well-being of those with median family incomes.

8. Gordon Tullock, *The Economics of Wealth and Poverty* (New York: New York University Press, 1986), 59.

9. Bruno S. Frey, "Why Do High Income People Participate More in Politics?" *Public Choice* 11 (Fall 1971): 101–5.

10. Robert H. Bremer, ed. *Children and Youth in America*, vol. II, Parts 7 and 8 (Cambridge, MA: Harvard University Press, 1971), 1438.

11. Ibid.

12. Ibid., 1442.
13. Ibid., 1443.
14. *Congressional Quarterly Almanac*, 1969: 843.
15. Ibid. When one congressman questioned "why the small taxpayers should be asked to subsidize a milk program for the children of . . . private schools which obtain students from very wealthy families," the sponsor of the legislation (Representative Poage, Chairman of the House Agriculture Committee) responded, "A child from the wealthiest home is just as subject to malnutrition as is a child from some other home."
16. Congressional Quarterly, *Congress and the Nation*, 1945–64 ed., Washington, DC, 1965: 740–41.
17. Lawrence M. Friedman, *Government and Slum Housing: A Century of Frustration* (Chicago: Rand McNally and Company, 1968), 95.
18. Housing policy generally consists of two parts; the first is establishing and enforcing housing codes. The second is providing subsidies for housing construction and/or rehabilitation. The above discussion is concerned with federal subsidies, the major federal approach. Housing codes have primarily been state and local government functions. Early tenement laws were directed at containing epidemics (cholera) and fires, each of which threatened the entire city, not just the slum areas. Later housing codes, whose effect was greatest in slum areas, were initiated by social reformers around the turn of the century. Although slum landlords opposed these measures, they were not an effective political force. They were small landlords, generally living in the slums themselves (Lawrence M. Friedman, Ibid, 33), and through magazines and newspapers they were portrayed as venal persons. The publicity generated by the social reformers resulted in the passage of housing codes. The enforcement of these codes, however, varied. Once these laws were passed, the reformers believed they had achieved their goal. They had little concern with the administration and enforcement of the codes. Modern housing codes were a prerequisite for cities to qualify for federal urban renewal subsidies.

    Housing code policy imposes costs on landlords to upgrade their buildings. Because there are no excess profits in slum housing (otherwise there would be a rush to invest in slums, rather than to abandon them), an increase in costs results in a decrease in supply of such housing. Although such a policy will halt the deterioration of housing in an area (if enforced) and thereby benefit the rest of the community, it will also eliminate slum housing. Unless subsidies are provided to house the displaced, they may then be worse off.

19. Ibid., 147–72.
20. James E. Krier, "The Rent Supplement Program of 1965: Out of the Ghetto, Into the . . . ?" *Stanford Law Review*, 19 (1967): 563.
21. Lawrence M. Friedman and James E. Krier, "A New Lease On Life: Section 23 Housing and the Poor," *Pennsylvania Law Review* 116 (1968): 612.
22. Ibid., 633.
23. This discussion is based on Winifred Bell, *Aid to Dependent Children* (New York: Columbia University Press, 1965).
24. Henry Aaron, *On Social Welfare* (Cambridge, MA: Abt Books, 1980): 72.
25. Ibid., 62.
26. George P. Shultz, "Reflections on Political Economy," in *The Economic Approach to Public Policy*, eds. Ryan C. Amacher, Robert D. Tollison, and Thomas D. Willett, (Ithaca, NY: Cornell University Press, 1976), 486.
27. Daniel P. Moynihan, *The Politics of a Guaranteed Income* (New York: Random House, 1973), 306.
28. Ibid., 311.
29. Ibid., 312.
30. Ibid., 325.
31. W. Lee Hansen and Burton A. Weisbrod, *Benefits, Costs, and Finance of Public Higher Education* (Chicago: Markham Publishing Co., 1969), 76.
32. Paul J. Feldstein, *Health Care Economics*, 6th ed. (Clifton Park, NY: Thomson Delmar Learning Co., 2004), 417.
33. Ibid., 386.
34. It is not difficult to think of other universal programs that have middle-income rather than low-income groups as their prime beneficiaries. For example, the interest deduction for home mortgages on the federal income tax benefits middle- and higher-income families rather than those with low incomes. Persons with higher incomes are more likely to itemize, and the deduction is worth more to someone in a higher income-tax bracket. The military draft was another universal program. Many children from middle-class and high-income families were able to avoid being drafted during the Vietnam War as they were able to take advantage of college deferments. Opposition to the war would have started much earlier had these deferments been unavailable to the middle class.
35. U.S. Department of Agriculture, National Agricultural Statistics Service, 2002 Census of Agriculture, http://www.nass.usda.gov/census/census02/volume1/us/index1.htm.

36. *Farm Programs: Information on Recipients of Federal Payments,* GAO-01-606, (Washington, DC: U.S. General Accounting Office, 2001), 14.

37. Brian M. Riedl, "Another Year at the Federal Trough: Farm Subsidies for the Rich, Famous, and Elected Jumped Again in 2002," The Heritage Foundation, *Backgrounder No. 1763,* May 24, 2004, http://www.heritage.org/Research/Budget/bg1763.cfm.

38. Farm subsidy recipient statistics are provided by the Environmental Working Group at http://www.ewg.org.

39. Nicolas Heidorn, "The Enduring Political Illusion of Farm Subsidies," *San Francisco Chronicle,* August 18, 2004, B9.

40. Dan Morgan, "Farm Subsidies May Not Face Limits: Lawmakers Would Have to Find Other Ways to Cut Costs," *Washington Post,* April 15, 2005, A23.

41. "New Farm Program Isn't Likely to Ease Crisis," *The Wall Street Journal,* December 20, 1985, 6.

42. Bruce Gardner, "Agriculture Relief Legislation in 1998: The Bell Tolls for Reform," *Regulation* 22 (1999): 31–34.

43. Riedl, "Another Year at the Federal Trough: Farm Subsidies for the Rich, Famous, and Elected Jumped Again in 2002."

44. John D. Donahue, "The Political Economy of Milk," *The Atlantic Monthly,* October 1983, 59–68.

45. U.S. Department of Agriculture, 2005, http://www.ers.usda.gov/briefing/farmincome/data/cr_t3.htm.

46. Although price supports are the overriding concern of dairy farmers, Donahue states, "[It is] too dull and confusing an issue for most voters to know or care much about it. Opposing the system would be likely to lose votes without winning any. Finally, pressing the matter means declaring war on powerful colleagues who have made political careers out of protecting price supports." Donahue, "The Political Economy of Milk," 63.

47. James H. Schulz, *The Economics of Aging,* 7th ed. (Westport, CT: Auburn House, 2001), chapter 5.

48. Edgar K. Browning, "Why the Social Insurance Budget Is Too Large in a Democracy," *Economic Inquiry* 13 (1975): 373–88.

49. Schulz, *Economics of Aging,* 192–13. See also, Robert Moffitt, "Trends in Social Security Wealth by Cohort," in *Economic Transfers in the United States,* ed. Marilyn Moon (Chicago: University of Chicago Press, 1984), 327–58; and D. Mark Wilson, "Who Pays the Payroll Tax? Understanding the Tax and Income Dynamics of the Social Security Program." Heritage Center for Data Analysis, March 3, 2000. http:// www.heritage.org.

50. Social Security Administration, *The Future of Social Security*, March 2005, http://www.ssa.gov/pubs/10055.pdf.

51. U.S. Census Bureau, 2005, http://www.census.gov/prod/2004pubs/p60-226.pdf.

52. John A. Brittain, *The Payroll Tax For Social Security* (Washington, DC: The Brookings Institution, 1972).

53. The earnings base on which the Social Security tax is applied was increased in recent years, thereby increasing its progressivity. The maximum wage taxable for Social Security was $90,000 in 2005.

54. One analysis of the Social Security system method of financing concluded, "The regressivity and other inequities of the payroll tax, rather than its stabilization and allocative-efficiency effects, are the grounds for considering it inferior to the personal income tax. The major differences that exist between the two taxes—the exemptions, the personal deductions, and the broader income concept under the personal income tax—argue in favor of the personal income tax rather than the payroll tax. The payroll tax bears too heavily on low-income persons and on those with heavy family responsibilities." Joseph A. Pechman, Henry J. Aaron, and Michael K. Taussig, *Social Security: Perspectives For Reform* (Washington, DC: The Brookings Institution, 1968), 188.

55. U.S. Census Bureau, 2005, http://www.census.gov/population/www/socdemo/voting.html.

56. U.S. Census Bureau, *America's Families and Living Arrangements, 2004*, http://www.census.gov/population/www/socdemo/hh-fam/cps2004.html.

57. Samuel H. Preston, "Children and the Elderly: Divergent Paths for America's Dependents," *Demography* 21 (1984): 447.

58. U.S. Census Bureau, *America's Families and Living Arrangements, 2004*, http://www.census.gov/population/www/socdemo/hh-fam/cps2004/tabAVG3.csv.

59. Donald O. Parsons, "Demographic Effects on Public Charity to the Aged," *Journal of Human Resources* 17, no. 1 (1982): 144–51.

60. Preston, "Children and the Elderly," 447.

61. Ibid.

62. Peter H. Schuck, "The Graying of Civil Rights Laws," *The Public Interest* 60 (Summer 1980): 69–93. This article is based on a larger article by the same author, "The Graying of Civil Rights Law: The Age Discrimination Act of 1975," *Yale Law Review* 89, no. 1 (1979): 27–93.

63. Schuck, "The Graying of Civil Rights Laws," 76–77.

64. Congressional Budget Office, S.1536 Older Americans Act Amendments of 2000, August 25, 2000, http://www.cbo.gov/showdoc.cfm?index=2359&sequence=0.

65. Schuck, "The Graying of Civil Rights Laws," 90.

66. Data for 2004 and estimates for 2015 come from Congressional Budget Office, *The Budget and Economic Outlook: Fiscal Years 2006 to 2015*, January 25, 2005, http://www.cbo.gov/showdoc.cfm?index=6060&sequence=4.

67. U.S. Special Committee on Aging, United States Senate, *Developments on Aging* (Washington, DC: U.S. Government Printing Office, 1984).

68. Patricia Ruggles and Marilyn Moon, "The Impact of Recent Legislative Changes in Benefit Programs for the Elderly," *The Gerontologist* 25, no. 2 (1985): 156.

69. Ibid., 159.

70. "Political Pressures Build to Assure Social Security Increases," *Wall Street Journal*, March 28, 1986, 1.

Under pressure to balance the budget and to limit cutbacks in projected expenditures for Medicare, congressional Republicans and Democrats changed the formula by which the aged receive cost-of-living adjustments. Congressional testimony by a group of economists stated that the Consumer Price Index overstates the amount of inflation in the economy. Therefore, limiting the cost-of-living adjustment to the Consumer Price Index minus one percent saved several hundred billion dollars.

71. Rent control can also be analyzed as a universal program. Rent control was legislated in a number of cities ostensibly to prevent sharp increases in rents from occurring when there has been a rapid increase in demand. The immediate beneficiaries of this legislation are renters, regardless of their incomes. The losers are landlords. Sharply increased rents represent a large increase in an obvious cost to renters. Thus, it is in the renters' economic interests to prevent this cost from being imposed. The key issue is whether renters can organize to effectively present their case to legislators. If renters can organize themselves then they represent, in terms of votes, more political support than landlords.

The longer-run effects of rent control, however, are a deterioration in the stock of housing and the elimination of rent controls on new housing. With the decrease over time in the number of rent-controlled housing units, the overall supply of housing is less than what it would otherwise have been, and the overall rental price is greater. There is less old housing available, a greater increase in new housing (because it is decontrolled), with consequently higher rents. One additional result is that with a decline in the supply of rent-controlled housing over time, those with lowest incomes are forced out of the area or must pay higher prices for housing.

72. Data from Congressional Budget Office, 2005, http://www.cbo.gov/showdoc.cfm?index=6060&sequence=4

73. Not all legislators need receive political support from each interest group that desires a particular legislative benefit. Through the process of logrolling, legislators receive backing for their own special-interest bills by voting for other legislators' special-interest legislation.

MEDICARE

After completing this chapter, the reader should be able to

- contrast Medicaid and Medicare,
- explain how Medicare satisfied two competing economic protagonists, AFL-CIO unions and the AMA,
- discuss why Part A and B of Medicare were financed by different taxes,
- identify who bears the burden of a payroll tax, and
- describe the "free choice of provider" provision and explain why it was removed from Medicaid but not Medicare.

Medicare is a universal program providing the same benefits to all the aged who contributed to the Social Security system (the eligibility requirements have been relaxed since it was enacted in 1965). At the time of its enactment there were two basic parts to Medicare: Part A is predominantly for hospital care, and Part B covers physician and outpatient services. Part A is financed by the establishment of a Medicare portion of the Social Security tax; Part B is a voluntary program in which the participants pay 25 percent of the premium and federal tax revenues subsidize the remainder. Both Parts A and B have deductibles and cost-sharing requirements. Medicaid is a means-tested program for the medically indigent of all ages that is administered by the states. The federal government contributes to the cost of Medicaid, and this amount varies from 50 to 80 percent of the cost of the program, depending on the state's per capita income. The federal government also sets minimum eligibility criteria and benefits, but each state may increase the eligibility of different population groups and increase the benefits received. Medicaid is financed from general taxes at both the federal and state levels.

Alternative hypotheses have been put forth about the passage and design of Medicare. One explanation involves the altruistic desire to help the elderly. There were (and still are) many poor elderly whose needs for medical care exceed those of the rest of the population.

Viewing Medicare as a charitable redistribution program does not satisfactorily answer certain questions, however. First, why was it necessary to enact two separate programs, Medicare and Medicaid, each with different and distinct financing mechanisms, to provide for the medical needs of all the aged on the one hand and the poor on the other (Medicaid is means tested while Medicare is not)? Second, how could the poor elderly be expected to pay the deductible and coinsurance requirements of Medicare, or to purchase the subsidized physician coverage (Part B)? Third, why were Medicare benefits established by Congress and the program administered by a federal agency, when Medicaid is a state-administered program with benefits that can vary by state? Further, why should Medicare Part A, which is in theory a redistributive program to aid a disadvantaged population, be financed by a regressive tax?

The case for Medicare as a charitable redistribution program might be made along the following lines. First, legislators may have lacked information on the effect of various provisions of the legislation. Second, the legislation may have been unduly influenced by certain powerful legislators to reflect their own preferences. And third, there may have been certain "political realities" that had to be accommodated. However, an explanation based on altruism and charity but relying on a number of explanations specific to that legislation is not as useful (nor generalizable to other redistributive programs) as an alternative, simpler, self-interest hypothesis. Further, how well can an assumption of altruism, modified by knowledge of the particular participants involved, predict likely legislative changes in Medicare?

The self-interest paradigm of legislation provides an alternative explanation for the development of Medicare. It also provides alternative predictions about the likely outcome of legislative changes to ensure the viability of Medicare.

The assumption of charity serves as a good explanation for Medicaid, over which there was little controversy. Medicaid is an in-kind subsidy, that is, medical services rather than cash, to the recipients who are defined as low-income persons of all ages who meet a strict means (income and asset) test. Medicaid was a continuation of previous welfare programs to provide medical services to the poor. Before Medicaid there was the Kerr-Mills legislation (1960), and before that a system of federally subsidized payments to providers. These medical assistance programs for the poor engendered little debate in Congress (although the generosity of benefit levels did).[1]

Thus, the motivations for the Medicaid and Medicare programs are different. Any income-related program, for which a means test is required, can be reasonably explained by the assumption of charity on the part of the middle class and producers lobbying for legislation to increase the demand for their services. The purpose of income-related programs is to help those who are less fortunate. These welfare programs are financed more equitably, namely through general taxes rather than through excise taxes (i.e., a specific tax on either goods and services or on labor). The poor are the principal beneficiaries of income-related programs. The generosity of the benefits and the method used to implement the means test reflect the society that bestows these programs. Medicaid benefits and eligibility were permitted to vary by state because the amount of charity the population is willing to subsidize varies by state income, the cost of providing charity (the costliness of medical care), attitudes toward charity, and so on.

Programs such as Medicare and Social Security, however, do not have as their primary purpose an altruistic motivation. These programs are "universal"; all persons within a particular group are eligible regardless of income. Universal redistributive programs are based on motivations similar to those of special-interest groups. The political process is used to transfer wealth from one group to another. It is within this framework that the legislative struggle over Medicare is examined.

The Passage of Medicare

The legislative fight over Medicare was emotional and lasted many years before being resolved in 1965. The legislation that emerged was the result of a number of compromises and differed from what was initially proposed.[2] Two parts of the Medicare legislation that were not changed, and that were the basis for much of the conflict, were basing eligibility on age (not income) and financing the program through an additional Social Security–type tax. These two aspects were in fact related. If a person paid into Social Security, then upon retirement he would be entitled to the program's benefits; it would be an "earned right." If, as the bill's opponents preferred, eligibility were based on a means test, then the appropriate financing mechanism would have been general tax revenues.

Attempts at compromise in the years before the passage of Medicare involved the structure of benefits; its proponents were even willing to endorse a catastrophic program. But a comprehensive catastrophic plan that was means tested, proposed by Senator Russell Long, (an opponent of Medicare) was defeated.[3] The one element for which there could be no compromise was the method of financing; it had to be financed by a separate Social Security–type tax. At one point, Medicare opponents proposed an increase in Social Security cash payments to retirees. Medicare proponents were opposed to these higher cash payments because they believed the increase in Social Security taxes to fund the cash payment would prevent later passage of Medicare, which would also have necessitated a similar tax increase.[4]

To understand the reasons for the conflict, why it lasted so long, and the final form of the legislation, one must know who the major interest groups were and how they perceived the proposed legislation would affect their economic interests. The battle over Medicare was a battle over economic self-interests.

Economic Interests

The major protagonists were health providers, spearheaded by the AMA, and the American Federation of Labor and Congress of Industrial Organizations (AFL-CIO) unions. Organizations representing the elderly also became active, stimulated by the AFL-CIO. There were many important participants, particularly Wilbur Mills, chairman of the House Ways and Means Committee, and Senator Robert Kerr, who, until his death in late 1962, was a strong opponent of Medicare. And finally, when President Johnson was elected in 1964, the resulting Democratic landslide changed the composition of Congress, thereby increasing the prospects for passage of Medicare.

Unions

The unions were in the forefront of the battle for Medicare.

> The executive committee of the AFL-CIO had decided early in 1957 to commit the 14 million-member labor federation to an all-out battle for Government health insurance. In contrast with earlier rounds, the AFL-CIO took on a leadership role. Government health insurance was pressed as labor's number one legislative priority, and organized labor became the rallying point for all those who favored the measure.[5]

Further,

> Partly at the urging of labor leaders, all the major contenders for the Democratic Presidential nomination (1960) lent their endorsements to the social security approach.[6]

Still another indication of the leadership and influence of the unions on the shape of the Medicare legislation is provided in the following discussion of the confusion among Medicare's supporters to an amendment proposed by Senator Long.

During the debate, several liberal senators who were uncertain about which way they should vote were told that the AFL-CIO was behind the amendment. When the story reached (Wilbur) Cohen, who was on hand outside the chamber, he rushed to a telephone and called Cruikshank (Director of the AFL-CIO's Department of Social Security) to ask if it was true. Cruikshank said it wasn't, and hurried over to the Capitol, where he found Douglas and Gore trying to rally the Medicare forces, and told them where the unions stood. Douglas and Gore passed the word around.[7]

The AFL-CIO's interest in this legislation was its desire to increase the wages of their working members. The AFL-CIO unions, such as the UAW, generally had the highest-paid employees and the most generous employer-paid health benefits. Retirees' health costs were paid by the employer (negotiated by the union) and represented a growing labor cost to the firm. Covering union retirees with Medicare would decrease employer payments. Medicare would substitute government financing of healthcare for the employers' health insurance payments. Reducing such employers' payments would lower the cost of labor to the firm. The released funds could then be used to increase workers' wages.

As a side note, retiree health benefits were not prefunded; they were paid out of current labor costs to the firm. The union and the employer negotiated a total labor cost package, which included payments to union retirees. The employer's interest is in the total cost of labor, not how it is divided among current or former union members. If, for example, 20 percent of those labor costs were paid for retirees' health costs, that meant current union workers would receive 20 percent less than if someone else (taxpayers) paid their retirees health costs. After eventually achieving Medicare coverage of their retirees, the union's policy goal was to have the government (taxpayers) cover the health costs of their union members under a comprehensive national health insurance system. If the firm no longer had to pay health benefits for employees, which is part of the cost of labor, then labor could receive higher wages.[8]

The unions' insistence on using the Social Security (payroll tax) mechanism to finance Medicare can be explained within the context of union self-interest. Although union members might have favored Social Security financing for noneconomic reasons, it is unlikely that this approach would have received such strong union support unless it was also consistent with the union's economic self-interest. Social Security financing would have determined eligibility for Medicare. All union retirees would therefore be eligible.

Basing eligibility on a means test would have excluded large numbers of retirees from those unions that were part of the AFL-CIO. From the unions' perspective, even though Social Security is a regressive tax with the heaviest burden falling on low-income workers, the unions' retirees would, at no additional cost, immediately become eligible to receive the benefits, as would the rest of the unions' workers when they retire.[9] (The Medicare Part A payroll tax was three tenths of one percent of earned income up to $6,000 income. Thus, this separate Social Security tax to fund Medicare Part A was regressive because the tax represented a greater portion of the wage for a low-income worker than a high-income worker.)

Although the unions insisted on a separate payroll tax up to a specified income limit for financing Part A of Medicare (hospital services), they were not opposed to using general federal taxes to finance Part B (physician services). The likely reason for this inconsistency is that eligibility for Part B was already determined by Part A. Therefore, the union's members would have been eligible because they contributed to Social Security.

Increased Social Security taxes on union employees to pay for Medicare (or for a comprehensive national health insurance program, such as the UAW desired would have cost the unionized employee less than the amount the employer was paying for health insurance on behalf of UAW members. Thus, there would be a subsidy from low wage–low health users in other industries to high wage–high health users, such as UAW employees. This type of cross-subsidy, which is clearly inequitable, has in fact occurred under "community rating" by Blue Cross in Michigan to UAW employees.[10]

The Aged

To pressure Congress into enacting Medicare, it was necessary for the AFL-CIO unions, the bill's proponents, to generate mass public support for Medicare among the aged and their supporters. Thus, the unions' strategy was to publicize Medicare's advantages to the aged and to organize the elderly into an effective political force. Wilbur Cohen had realized the immense political potential of this group. Referring to a 1952 Medicare bill of which he was coauthor, he said,

> At the time there were between twelve and thirteen million people over sixty-five, and every day there were a thousand more, almost all of whom were eligible to vote, and most of whom did. That's a massive political bloc. Generally speaking, older people are conservatives, but not when it comes to Social Security increases or government participation in health care.[11]

Self-interest transcends political beliefs. As the proposed beneficiaries of Medicare, the aged (and their children many of whom would have been financially responsible for their care) realized early the benefits to themselves. (Because the public debate over Medicare was in broad terms, proponents of Medicare became concerned that the aged believed the bill was more comprehensive than it really was.)[12]

The unions were instrumental in organizing the aged.

> A third project, aided by the [Democratic] White House and the Democratic National Committee as well, involved an effort to mobilize elderly people themselves in behalf of Medicare. . . . Starting with a nucleus of union retiree organizations . . . comprising several hundred thousand pensioners, the organizers of the National Council [of Senior Citizens] were able within a few months to build a loose confederation of senior-citizen groups (mostly union, golden-age, senior-center, and church groups) numbering about one million persons. Not only did the National Council establish itself as a spokesman for the elderly, but it was able to stimulate local political action through its various member organizations.[13]

It was ironic that Medicare's proponents favored limiting eligibility to only those aged already receiving Social Security, proposing limited benefits, and financing the program by a regressive tax. The opponents had countered with a more comprehensive set of benefits, to just the medically needy, proposing that the method of financing be based on general tax revenues, which is a more progressive form of taxation. Thus, self-interest was a more important determinant of the design of Medicare than altruism.[14]

Medicare became a very visible issue, in contrast to most congressional legislation. Representatives' votes and their positions on Medicare became known to their constituents. In each of the several congressional elections leading up to the landslide presidential election of 1964, it was believed that the aged and their supporters voted based on their representatives' positions on Medicare.

> President Kennedy was also impressed by the analysis of the election returns, and . . . decided to make a push for passage of the Medicare bill in 1962. "With a pivotal congressional election coming up this fall, [reported the New York Times] it was patent the Democrats hoped to claim a major achievement if the bill passed, or a campaign issue with real bite if it failed."[15]

In the congressional elections of 1962 the Democrats did much better than expected. They did not lose any congressional seats by candidates who campaigned for Medicare.[16]

American Medical Association

The passage of Medicare was viewed as a defeat for a powerful interest group, the AMA. Although other health groups such as the AHA were also opposed, the opposition was led by the AMA, which had been successful in defeating President Truman's proposal for national health insurance earlier. The AMA tried very hard to defeat Medicare; it hired public relations firms, contributed large sums of money in support of its position and to publicize its viewpoint to the public, and galvanized the support of its physician members around the country to present the AMA's viewpoint to legislators, patients, and local organizations.

The political power of the AMA was also based on legislators' fears that physicians would withhold their services if legislation adversely affecting physician interests was enacted. In 1962, 44 physicians at a hospital in New Jersey signed a petition stating that they would "refuse to participate in the care of patients under the King-Anderson bill or similar legislation."[17] (King-Anderson was an earlier version of Medicare.) Other physician groups around the country stated their support for the New Jersey physicians. Shortly thereafter, a provincial medical society in Canada refused to provide care in other than designated emergency centers after the provincial government imposed a medical plan that the physicians had opposed.[18] The fear that physicians would not participate in any Medicare legislation was real. As an interest group, the AMA was correctly viewed as being politically very powerful.

And yet, in retrospect, after Medicare was enacted over the opposition of the AMA, physicians were among its greatest beneficiaries.

The AMA believed its economic interests were threatened in two ways: first, that the government would set fees for physicians, and second, that the Medicare legislation would, over time, be extended to cover other nonneedy population groups. The AMA was not opposed to having subsidies provided on behalf of those who could not afford to pay for medical care. As an alternative to the Medicare proposals, the AMA eventually developed its own proposal for helping the medically indigent; it favored a tax-credit approach that varied according to a person's income. General tax revenues were proposed as the funding source for the tax credit.

Government subsidies for the medically needy would increase demand for physician services and result in increased physicians' incomes. As long as physicians could charge these subsidized patients the same fees they charged their other patients, their incomes would increase. Thus, it was essential to physicians that any legislation enable them to charge what they wanted—what the market would bear. The code name for such a pricing strategy was the physician's "usual and customary fee."

Extending government subsidies to population groups other than the medically indigent, however, would merely substitute government expenditures for the patient's expenditures. There would be little increased demand from this group while the government would become a larger payer of physician services. And as the cost of the program to the government increased, the government would try and control its expenditures by regulating physician fees. The AMA was also concerned that the concept of universality would be applied to other population groups in the future. The AMA viewed Medicare as a beginning step in the direction of a nationalized health service, similar to what existed in Great Britain at that time. If this occurred in the United States, physician incomes would be much lower.[19]

Subsidies to low-income groups are in the providers' economic interest (as long as the method of payment is according to the providers' preferences). In fact, the demand for government subsidies to pay for medical services for the medically indigent often originates from the providers themselves. For example, the main proponents for federal subsidies for "uncompensated care," which is the lack of (or inadequate) reimbursement for hospital care by certain population groups, is led by those hospitals most affected by it.[20]

If the government were to become responsible for the payment of a larger population group, the AMA feared that the government would want to become more involved in determining physicians' fees and, consequently, physicians' incomes. (The AMA's concern became a reality in the early 1970s with the establishment of the Medicare Economic Index, which set limits on physicians' fee increases.)

Higher-income patients were being charged the highest price physicians believed the patients could bear. If high-income aged patients were included in a government plan, then the price the government would pay the physician would be similar to its payment for low-income patients. A government fee that reimbursed the physician one price regardless of the patient's income would be less than the fee the physician charged the higher-income patient. It would be more to the physicians' interest if they could still charge the higher-income patient as they wished, while the government reimbursed them for care to those who currently could not afford physician services or for whom a physician was providing care at a low fee.

Charging the highest price the patient could bear is a profit-maximizing strategy. Such a pricing strategy would also imply that the physician would charge some patients more than others, in other words, the physician would price-discriminate. This does not imply that every physician always does this or even thinks in this way. There were even some physicians, although relatively few, who favored the Medicare legislation.

The continuance of a profit-maximizing pricing strategy, however, is a useful assumption for predicting the AMA's political positions, which represent the economic interests of its physicians.[21]

The AMA defeat occurred over the financing, hence eligibility, issue. Medicare Part A was financed by an addition to the Social Security tax, which ensured that all aged who had contributed to Social Security, regardless of their incomes, would be entitled to the programs' benefits. Thus, Medicare covered all aged receiving Social Security, not just the needy aged, which the AMA preferred. Except for this defeat, the AMA was victorious on all other issues.[22]

First, physicians were to be reimbursed according to their "usual and customary" fees for Medicare patients. Second, they were not required to participate in the program. If the physician participated, that is, accepted assignment, the government would pay the physician through an intermediary in the above manner. If the physician decided not to participate, then the physician could bill the aged person directly. The aged person would then have to seek reimbursement from the government, whose payment was less than the physician's fee. In this manner, physicians were free to decide which elderly patients to accept on "assignment" and which to bill directly.

Leaving the decision up to the individual physician whether or not to take assignment on a claim-by-claim basis enabled the physician to price-discriminate; the physician would accept the Medicare payment as payment-in-full for low-income patients, but for patients who had higher incomes, the physician could charge a higher fee. The ability to accept assignment on their own terms allowed physicians to continue charging according to ability to pay.[23]

Another important economic interest of physicians has always been the concept of "free choice" of provider, which the government also accepted. To physicians free choice means that no physician can be excluded from participating in any method of delivering medical services. Rather than being pro-competitive, free choice in medicine has been used to limit price competition among providers.[24]

An insurance company, for example, could not offer a policy at a lower premium by using a limited or closed panel of physicians who would charge a lower price. Under organized medicine's definition of "free choice," the insurance company would have to permit patients to go to any physician. Physicians would have no incentive to join an insurer's limited provider network by reducing their fees in the expectation that they would receive a greater volume of that insurer's patients if the insurer had to allow its enrollees go to any physician the patient chose.

Both PPOs and HMOs violate the AMA's free-choice concept, which explains why these organizations have been so opposed by organized medicine. The HMOs and PPOs compete for patients on the basis of lower premiums, increased benefits, or both. The patient in return has to limit her use of providers to only those participating in the PPO or HMO. By mandating the AMA's definition of free choice of provider under Medicare and Medicaid, the development of these alternative delivery systems was held back. Price competition between these delivery systems and private physicians and hospitals was precluded.

In 1981, as part of the Omnibus Reconciliation Act, the free choice of provider provision was removed from the Medicaid program. As a trade-off to save federal matching dollars the Reagan administration gave the states greater flexibility to manage their programs. Until 1981, states could not take bids from groups of physicians for the care of the state's Medicaid population. Nor were the states permitted to enroll Medicaid patients in HMOs. With the removal of the free-choice provision, states, starting with California, took bids from providers and negotiated contracts with HMOs for the care of the Medicaid population.

Although the free-choice provision was removed for Medicaid recipients, it remained in effect (and still is in effect) for Medicare beneficiaries. The aged now have the opportunity to join HMOs; however, unlike Medicaid recipients, they cannot be required to join. This difference in choices available to beneficiaries of these two programs reflects society's attitude toward charity. According to opinion polls, "The public is enthusiastic (66 percent) about requiring low income people to use less costly clinics or HMOs."[25] Most Americans, however, do not want to be subject to these requirements themselves.

Thus, although physicians opposed the financing and eligibility requirements of Medicare, they were able to structure the provider payment and participation aspects according to their economic interests. For those aged who were medically indigent, physicians would participate and receive their usual and customary fees, through their own physician-controlled fiscal intermediary, Blue Shield. Thus, there was no interference by the government in the scrutiny or setting of physician fees. When physicians believed elderly patients could pay more than the usual and customary fee, they did not accept assignment and charged these patients a higher fee.

Other Provider Interest Groups

The other provider interest groups that were important participants in the struggle over Medicare were the hospitals, represented by the AHA; Blue Cross organizations, which had been started by and were controlled by hospitals; and the commercial insurance companies.

Hospital utilization rates for the aged were greater than for any other age group. When the aged could not pay the hospital—and many of them did not have hospital insurance—it was not possible for community, not-for-profit hospitals to simply turn them away. Hospitals, however, could not recover their costs for the care of the aged. Hospitals bore the brunt of the problem of the medically indigent elderly, and many hospitals viewed these bad debts as a threat to the financial survival of the community hospital. For a number of years the AHA formed special committees to explore approaches to alleviating this growing financial problem.[26]

Up until 1962, the AHA had been a strong supporter of the AMA's position. However, as the problem of hospital bad debts for the aged increased, the AHA began to distance itself from the AMA. In 1962 the AHA declared that federal help in resolving this issue was necessary and that the method of financing (Social Security taxes) was secondary to that concern.[27] Although the AHA was willing to have a program funded by Social Security taxes, it still favored subsidies only to low-income aged, and it wanted these subsidies funneled through Blue Cross. The AHA was concerned, as was the AMA, that the government not pay hospitals directly.

The AHA was also quite successful in designing hospital payment to their liking under Medicare. Hospitals were to be paid their costs (whatever they were) "plus 2 percent." Hospitals also received an extra differential for nursing care to Medicare patients. Depreciation rules for hospitals were rewritten so that hospitals were to be reimbursed for assets that were already depreciated and for assets that were donated. Needless to say, like any cost-plus arrangement, there were no incentives to keep hospital costs from rising. Not only would hospitals receive their costs, but they would also receive an additional 2 percent. The incentive was to increase their costs. The effect of the legislation on hospitals was an embarrassment of riches. Their net income (as a percentage of total revenue) and their cash flow were greater than ever.[28]

Before Medicare, Blue Cross found itself in difficulty competing with the commercial insurance companies because of the aged. Blue Cross had been using a "community rating" approach for setting its premiums; all age groups, regardless of their utilization experience, were charged the same premiums. Because the aged had higher-use rates than younger populations, the younger groups were subsidizing the aged. As these subsidies increased, younger groups found that commercial insurance companies were designing insurance programs that charged premiums based on each group's experience (referred to as "experience rating"). As younger groups left the Blue Cross organizations, the community rates increased, which led to more young groups leaving. It was an unstable situation for Blue Cross.

The commercial insurance companies and Blue Cross also believed that by becoming the intermediaries between medical providers, hospitals and physicians, and the government, they would have a new source of revenue. The Medicare program would be administered by these third parties. The outcome of the legislation permitted hospitals and physicians to select the intermediaries. The winners in this phase were again the health interest groups.

The Redistributive Effects of Medicare and Medicaid

The direct beneficiaries of Medicare were the aged, both the poor and the nonpoor (including their families whose financial responsibilities were thereby lessened). Benefiting indirectly were the health providers, physicians, and hospitals, as well as union members, whose wages increased when union retiree's health costs were no longer paid out of current labor costs. The benefits to the aged were very obvious. The redistribution of wealth to the providers and union members were not. The costs of providing benefits to these groups were borne (and still are) by the younger, working generations.

The Aged

The aged clearly benefited, although some more so than others. They received increased access to medical services. Physician visits and hospital use by the aged rose. It has also been suggested that life expectancy has increased as a direct result of Medicare.[29]

A universal program that treats persons of different incomes alike will not result in equal use of services. Medicare uses deductibles and copayments. The aged also have to pay a premium to participate in Part B of Medicare. Thus, to low-income aged, the required out-of-pocket expenditures represent a greater barrier to the use of those services than to higher-income aged. Medicare data show that after the enactment of Medicare high-income aged used more physician services than did low-income aged. The data also show that blacks used more services from hospital outpatient departments than whites, whereas whites used more services from private physicians. Even after controlling for health status, higher-income aged used more physician services than those aged with lower incomes. In 1969, of those aged whose health was considered "poor," the highest-income aged had 60 percent more physician visits than the lowest-income aged.[30]

Those aged who could not afford the Medicare deductibles and copayments or who could not pay for services not covered by Medicare, generally chronic and long-term-care services, had to fall back on Medicaid, a means-tested program. States used varying levels of benefits and eligibility rules when they established their Medicaid programs. The federal government pays matching funds, but it is a state-administered and state-designed program. Initially, some states were very generous in their benefits and eligibility requirements. However, as the cost of the program began to increase, states became more restrictive. To qualify for Medicaid, an aged person cannot have more than several thousand dollars in assets, excluding a home. The effect of this requirement is that many aged have had to "spend down" to this limit, in effect bankrupting themselves, to qualify for Medicaid.

Many middle-class elderly people, and their children, are shocked to learn that if they or their spouses require long-term care, they must rid themselves of all their hard-earned assets to meet the Medicaid means test. The long and emotional fight over the use of a means-tested versus a universal program has not prevented many low- and middle-income elderly from having to rely on a means-tested program.

Physicians and Hospitals

Was it possible to anticipate the financial consequences of a universal redistributive system designed according to provider preferences? Medicare (without Part B) was estimated to cost less than $2 billion a year. In a statement that could probably match the accuracy of "Peace in our time," Robert Myers, the chief actuary for the Social Security Administration, testified that "according to our estimates . . . the financing provided in the bill . . . will be sufficient to finance the proposal for all time to come."[31] Federal expenditures for both Medicare Parts A and B and Medicaid, which was also designed according to provider preferences, exceed $400 billion a year.[32]

According to Wilbur Cohen, one of the major architects of Medicare, the rapid rise in federal expenditures for these programs, the unnecessary services, and the inefficiency and waste of the system were unforeseen.[33] The development of new technology could not have been anticipated. However, it is difficult to believe that providing universal coverage for a large population group, reducing their out-of-pocket prices for medical services, and placing limited constraints on the providers would not have a major effect on the rise in prices and expenditures. If hospitals were paid their costs plus 2 percent, physicians were to be paid their usual and customary fees, and there were limited, if any, controls on utilization, costs, or fees, what would constrain utilization and expenditures from rising?[34]

Although physicians had the medical responsibility for the patient's care, physicians were not fiscally accountable for that care. In addition to providing needed hospital care, hospitals also served as substitutes for the home and for nursing homes. Because hospitals were well reimbursed for their services, who objected if a patient preferred to stay a few extra days? If it was difficult to care for a patient at home, the physician would approve a longer stay in the hospital. If the hospital was not fully occupied, longer hospital stays would also be beneficial to the hospital.

During this period, the late 1960s and 1970s, private health insurance coverage among the working population was also increasing. As the cost of hospital care increased, so did the demand for insurance to protect against these high costs. (Less than 10 percent of hospital expenses are paid for by patients directly.) And as more of the hospital bill was reimbursed in full, the constraints limiting hospital cost increases became fewer and fewer.

Physicians and hospitals, and those employed by the hospitals, fared well as a result of Medicare and Medicaid.

The Working Nonaged

The working nonaged paid for Medicare and Medicaid in two ways: first, they paid higher payroll taxes to finance Medicare Part A and higher income taxes to pay for Medicare Part B, and second, they paid higher prices for medical services. Medicare stimulated demand for medical services by the aged, which led physicians and hospitals to increase their prices. These increased prices and expenditures were also passed on to the private sector. Consequently, employees paid higher premiums for their own health insurance. These increased prices for medical services led to a decrease in demand for health services by the nonaged.[35] The uninsured as well as those with the least comprehensive insurance policies were also those workers with the lowest-paying jobs.

Insurance premiums for medical services in the private sector increased as medical prices and utilization increased. Although the burden of these higher premiums affected everyone, their impact was proportionately greater on those with low incomes. Higher-income employees and unions with higher-income members did not bear as large a burden. Employer-purchased insurance is considered a nontaxable fringe benefit to employees. Had the employee received the fringe benefit in cash, for those higher-income employees in higher marginal tax brackets, a greater portion of it would have been taxed away. As the employer paid increased premiums for health insurance to keep up with rising medical care prices, this was not as great a loss to higher-income employees receiving tax-free benefits. Thus, higher-income employees did not bear the full cost of increased medical prices.

The method used to directly finance Medicare also placed a greater burden on low-income employees. When Medicare is viewed as a redistributive program based on economic interests rather than charity, the method insisted on for financing makes more sense. Medicare was financed by a separate payroll tax up to a maximum income limit. Both the employees' and employers' Social Security taxes were increased. However, as noted earlier, regardless of whether the tax is placed on the employee or on the employer, the effect is the same. The tax is borne by the employee.[36] The advantage of placing part of the tax on the employer is to disguise its cost to the employee; *it is not as visible.* Employees are unaware that they are also bearing the employer portion of the tax. The working-age population bears the cost of the Medicare program as it does the Social Security system.

The use of a payroll tax, such as used to finance Medicare Part A, is a clever method of financing a program for which the motivation is based on the desire for an intergenerational transfer of wealth rather than charity for the poor. The original group of aged that became eligible for Medicare had never contributed to the cost of the program. Subsequent aged have, on average, incurred higher Medicare Part A expenses than they contributed to the Medicare payroll tax when they were employed. The benefit-to-cost ratio is very different for future retirees compared to current or near-aged. Representing the tax as an entitlement for future retirees tends to blur the burden of this method of financing. Future retirees are unlikely to receive the same benefits as current or past retirees as the costs of medical care increase rapidly and the number of employees per aged decline. Rather than just increase the tax on the working population, the burden would become too great, and benefits to the aged will have to be reduced.

An increase in the Social Security tax to finance Medicare not only has this intergenerational effect but also places the heaviest burden on low-income employees. A fixed dollar amount (the Social Security tax) on a lower income represents a greater percentage of that income than if the tax were proportional to income. Hence Social Security is a regressive tax; lower-income employees pay a greater portion of their income than do higher-income employees. (Currently, the Medicare payroll tax has been increased to become a fixed portion of all earned income. Although this has increased the progressivity of the tax, it is still regressive because unearned income is not taxed.)

Another adverse effect of financing Medicare through an increase in Social Security taxes is that it raises the cost of labor—low-wage labor in particular—to employers. Employers cannot shift the entire payroll tax back to those employees whose wages are at or near the minimum wage. The resultant effect is a decrease in the quantity of low-wage labor demanded.

Thus, the method selected for financing Medicare placed a proportionately greater burden on the lowest-income employees; they pay a greater percentage of their income to finance the program, they have to pay increased prices for medical care, and their insurance coverage is more limited. These consequences are inconsistent with any program whose purpose could be considered charitable.

The Medically Indigent

Paradoxically, the one group also adversely affected by Medicare or any universal redistributive program is the poor. There are two reasons for this. First, the explosion in medical and hospital prices, and consequently in insurance premiums, resulting from the Medicare program has made it more difficult for the poor and near-poor, who are not covered by Medicaid, to receive care. At times these groups became medically indigent and qualified for Medicaid. However, not all of these groups sought Medicaid assistance or were eligible. Because Medicaid is administered by each state, there are wide variations in eligibility requirements; in some states, people may lose all of their eligibility if their income rises slightly above the cutoff level. Eligibility is not graduated according to income levels. In 2003, 57.9 percent of those below the federal poverty level were not covered by Medicaid because of differences in eligibility among states.[37]

Perhaps the major impact of Medicare on the medically indigent is the lost opportunity of what might have been done. In 2003 federal and state expenditures under Medicare and Medicaid exceeded $550 billion a year.[38] Both the aged and many of the poor benefited from the hundreds of billions of dollars spent on Medicare and Medicaid. However, a significant portion of government expenditures under Medicare are used by those in the middle- and high-income groups.[39] A more limited program that did not provide such large subsidies to middle- and high-income aged could have been redirected toward the poor. A federal program that emphasized the poor would have cost less, would have led to smaller increases in demand, and would not have caused rapid price increases.

Concluding Comments

The purpose of this chapter has been to discuss alternative motivations underlying the passage of Medicare and Medicaid. The charity motivation assumes that the purpose of these redistributive programs was society's desire to help the less fortunate. The self-interest paradigm views Medicaid as the result of middle-class charitable intentions and producer interests; it is directed solely at the poor. Medicare, however, is consistent with other self-interest legislation. The distribution of benefits and the burden of financing those benefits were based on the amount of political support— money and votes—available from the various groups. Members of Congress, in their desire to maximize their political support, redistributed wealth from those with little political support (namely, low-income workers and future generations) to those with more (the aged, their supporters, and the unions). Although the middle class may have been initially motivated by charity to assist the medically indigent, Medicare, as designed by Congress, was not structured for that purpose. Separate legislation, Medicaid, which was a continuation of previous welfare policy, was enacted to serve the needs of the poor.

The beneficiaries of Medicare were the aged, the poor and nonpoor (including their families whose financial responsibility was thereby lessened), health providers (particularly physicians and hospitals), and AFL-CIO union members. The benefits to the aged were very obvious: care at reduced prices. The redistribution of wealth to the providers was not meant to be obvious, nor was it initially so. These gains to providers were (and are) borne by the younger, working generations who pay increased taxes as well as higher premiums for health insurance.

There are several reasons for attempting to distinguish between alternative motivations describing the passage of Medicare and Medicaid. The first is to increase our understanding of why redistributive legislation occurs and the resulting effects on equity and economic efficiency. Regardless of the stated intent of such legislation, equity and efficiency were not the legislature's real intent. Separating the charitable motivation from universal redistributive programs clarifies the debate on how to best improve the problems inherent in Medicare and Medicaid. Should the medically indigent be the primary beneficiaries of these two programs? Those opposed to restructuring Medicare along the lines of a graduated means-tested program have appeared more virtuous than their opponents; they have claimed that the opponents want to remove the aged's "earned right." Even though the aged did not initially contribute to Medicare, the aged receive huge subsidies even today for Medicare Part A, and they only pay 25 percent of the cost of Medicare Part B. (And the aged receive another subsidy for prescription drugs as a result of the recently enacted prescription drug program, discussed in Chapter 11.) The consequences of maintaining the system to the poor, the young, and current workers have been neglected in this debate.

The second reason for differentiating between alternative theories is to distinguish between the true versus the stated intent of legislation. Understanding the actual intent of legislation provides one with an increased ability to predict legislative change.

If the motivation underlying Medicare and Medicaid were charity, a greater amount of charity could have been provided to those most in need, of all ages, if the funds for Medicare and Medicaid had been combined. A more comprehensive set of benefits could have been provided and a graduated means test could have been used. The working poor could also have been included and a more equitable financing mechanism could have been adopted. The efficiency by which the subsidies were provided could have been improved by greater use of managed care plans. Instead, the rapid growth in Medicare and Medicaid expenditures decreased the government's financial ability and the middle class' desire to provide more funds for the medically indigent.

There was, and is, insufficient political support for an efficient and equitably financed program for the medically indigent. Programs for the indigent are not designed by malevolent bureaucrats or politicians. Instead, they reflect the preferences of the middle class and the providers of those services. This is the reason true welfare programs (those that serve only the poor) are but a small proportion of all redistributive programs and, unlike universal programs, are less controversial when reductions are proposed.

Study Questions

1. Contrast Medicaid and Medicare in terms of their intended beneficiaries, the basis of each program's political support, and each program's method of financing.
2. How did the design of Medicare satisfy the two competing economic protagonists, namely, the AFL-CIO unions and the AMA?
3. Why was Medicare Part A financed by a regressive payroll tax and Medicare Part B financed through a progressive tax, namely general tax revenues?
4. Who bears the burden of a payroll tax? Why is half of the Medicare payroll tax imposed on the employer?
5. Describe the "free choice of provider" provision and explain why it was removed from Medicaid but not Medicare. Is this consistent with the public interest theory?
6. Using the two different theories of government, explain why attempts to reduce the rate of increase in Medicare and Medicaid expenditures will or will not treat both of these programs equally.

Notes

1. Robert Stevens and Rosemary Stevens, *Welfare Medicine in America: A Case Study of Medicaid* (New York: The Free Press, 1974), particularly 26–32.
2. For a legislative history of Medicare, see Eugene Feingold, *Medicare: Policy and Politics* (San Francisco: Chandler Publishing Co., 1966). See also, Richard Harris, *A Sacred Trust* (Baltimore, MD: Penguin Books, 1966); Theodore R. Marmor, *The Politics of Medicare* (New York: A. de Gruyter, 2000); In 1996 the Health

Care Financing Administration held an academic conference at the LBJ Presidential Library in Austin, Texas to commemorate the 30th anniversary of the implementation of Medicare. These papers are available online at http://www.ssa.gov/history/30thMedicare .html; *Legislative History of the Medicare Program to 2000*, Social Security Bulletin, Annual Statistical Supplement, 2000. This is a chronological list of the major changes in law governing various aspects of the Medicare program. It is available online at http://www.ssa.gov/history/pdf/hlth_care.pdf. [Sue A. Blevins, *Medicare's Midlife Crisis* (Washington, DC: CATO, 2001); and R. M. Ball, "What Medicare's Architects Had in Mind." *Health Affairs* 14, no. 4 (1995): 62–72.]

3. Feingold, *Medicare: Policy and Politics*, 119, 145–46. The Johnson administration opposed the Long plan on grounds that it violated "the principle of Social Security."

4. Ibid., 136.

5. Peter A. Corning, *The Evolution of Medicare . . . from Idea to Law*, Office of Research and Statistics, Social Security Administration Research Report No. 29 (Washington, DC: U.S. Government Printing Office, 1969), 78. This research report provides a survey of the development of the Medicare program in a larger historical context. It is available online at http://www.ssa.gov/history/corning.html.

6. Ibid., 83. Other indications of the unions' activity are the following: "The AFL-CIO had made a broad grassroots effort to carry the issue (the Forand bill) to the voters during the 1958 midterm elections" (82). Further, "On the other side, organized labor and its allies were equally busy promoting the bill. One project involved mobilization of local pressure in the districts of Ways and Means Committee members. Another involved helping a group of physicians organize in behalf of Medicare" (91).

7. Ibid., 211.

8. Few, if any, of the books detailing the history of Medicare discuss the economic interest of the unions as a reason for their strong support of Medicare and the reason for using the Social Security method of financing. By omitting the economic interests of the unions, the reader is left with the impression that the unions had no economic interests and were only concerned with the needy aged.

9. Marmor provides another explanation for the design of Medicare. It is based on society's lack of generosity. By tying eligibility to Social Security contributions it is implied that these contributions confer "rights" and that the program would not be viewed as a giveaway

(Marmor, *The Politics of Medicare*, 21). Some of the original architects of Medicare believed Medicare was an initial step toward a more comprehensive health program (single-payer system) that would include more population groups (Marmor, 20, 23, 61). Single-payer proponents have continued to propose expanding Medicare eligibility by including more population groups. The Medicare strategy was successful because singling out the aged generated great public sympathy (including the political support of children of the aged) while the real political fight was between the unions and the AMA over their economic interests.

10. Paul J. Feldstein, *Health Care Economics*, 6th ed. (New York: Delmar Publishing Co., 2004), 199–202.

11. Harris, *A Sacred Trust*, 64.

12. Marmor, *The Politics of Medicare*, 112.

13. Corning, *The Evolution of Medicare*, 91.

14. Marmor claims that the reason for opposing the more charitable plan was that Medicare's advocates did not believe states would implement the more generous plan (35). It is unlikely that this was the cause of the basic differences between the opposing sides. This explanation neglects the economic interests of the unions and the nonneedy aged. Because the basic conflict was over eligibility, with the emphasis on Social Security financing, it appears that it would have been easier to come to agreement over an implementation system.

15. Harris, *A Sacred Trust*, 138.

16. Ibid., 149.

17. Feingold, *Medicare: Policy and Politics*, 121.

18. Ibid., 122–23.

19. "The reformers' fundamental premise had always been that Medicare was only 'a beginning,' with increments of change set for the future." Marmor, *The Politics of Medicare*, 61.

20. As would be expected, according to the hospital advocates of federal subsidies for uncompensated care, any such subsidies should be given directly to those hospitals providing such care. Such a policy would be more to the economic interest of those hospitals than subsidies that would enable the payer of those services, that is, the State Medicaid program or the aged person, to purchase all their medical services through an HMO that would provide the same level of services to the medically indigent but use fewer hospital services in doing so.

21. For a discussion of price discrimination as practiced in medicine, and organized medicine's attempts to maintain it, see Reuben

Kessel, "Price Discrimination in Medicine," *Journal of Law and Economics*, (1) October 1958.

Under Medicare, each physician submitted his fees to a fiscal intermediary, such as Blue Shield. Physicians were able to update their fee profile each year. This was the same procedure used by physicians with privately insured patients participating in the Blue Shield program. As in the case of patients who had private Blue Shield coverage, physicians could participate on a claim-by-claim basis.

22. Coverage for nonhospital physician services was not initially included in the Medicare proposals. When it became clear that Medicare was going to pass the House Ways and Means Committee, House Republicans offered a plan (the Byrnes Bill) that included more comprehensive benefits; however, participation among the elderly was to be voluntary and the benefits were to be financed by general taxes. Not to be embarrassed by voting for a bill that was more limited, Chairman Mills added a physician component to Medicare (Part B) along the lines of the Republican proposal. Feingold, *Medicare: Policy and Politics*, 142.

Hospital-based physician specialists, such as anesthesiologists, radiologists, and pathologists, were also reimbursed according to the preferences of those physicians (Part B of Medicare) rather than being included in Medicare Part A, which was the administration's proposal and also hospital's preference. Feingold, *Medicare: Policy and Politics*, 143–45.

23. Lynn Paringer, "Medicare Assignment Rates of Physicians: Their Responses to Changes in Reimbursement Policy," *Health Care Financing Review*, no. 1 (Winter 1980) 75–89.

24. Charles D. Weller, " 'Free Choice' as a Restraint of Trade in American Health Care Delivery and Insurance," *Iowa Law Review* 69 (1984): 1351–92.

25. "Though polls show public support for the Medicaid program, in practice, eligibility for Medicaid is closely linked to the nation's welfare programs, and in striking contrast to Medicare, welfare is an area in which most Americans (71 percent) want no additional spending." Robert J. Blendon and Drew E. Altman, "Public Attitudes About Health Care Costs," *New England Journal of Medicine* 311 (1984): 614.

26. Corning, *The Evolution of Medicare*, 78–9.

27. Ibid., 92.

28. Paul J. Feldstein and Saul Waldman, "Financial Position of Hospitals in the Early Medicare Period," *Social Security Bulletin* 31

(1968): 18–23. See also, Karen Davis, "Hospital Costs and the Medicare Program," *Social Security Bulletin* 36 (1973): 18–36.

As federal reimbursement to hospitals for treating Medicare patients became less generous, the AHA proposed (1984) that hospitals be allowed to participate on the same conditions as physicians, namely on a case-by-case basis. Congress refused to go along with this. Such a proposal was opposed by aged organizations since its effect would be an increase in hospital charges to the nonpoor aged.

29. Karen Davis, "What Medicaid and Medicare Did—and Did not—Achieve," *Hospitals*, August 1, 1985, 41–42.

30. Karen Davis, "Equal Treatment and Unequal Benefits: The Medicare Program," *Milbank Memorial Fund Quarterly* 53 (1975), 457, 468–69. See also, Karen Davis, *National Health Insurance: Benefits, Costs and Consequences* (Washington, DC: The Brookings Institution, 1975), 85.

31. Testimony of Robert Myers, *Hearings Before the Committee on Ways and Means on HR 3920*, House of Representatives, 88th Congress Part 1 (Washington, DC: U.S. Government Printing Office, 1964), 58. Also see the insert between 28–29.

32. Federal expenditures in 2003 for Medicare Part A were $155 billion, Medicare Part B were $126 billion and Medicaid were $161 billion. Centers for Medicare and Medicaid Services, 2004 Annual Report of the Board of Trustees of the Federal Hospital Insurance and Federal Supplementary Medical Insurance Trust Funds, http://www.cms.hhs.gov/publications/trusteesreport/2004/. For Medicaid, see Congressional Budget Office, *The Budget and Economic Outlook: An Update*, September 7, 2004, at http://www.cbo.gov/showdoc.cfm?index=1944&sequence=0.

33. Wilbur J. Cohen, "Medicare, Medicaid: 10 Lessons Learned," *Hospitals*, August 1, 1985, 44–7.

34. It is likely that proponents of a single-payer system anticipated rapidly rising Medicare expenditures and hoped to use the rapid increase in expenditures as a justification for greater government control over costs and expenditures in both the public and private health sectors.

35. John Rafferty, "Enfranchisement and Rationing: Effects of Medicare on Discretionary Use," *Health Services Research* 10, no. 1 (1975): 51–62.

36. John A. Brittain, *The Payroll Tax For Social Security* (Washington, DC: The Brookings Institution, 1972).

37. U.S. Census Bureau, *Health Insurance Coverage in the United*

States: 2003, P60-226, Tables HI02 and HI03, http://ferret.bls .census.gov/macro/032004/health/toc.htm.

38. Centers for Medicare and Medicaid Services, Office of the Actuary: National Health Statistics Group, http://www.cms.hhs.gov/statistics/nhe/default.asp.

39. Previous research indicated that more than 50 percent of Medicare expenditures went to middle- and high-income aged. Mark McClellan and J. Skinner, "Medicare Reform: Who Pays and Who Benefits?" *Health Affairs* 18, no. 1 (1999): 48–62. More recent research claims that a majority of such expenditures go to those aged with lower incomes. Centers for Medicare and Medicaid Services, *Medicare Current Beneficiary Survey*, http://www.cms.hhs .gov/mcbs/CMSsrc/2002/sec4.pdf. The same data are discussed by Jay Bhattacharya and Darius Lakdawalla, *Does Medicare Benefit the Poor? New Answers to an Old Question*, NBER Working Paper No. 9280 (Cambridge, MA: National Bureau Of Economic Research, 2002.)

10

REDISTRIBUTIVE HEALTH LEGISLATION, MID-1980s TO 2000

After completing this chapter, the reader should be able to

- explain why the Medicare Catastrophic Act was enacted in 1988 and repealed in 1989,
- explain why President Clinton placed healthcare reform at the top of his policy agenda,
- list and explain which groups were in favor of an employer mandate,
- discuss why automobile companies and the UAW were in favor of the Clinton health reform plan,
- explain why President Clinton's healthcare reform plan failed,
- identify the main health insurance issues addressed by HIPAA,
- describe how ideological conflicts were resolved in SCHIP,
- assess why the Commission on the Future of Medicare was unable to develop a bipartisan consensus to reform Medicare, and
- name the groups that would be most affected by Medicare reform that proposes to reduce the rate of increase in Medicare expenditures.

Redistributive legislation creates winners and losers, but the losers have a greater motivation to protest. Winners are unlikely to be as aware of the benefits as losers are to their losses. The winners are either less well organized, such as the uninsured, or they lack the public support offered by potential losers. This chapter discusses several major legislative initiatives and the reasons why they were enacted or failed to become law. The importance of interest groups and the political support (or lack thereof) by the middle class was crucial to the outcome of these health initiatives. Equity and efficiency considerations were apparently irrelevant to the decision-making process.

The Medicare Catastrophic Coverage Act of 1988

In 1988 Congress, by an overwhelmingly majority, enacted the Medicare Catastrophic Coverage Act (MCCA). The 1988 legislation had bipartisan support in Congress and had received overwhelming approval from the public and from interest groups. The American Association of Retired Persons (AARP), generally considered to be the lobby group representing the aged's interests, was also supportive of the act. In 1989, one year later, Congress repealed the act.[1]

The MCCA was meant to correct a major shortcoming of the original Medicare Act by providing coverage for catastrophic expenses incurred by the aged. Chronically ill patients could incur many thousands of dollars of out-of-pocket expenses in the form of deductibles; copayments; and fees for uncovered services, such as prescription drugs. Under Medicare Part A (hospital coverage) all Medicare beneficiaries admitted to the hospital had to pay the same large deductible ($560 in 1988). If they were admitted to the hospital several times during the year, they were financially liable for the same deductible each time. Medicare Part B (physician and outpatient services), which was a voluntary program, although almost all the aged participated, required the aged to pay a monthly premium (equal to one-fourth of the cost of Part B), a $100 deductible, and a coinsurance of 20 percent of Medicare's fee for each physician or outpatient visit.

Unlike private health insurance, Medicare did not have a "stop-loss" benefit, which limits a beneficiary's out-of-pocket medical expenditure. The lack of stop-loss coverage was a financial hardship and forced many elderly to spend their limited resources and then become eligible for Medicaid. Middle- and high-income aged purchased supplementary (Medigap) coverage that covered most of their out-of-pocket payments.

The new legislation provided for unlimited annual hospital coverage for catastrophic illnesses (the aged would have to pay the $560 hospital deductible only once), 150 days of skilled nursing care, unlimited hospice care, and 38 days of home health care. Out-of-pocket expenses for Medicare Part B (physician and outpatient services) were capped at $1,370 (for 1990). In addition, new benefits were added to Medicare; mammography screening, respite care, and outpatient prescription drug coverage were to be phased in (with a deductible and copayment). The act was a very generous expansion of Medicare's benefits.

The AARP, the lobby group for the aged, had proposed adding an outpatient prescription drug benefit to the bill and once this occurred, they became a strong advocate of the new legislation. Congress, believing the AARP had the support of the aged, enacted the bill.

A change in federal budget policy caused Congress to use an innovative approach for financing these new benefits, which would prove to be the undoing of the MCCA.

In response to large federal deficits during the 1980s, Congress adopted a new budgeting process that was intended to limit Congress' generosity in providing new redistributive benefits. The costs of financing new benefits had to be made explicit; the expenditures expected to finance the new benefit and how those expenditures were to be raised were required to be spelled out. Thus, there was no way for Congress to avoid identifying those groups that would have to finance new benefits provided to other groups. The cost side of redistributive legislation, previously invisible, became obvious. Identifying legislative losers and the amount of their increased taxes was expected to limit Congress' tendency toward deficit financing.

President Reagan and the Democrats (who controlled both houses of Congress) were concerned with the large federal deficits and insisted that the new Medicare benefit not increase the deficit; further, both the president and Congressional leaders decided that the cost would be borne solely by Medicare beneficiaries. Requiring the aged to pay the full cost of new benefits was a break from the past; previously, Medicare benefits were heavily subsidized. In addition, for the first time, the aged were required to pay an *income-related* premium, which is a more equitable method of financing.

The aged with low incomes, who were not on Medicaid, would have benefited most from the MCCA. Had the new benefit been financed by a flat increase in the Part B premium, it would have been a financial hardship to the very group the act was intended to benefit. (An equal increase in the premium for all the aged would be similar to a regressive tax in that the increased premium represents a greater percentage of income for those with low incomes than from aged with higher incomes.) Those same aged who were supposed to benefit from the benefit would be unable to afford to pay the premium to receive the benefit.

The MCCA was to be financed by a $4 monthly premium for the catastrophic coverage; a monthly premium of $1.94 for the drug coverage, which would have a $550 deductible and a 50 percent copay; and a new income-related supplementary premium that could go as high as $800 per person or $1,600 per couple annually.

In another controversial change from the past, to ensure the fiscal solvency of the program, Medicare beneficiaries would have to pay the increased premiums *before* receiving their new benefits, which would be phased in over time.

During Congress' discussions before the bill's passage, the aged were unaware of the details of the new bill and its method of financing.

Congress had acted rationally, believing that by providing increased benefits to the aged, they would be rewarded at election time. Unfortunately, they acted on poor information. Although public hearings were held, the details and cost of the legislation were not clearly understood. An important function of lobbyists is to make sure legislators understand the position of their constituents and to represent their constituent's interests. Legislators believed the aged were in favor of the legislation because the AARP supported the legislation. However, the AARP has a large and profitable prescription drug business and the new drug benefit, which was the basis of their support for the legislation, would have increased the AARP's profits. The AARP had placed its own interests above those of its constituents, the aged.

As the redistributive effects of the MCCA became well known, opposition to change among the losers increased and their lobbying against the legislation intensified. The main opposition to the new bill and its method of financing came from higher-income aged who believed they were worse off under the new act because they would have to pay increased Medicare premiums for benefits they were already receiving through Medigap policies or from their employer's retirement plan. About 75 percent of the aged, mainly the middle- and high-income aged, had purchased supplementary insurance policies or received through private retirement programs many of the same benefits that were in the new legislation. (The new MCCA would have protected only about 25 percent of Medicare beneficiaries from catastrophic medical expenses.)

A growing backlash developed among senior citizen's organizations as the aged realized they would have to buy additional Medicare benefits, whether they wanted them or not, and, more importantly, they would have to pay an income-related surcharge that exceeded the value of the additional benefits. Senior citizens flooded congressional offices with angry letters and phone calls demanding that the bill be repealed.

The AARP continued to support the bill, maintaining that opposition to the bill was based on inadequate knowledge. However, local AARP chapters began to come out against the bill.

As opposition to the new bill increased, Congress was shocked, believing AARP support for the bill meant that they would receive the aged's gratitude for increased Medicare benefits. Instead, when legislators returned to their districts for town meetings, the aged were outraged at them. The climax of the opposition was extensively reported in the media.

A quote from the *Chicago Tribune* tells what happened:

"Congressman Dan Rostenkowski, one of the most powerful politicians in the United States, was booed and chased down a Chicago street Thursday morning by a group of senior citizens after he refused to talk with them about federal health insurance. Eventually, the six-foot four-inch Rostenkowski cut through a gas station, broke into a sprint and escaped into his car, which minutes earlier had one of the elderly protesters, Leona Kozien, draped over the hood."[2]

Congress got the message. After being enacted in 1988, the act was quickly repealed in 1989, a rarity in American politics.

Congress learned several important lessons from the repeal of the MCCA. Legislators became very cautious when considering new health reform proposals. Legislators believed they were misled by various interest groups, such as the AARP. Next time they would move more slowly to be certain of the political support behind their proposals. Second, instead of financing new benefits for the aged by having higher-income aged subsidize low-income aged, Congress would return to its previous approach for gaining senior's political support, providing them with increased benefits without having them bear the full cost of those benefits.

President Clinton's Proposal for Healthcare Reform, 1993 to 1994

Healthcare reform reemerged as a popular political issue in 1992 when a relative unknown, Harris Wofford, defeated a well-known Republican in a special election held in November 1991 to fill the unexpired term of the late Senator John Heinz, who had died in an airplane crash. Richard Thornburgh, a former two-term governor, resigned as U.S. Attorney General under President Bush to run for the U.S. Senate in Pennsylvania. He was expected to win the election easily. Wofford campaigned on the issue of healthcare reform and scored an upset victory.

Opinion polls indicated that the public was very supportive of health reform, an issue on which politicians from both political parties sought to capitalize. It was not clear, however, what health reform meant. Unions, large employers, and the middle class assumed they would keep their current coverage and would not have to pay increased premiums or additional taxes.

Although elected with only 43 percent of the popular vote, and with the Democrats in control of both houses of Congress, President Clinton believed he had both a strong public mandate and the means to reform the healthcare system.

Immediately upon taking office in January 1993, President Clinton announced the formation of a task force, headed by Hillary Clinton, to develop a proposal for healthcare reform. A large task force was formed to develop President Clinton's health plan. The administration kept membership on the task force and its deliberations secret, raising suspicions among many as to whether some interest groups would have greater influence over its deliberations than others. President Clinton wanted the task force to develop a detailed plan within 100 days so that the Congress could act on reforming one-seventh of the U.S. economy before the end of his first year in office. The complexity of the task, the administration's negotiations over the federal budget, and other factors delayed the administration's unveiling of its health plan until late in the year.

Given the high degree of public support for health reform, legislators within each of the political parties decided not to wait for the president to introduce his health plan; they introduced their own. About 100 House Democrats introduced a "single-payer" plan, while a similar number of Republicans introduced an "individual mandate," requiring all persons to have health insurance and subsidizing those with low incomes.[3] These competing plans differed with regard to the role of health insurers, the use of an employer mandate, and, more importantly, spending limits with implicit price controls. These different legislative proposals indicated Congress' deep divisions on health reform. The ideological differences in Congress on government's role in healthcare were huge.

President Clinton's very complex healthcare reform proposal, the Health Security Act, was driven by several factors. First, the president required the plan to provide for *universal coverage*; however, to achieve its goal of universal coverage, President Clinton needed to raise additional funds. The president was politically sensitive about additional taxes to pay for its health plan. Congress was against additional taxes; consequently, only increased cigarette taxes were proposed. Second, to be able to state that universal coverage could be achieved without increased income taxes, the Clinton administration proposed several redistributive mechanisms, the most important being an *employer mandate*.[4] (President Nixon had previously proposed a variant of an employer health insurance mandate in the early 1970s.) Employers would be required to pay 80 percent of their employees' health insurance premiums, and the employees would pay the remaining 20 percent. Subsidies would be provided to small firms and firms with low-wage employees.

Third, health insurance *premium increases would be limited by annual spending caps.* These caps would be equal to the inflation rate plus population growth, a rate of increase that was much lower than had been occurring and lower than any industrial country had been able to achieve on a sustained basis. Although the government would not directly institute price controls on hospitals and physicians, private insurance firms would be required to do so if they were to remain within their spending limits; otherwise they would have to ration care to their enrollees. Large *regional "health alliances"* (purchasing pools) and *national boards* were to be established, whose role, in large part, was to help control the introduction of new technology and premium increases. These alliances would collect insurance premiums from employers and individuals within a large geographic region and negotiate directly with private insurers.

After presenting his proposal, President Clinton threatened to veto any legislation that did not provide universal coverage.

The employer mandate had certain political advantages. Although it was equivalent to a tax on employers, the administration did not consider it to be a tax and therefore did not include these premiums as part of its budget to finance the plan. Requiring employers to purchase health insurance for their low-income employees reduces the number of uninsured, and decreases federal and state government expenditures for Medicaid, which is what the uninsured would otherwise have relied on.

Large employers and their unions, such as the auto industry and its union, the UAW, favored an employer mandate and spending caps. The auto industry had an older workforce and had incurred huge liabilities to pay for its retirees' health benefits. These firms' obligations to retirees and current employees would have been limited, while industries with younger employees and no retiree health benefits would have been burdened with larger costs. The Clinton plan set a maximum limit on the percentage of payroll taxes that each company was to pay under the employer mandate (about 11 percent). Because the auto companies were paying between 15 to 18 percent of payroll for their employees' health benefits, union members would be effectively rewarded with a 3 to 5 percent wage increase. Organized labor was concerned that rapidly rising healthcare costs were resulting in lower wage increases and higher employee cost sharing. Their higher health benefit costs would be shifted to the government (in reality to other firms and employees). More importantly, annual spending limits would have held down future employee and retiree medical cost increases, thereby saving money for the auto industry and permitting greater wage increases for union members.

Furthermore, an employer mandate would primarily affect low-wage firms whose employees did not have health insurance. The cost of low-wage labor would increase, thereby making them less competitive against higher-paid union labor. Large firms in competition with small firms favored the employer mandate as a means of increasing the costs, hence prices, of their competitors.

The Health Insurance Association of America (HIAA) favored an employer mandate because it would increase the demand for private health insurance (but strongly opposed the diminished role for health insurers in the Clinton plan). Hospital and physician associations also favored an employer mandate because it would provide coverage for the uninsured and shift low-wage employees and their families away from Medicaid onto private insurance, which paid higher fees.

According to various polls, the middle class also favored an employer mandate, believing the employer would bear the cost of the program. In this way the middle class could believe they would not have to tax themselves to provide coverage to those with low incomes. Presumably, the employer would bear the burden. It was to enforce this deception that the employer was obligated to pay 80 percent of the premium and the employee the remaining 20 percent. The visibility of the burden fell on the employer, even though, in reality, most of the cost would be shifted to the employee in the form of lower wages. (Polls also showed that the middle class was less supportive of an employer mandate if it meant the higher cost of labor would lead to a large loss of jobs. For this reason, both opponents and proponents of an employer mandate produced studies on job loss to support their viewpoint.)

The National Federation of Independent Business (NFIB), representing 600,000 small businesses, was the major interest group opposing the employer mandate and universal coverage. Most large employers already offered health insurance to their employees; thus, small businesses would be most affected by the increased cost to employers and employees, many of whom were low-wage workers. They were concerned that an employer mandate would increase their labor cost; employers would not be able to pass all their costs onto the employees, particularly for those at or near the minimum wage; they would have to lay off employees; and their profits would decrease. Small businesses, which are located in all Congressional districts, proved to be very effective lobbyists opposed to the employer mandate.

Although President Clinton offered subsidies to small businesses to induce them to support his plan, small business owners distrusted government and did not believe government subsidy promises would be kept, particularly given the huge federal deficit.

Mandated employer health insurance, however, would not meet any of the middle-class objectives, nor the objective of those desiring a less rapid increase in medical expenditures. In fact, by itself, an employer mandate would cause a more rapid increase in medical expenditures because it would increase the demand for medical services. Therefore, President Clinton's employer mandate had to be combined with spending caps, regional alliances, and national technology evaluation boards to meet the objectives of these other groups.

Interest-Group Lobbying

The Clinton plan was a major redistributive proposal. As such it would have resulted in many winners and losers. Although some interest groups agreed with certain parts of the Clinton plan, they were opposed by other interest groups. The different components of the plan drew different opponents. It intensified lobbying by interest groups and caused constituencies within an interest group to take opposing positions. Large trade associations, such as the AMA, health insurers, and the Chamber of Commerce, could no longer speak on behalf of all their members.

To receive the political support of certain organized groups, the administration included specific benefits for those groups. For example, to assist those companies with large unfunded retiree medical liabilities, the government proposed to pay for 80 percent of those costs. Over the opposition of HMOs who claimed it would limit their ability to control costs, the AMA was rewarded with an "any willing provider" amendment, which would enable physicians unaligned with closed panel plans to have access to patients in closed panels. (Kaiser was, however, able to exempt itself from this provision, thereby angering other HMOs.) The AMA was also promised exemptions from the antitrust laws, which would have allowed physicians to negotiate collectively with HMOs, as well as relief from large malpractice awards. Chiropractors, who gave $1.9 million to the Democrats in 1993, received permission under the Clinton health plan to receive payment for performing x-rays, something that was previously denied to them under Medicare. To secure the support of nurses, a provision was included that would remove barriers limiting the role of advanced-practice nurses. And the aged were promised new benefits, including a prescription drug benefit.

The AMA opposed Clinton plan's spending limits, fearful that they would result in a loss of physician autonomy and decision making. The AMA initially favored an employer mandate but was opposed by state medical societies. Lobby groups also threatened other lobby groups that supported elements they opposed; for example, the NFIB threatened the AMA over its initial support of the employer mandate, stating that the NFIB would favor government controls on physician fees. Large managed care insurers wanted to be able to choose their own participating physicians, while medical societies wanted all physicians to be able to participate in an insurer's provider network. Physicians also differed among themselves on the issue of closed provider panels.

Large and small health insurers also disagreed on aspects of the Clinton plan. The huge purchasing power that would be accumulated by the regional purchasing alliances would enable them to decide the number and types of health plans with which it wished to contract. Large insurers believed the health alliances would contract with them, while small insurers believed they would be excluded. The HIAA proved to be a very effective opponent of the Clinton health plan. Although the HIAA, representing smaller insurers, favored an employer mandate and universal coverage (it would have increased the demand for health insurance), it opposed those aspects of the plan that would limit employees' choice of a health insurance plan. Concerned for the survival of its member health plans, the HIAA introduced a series of television ads claiming that the government, not the individual, would choose the health plan and its benefits. Two characters, Harry and Louise, were used to dramatize their concern over loss of health plan choice. These ads received a great deal of publicity as the news media kept replaying them.

Large businesses favoring an employer mandate were opposed by small businesses; thus, the Chamber of Commerce could not speak on behalf of all businesses.

Proponents of redistributive legislation typically offer subsidies or benefits to a few groups to gain their support. However, the Clinton plan's redistributive effects were so large that subsidies could not be offered to all those adversely affected by some part of the legislation.

Many other interest groups lobbied for changes to protect or enhance their own economic interests. For example, legislators from tobacco districts were opposed to large increases in the cigarette tax, which was the only explicit tax the Clinton health plan relied on to provide subsidies to low-wage employees.

The Congressional Budget Office

Many legislators were skeptical that the new health plan could cover all the uninsured and subsidize low-wage employees by simply raising the cigarette tax. The health plan's cost estimates were sharply debated, as were the sources of funding.

The Congressional Budget Office (CBO) became very influential in the debate over the Clinton plan. In response to large federal deficits and legislators' proclivity for enacting new and expanded spending programs without specifying how they would be financed, Congress enacted the 1990 Budget Enforcement Act, which established limits on discretionary spending for 1991 to 1995. New federal programs that increased federal spending or reduced federal revenues (tax reductions) had to be paid for through increased taxes or other spending reductions. These were known as the "pay-as-you-go" (or paygo) rules, which could only be waived by a super majority of 60 Senators. The CBO was given the task of costing out ("scoring") new legislative proposals to determine whether they met the pay-as-you-go rules.

In an important announcement with significant political implications, CBO ruled that the cost of the Clinton plan would be higher than the administration estimated and that it would increase the deficit. Additional funds would be needed to pay for it.

The CBO also claimed that the proposed mandatory employer contributions to pay for the plan were equivalent to a tax, a term the administration tried to avoid, and these revenues had to be included as part of the administration's budget.

The Congress

Congress reflected the division of opinion among interest groups and the public. Given the president's demand for universal coverage, a Republican minority party opposed to a major reform bill, and a Democratic party that was severely divided, Congress found it impossible to craft a compromise bill.

Polarization among the parties had been increasing, particularly in the House of Representatives. Democrats controlled the presidency and both Houses of Congress. Believing they did not need Republican support to enact legislation that would transform a major portion of the economy, Democrats in the House did not attempt to develop legislation that had strong bipartisan support.[5] Instead, the strategy was to attempt comprehensive reform of the healthcare system through a minimum winning coalition of Democrats rather than a more consensual coalition among Democrats and Republicans. A bipartisan coalition would have meant losing the support of their own strong liberal base, resulting in incremental rather than comprehensive reform, which was the goal of President Clinton and the bill's proponents.

Democrats divided according to the "centrists," who favored expanding coverage within the existing system, and the liberals, who favored a government-run single-payer system, similar to the Canadian system. Democratic liberals in the House wanted a single-payer system. Moderate Democrats, of similar number, favored a plan without universal coverage. Liberal democrats were opposed to incremental reform, believing that if the number of uninsured were reduced, there would be less political pressure to achieve universal coverage.

House Republicans decided to oppose the Clinton plan and use their opposition as an election issue; believing their opposition would provide them with greater political support than if they helped it to pass. It was easier for Republicans to agree on an opposition strategy than on a health reform bill. (The Republican strategy enabled them to gain control of the House of Representatives in the 1994 election.)

The Congressional committee structure further served to delay and change the Clinton plan once it was introduced. Jurisdictional fights over which committee would oversee the Clinton plan resulted in the bill going to committees whose chairs proposed drastic changes. Although the Democrats controlled both houses of Congress, they could not agree on a health reform bill.[6] They disagreed on an employer mandate, whether the benefits were sufficiently comprehensive, whether cost-control limits should be included, whether abortion should be a covered benefit, and whether a single-payer plan should be substituted for the Clinton plan.

Divided Democrats could not outweigh a unified Republican opposition. The bill failed to receive a majority in either the House or Senate.

The Public

The public, while favoring health reform, assumed they would keep the coverage they had, without paying more for it. But the public was unfamiliar with the details of the Clinton health plan. As more information about the health plan became available, public skepticism increased and political support declined. The administration acknowledged at one point that, in fact, 40 percent of the middle class would have to pay more than they did currently. Middle-income families, particularly families with two wage earners, would pay much larger premiums than previously. Redistribution began to be seen as hurting rather than helping middle-income groups. The complexity of the health plan—national boards were proposed to control new technology—and the role of the regional alliances to allocate healthcare funds concerned those who were fearful of government intrusion in their healthcare. There was a concern, reinforced by television ads paid for by HIAA, that with coverage of everyone, more comprehensive benefits, and limits on medical expenditure increases, "rationing" would occur.

The middle class started to believe that the drastic overhaul of the health system President Clinton proposed was not necessary to alleviate their concerns. The majority of the public had health insurance and was concerned that with a far-reaching reform of the country's healthcare system they would lose what they were familiar and pleased with, in exchange for an unknown system that would be more costly and might limit their choices. Although incremental reform would also have been redistributive, it would not have had such large redistributive effects on important interest groups and would not have changed the basic system with which the public was familiar.

The declining support by the middle class was not lost on legislators, who believed they did not have to vote for major change. Given divided public opinion, a weak president (who had been elected with only 43 percent of the popular vote) making strong demands that he would veto legislation without universal coverage (which discouraged incremental reform), and a divided Democratic party, it was not surprising that comprehensive health reform failed.

In Retrospect

The Clinton healthcare plan was an attempt to enact a broad, visible, redistributive program. President Clinton proposed a major restructuring of the healthcare system; it was an all or nothing approach as he promised to veto anything less than universal coverage. Universal coverage, employer mandates, spending limits with implicit price controls, and regional purchasing alliances were key aspects of the plan that caused different interest groups to oppose specific parts of the plan. Each of these components of health reform entailed extensive regulation together with winners and losers. Additional funds (taxes) would have been required, the benefit coverage would have to be specified, and controls would have to be implemented to control spending. A new large bureaucracy would have to be created.

Any visible redistributive program had to receive the political support of a majority of the middle class. They had to perceive benefits in excess of their costs. Thus, the Clinton health plan promised universal health insurance, with a very comprehensive set of medical benefits and no decrease in access to care or in the quality of care, without having to raise income taxes or place a large financial burden on the public. It sounded too good to be true.

Any major restructuring of the health system would also have redistributive effects on organized groups, such as different provider associations, insurers, unions, large businesses, and small business associations. Each major group would attempt to economically benefit from the plan.

President Clinton's healthcare proposal attempted to satisfy all of the above groups and achieve universal coverage for everyone. To accomplish these conflicting goals, a very complex plan (longer than 1,300 pages) was proposed.

The design of the Clinton plan failed on both counts. As the middle class became more aware of the details of the Clinton plan, they began to perceive that they might not benefit and, in fact, might have to pay more. And groups with a concentrated interest were willing to expend political support to change or defeat parts of the proposed legislation.[7]

The president's veto threat restricted members of his own party from developing less comprehensive legislation that could have been approved by the Congress. Given the pay-as-you-go budget rules, the divisions in the Congress (even within his own party), the complexity of the Clinton plan, the short period Congress had to work on the plan, opposition to key parts of the plan by influential interest groups, and an inability to provide the middle class with any new benefits or lower costs, the Clinton plan had little likelihood of success. An opportunity for incremental change was lost.

President Clinton accused "special interests" of opposing his health plan. In fact, some special interests were for and others were against the plan. Many producer groups, such as companies with unfunded medical retiree liabilities, unions with high medical premiums relative to their wages, physicians opposed to managed care, and nurses who wanted more independent practice, were major beneficiaries of the proposed legislation.

The real reason why President Clinton's proposal failed was that public support for a radical restructuring of the healthcare system declined. Although the public wanted health reform that included universal coverage, as indicated by the polls at that time, middle- and higher-income groups wanted something for nothing—traditional indemnity insurance, comprehensive benefits, the latest medical technology, free access to all healthcare providers, the security of not losing their insurance—and they would like someone else to pay for it. It was an unrealistic and impossible package for any legislator to deliver.

The public was sending contradictory messages. The president and legislators did not seem to realize that the demand for universal coverage was not paramount, and the middle class was not willing to sacrifice other goals to have the government cover more of the uninsured. In fact, most of the middle class was satisfied with the quality and availability of their care; they just did not want to pay more. Radically changing the system to cover the 15 percent who were uninsured made the 85 percent with coverage apprehensive that their taxes and government controls would increase and access and quality to decrease. In the end, they did not perceive any new benefits for themselves,

The difficulty in enacting national health insurance in this country does not come from the special interests as much as it is comes from the middle class. Achieving change requires making a trade-off. To receive a lower rate of premium increases, the public must be willing to accept some restrictions, such as giving up choice of provider, access to care, and/or access to new medical technology. It is difficult for politicians to rationally discuss these choices with the public because it means that they cannot then provide the public with benefits in excess of their costs.

Congress, closely attuned to the public and no longer fearful of losing public support, opposed the Clinton plan.

The Health Insurance Portability and Accountability Act of 1996

After the Clinton healthcare plan was rejected, Congress was reluctant to attempt any far-reaching, complicated, reform of the healthcare system. Congress realized that it was too difficult to enact a broad-based health plan that would satisfy the conflicting interests of all those with a concentrated interest in health reform. Instead, they focused on specific issues of concern to the middle class. Specifically, the middle class, those with health insurance, was concerned with maintaining their coverage and not losing it.

In 1996, the Republicans had taken control over both the House of Representatives and the U.S. Senate. Although Republicans in the House were able to strongly influence the type of bill that would be sent to the Senate, the filibuster rules in the Senate made it necessary for Republicans to compromise with Democrats when bills came up for a vote. President Clinton, having failed to have his reform plan enacted, was anxious to work with the Republicans and sign some health legislation, even though it was much smaller in scope than his grandiose attempt.

To alleviate certain middle-class health insurance concerns, Congress enacted HIPAA. This legislation was considered to be highly significant in that the federal government became more involved in regulating and setting standards for private health insurance.

Many states already regulate most insurers, guaranteeing portability and limiting insurers' ability to charge very high premiums. However, under the 1974 Employee Retirement Income Security Act (ERISA), states cannot regulate the health plans of businesses that self-insure. (About 44 million Americans were covered by ERISA plans.) The HIPAA bill would apply to all plans, including those exempt from state regulation under ERISA.

One may view HIPAA as an extension of Congress' role in regulating the private health insurance market.[8] In 1990, Congress set standards for Medigap (Medicare supplemental) policies. Many elderly purchased Medigap insurance policies that covered the deductibles, coinsurance, and open-ended liabilities that exist in Medicare. A large variety of these types of policies were being sold to the aged. To reduce the confusion to the aged, Congress enacted legislation that reduced the types of Medigap policies that could be offered to ten, different, standardized plans.

Similar to the 1990 Medigap legislation, which did not increase access to medical services by those aged who could not afford Medigap insurance, HIPAA's purpose was not to increase access to medical services by those who could not afford private health insurance.[9]

The HIPAA bill addressed four middle-class concerns with their private health insurance. First, HIPAA limited the waiting period for preexisting exclusions to no more than 12 months. Previously, if a person had sought medical advice or had been diagnosed or treated for an illness (e.g., heart disease) in the previous six months, an insurance company could either deny coverage for that illness or extend insurance coverage only after a long waiting period. Employees who had health insurance were also concerned that they or their family members would not have their insurance coverage renewed if they had a preexisting condition. By limiting the preexisting exclusion period to a maximum of 12 months, employees would be able to have complete insurance coverage for themselves and their family members.

Second, and related to the above maximum waiting period, HIPAA increased job "portability." If a person had been insured for at least 18 months of continuous health insurance coverage, then she would have met the preexisting waiting period should she then decide to change jobs. The employee (and her family members) would not have to meet any new preexisting condition waiting period and would be immediately eligible for insurance at her next job as long as the new company provides insurance. (This is referred to as "guaranteed availability.") Previously, employees had been fearful of changing jobs if it meant that they or a family member would be subject to a new waiting period for preexisting conditions or be denied insurance. (A new, controversial, rule permitted individuals who were previously insured as part of an employer group to move to the "individual" market and continue to be insured.)

Third, HIPAA required insurance companies to offer *guaranteed renewability* of a firm's health insurance. Previously, if a firm's employees had high claims expenses (relative to the premium paid) an insurer did not have to renew the firm's insurance. Yet HIPAA required insurers to offer renewability of all of the insurer's products. Individuals who were insured as part of the "individual" market were also guaranteed renewability.

Fourth, HIPAA required insurers that sell policies to small employers to offer their products to small firms (2 to 50 employees) and to all members of that firm, subject only to the 12-month waiting period for preexisting conditions. (This is referred to as "guaranteed issue.") Previously, small firms found it difficult to purchase certain types of insurance or any insurance because insurers believed they might be subject to adverse selection (the small firm buys insurance because it is at high risk). Previously, insurers were also able to exclude certain employees from being insured.

During the first Bush Administration, President Bush had proposed several aspects of HIPAA, described above. However, Democrats at that time believed enacting such legislation would lessen the public's interest in having more broad-based health reform. After President Clinton was elected, and once the Clinton plan failed, legislators were more willing to enact limited reforms to address middle-class concerns.

The HIPAA legislation included a number of other features. The deductibility of health insurance for the self-employed was increased; previously they could deduct only 30 percent. Under HIPAA, that percentage gradually increased, eventually reaching 80 percent in 2006 and thereafter. (This percentage deduction was still less than if they were a worker in an employer group, in which case 100 percent of the premium could be paid with before-tax income. Also, HIPAA provided tax breaks to increase the use of long-term-care insurance. Long-term-care insurance was to be treated the same as health insurance. Employer contributions for long-term-care insurance to benefit the employee, spouse, or dependents, were excluded from the employee's taxable income. (Tax-exempt employer contributions provide a greater benefit to those in higher income-tax brackets.) Further, to raise revenue under HIPAA, many additional elements were included, such as those relating to fraud and abuse, taxes on expatriates, and so on.

Two very controversial aspects almost derailed the bill. The HIAA was opposed to provisions in the bill that would have required insurers to provide employees leaving group health plans with the same policy they had while in the group. The HIAA, representing 210 small insurers, believed the cost of the reforms would have a bigger impact on their premiums than on premiums of large health insurers, who favored the changes. The HIAA claimed that the requirement to cover people moving from group to individual coverage would cause premiums to increase in the individual market, leading to a drop in coverage by other individuals. They believed individuals leaving an employer plan and buying an individual plan were more likely to be sick (adverse selection) and thus more expensive to insure. Healthy individuals leaving a group plan were more likely to forego buying an expensive policy. Insurers did not want to provide the same group-policy benefits to an individual. To satisfy insurer's objections, Congress permitted them to design the types of plans they would offer. Insurers could offer their current menu of individual policies, which might include high-deductible plans.

The most controversial issue that delayed Senate agreement on the bill was the medical savings account (MSA), which was an ideological issue. Republicans in the House, against the opposition of Democrats, included MSAs in the bill passed by the House.[10] They viewed the inclusion of MSAs as an opportunity to move away from the employer-based healthcare system toward a system based on individual responsibility that relied on individual incentives. (An MSA allowed individuals with high-deductible health insurance plans to set up tax-deductible savings accounts to use for medical expenses.) Senator Kennedy objected to MSAs, which were not included in the Senate bill but were in the House bill. A compromise was eventually reached that resulted in permitting MSAs in a pilot project limited to 750,000 people for four years. After the trial period Congress would vote on whether to expand the program. Only workers in firms with 50 or fewer employees, those who are self-insured, or the uninsured would be eligible for the MSAs. The uncertainty of the continued existence of an MSA product, the limited market eligible for such a product, and the higher marketing costs involved in reaching those eligible, led to a lack of insurer interest in marketing MSAs.

Republican Senator Nancy Kassebaum and Democratic Senator Edward Kennedy, cosponsors of HIPAA, wanted to ensure that the bipartisan coalition behind the bill would remain intact and that the bill would pass. Thus, they agreed to oppose all unrelated provisions that legislators wanted to include in a bill likely to be enacted.

The Republicans in the House included several provisions in their bill that Democrats opposed. Two such provisions were limits on monetary damages in medical malpractice lawsuits, which was favored by the AMA, and reducing states' regulatory authority over insurance plans purchased by small business pools, which was favored by small businesses to reduce their health insurance costs. These provisions were eliminated in the House Senate conference committee reconciling the House and Senate versions of the bill. In the Senate, Republican Pete Domenici failed to include a provision to have severe mental illness treated similar to other major physical illnesses in any insurance plan.

Yet HIPAA did little for the estimated (at that time) 43 million people without health insurance, who had been the focus of President Clinton's healthcare reform proposal. Instead, the bill was meant to protect those who already had health insurance from losing it. The HIPAA was meant to give the middle class a sense of security.

The Balanced Budget Act of 1997

The Balanced Budget Act (BBA) of 1997 resulted in three important redistributive actions: several short-term changes were made to Medicare, thereby postponing the expected 2001 bankruptcy of the Medicare (Part A) Trust Fund; a Commission on the Future of Medicare was established to address the long-term solvency of Medicare; and a new program was initiated to cover uninsured children who were not eligible for Medicaid (SCHIP). Each initiative is discussed below.[11]

To gain control of the Congress in the 1994 congressional elections, Republicans promoted their "Contract with America." The contract included ten items, one of which was to balance the federal budget by the year 2002. After winning a majority in the House (and the Senate), the Republican House leadership believed they were committed to fulfilling their campaign pledges, otherwise the public would consider them to be no different from the Democrats and vote them out at the next election. Once House Republicans calculated what they would have to do to balance the budget in seven years, it became obvious they would have to reduce the rate of growth in Medicare and Medicaid spending.

Had it not been for their pledge to balance the budget by the year 2002, House Republicans would have found it politically popular to delay any serious changes to the Medicare system. Because the Democrats and the Clinton Administration were not bound by the Republicans' balanced budget pledge, their position was to minimize the burden of reducing the rate of increase in Medicare spending on its current beneficiaries, namely, the current aged and healthcare providers. The House Republican plan was approved along a party-line vote.[12] By attacking the proposed reductions as too large, the Democrats hoped to force the Republicans to either renege on their pledge to balance the budget by the year 2002 or drop their proposed tax cuts. (Tax reductions were another part of the House Republicans' contract.)

Each political party attempted to define the terms of the debate over Medicare. The Republicans did not want to use the phrase "cutting Medicare spending to reduce the federal budget deficit" as a reason for their proposed changes. Polls indicated that the public was opposed to this justification for reducing the rate of increase in Medicare spending. Instead, using a routine report issued by the Trustees of Medicare Part A (hospital care) projecting bankruptcy of the Part A Trust Fund in the year 2001, the Republicans claimed their proposals were needed to "save," "protect," and "strengthen" Medicare for future generations without asking any beneficiaries, except for the richest, to pay more. (Only those aged couples with more than $125,000 income or individuals with more than $75,000 income would be expected to pay an additional premium. It was estimated that only 3 percent of the aged would be adversely affected by these higher premiums.)[13] The Republicans claimed that they were merely reducing the annual rate of increase in Medicare spending from 10 percent to 6.5 percent.

The Democrats criticized the Republican plan for "cutting" Medicare by $270 billion over seven years to provide $250 billion in "tax cuts" for the rich.

The budget differences between the Republican-controlled Congress and President Clinton led to a stalemate in the fall of 1995. President Clinton vetoed the BBA of 1995, which then led to a government shutdown in late 1995. Fearing that they were losing public support (opinion polls blamed the Republicans for the government shutdown), the Republicans agreed to drop deep spending cuts and their Medicare proposal and the government reopened.

During the 1996 election the Democrats continued to claim that Republicans were trying to cut Medicare spending to provide tax cuts for the wealthy. The House Republicans ended up losing three seats but still retained a slim, nine-vote majority. However, they blamed their losses on the Medicare issue. As a result, their enthusiasm for making drastic changes to ensure the long-term solvency of Medicare declined.

Republicans decided that before they would make any changes to Medicare they needed support from Democrats and President Clinton.

The 1997 BBA was a consensus bill.[14] The Republican congress, fearful of being attacked by their opponents as trying to destroy Medicare, decided a compromise bill was a way to defuse Medicare as a political issue. Also making a compromise easier was the strength of the economy, which led to smaller forecasts of budget deficits; thus, much smaller reductions were needed in the rate of increase in Medicare Part B spending. The Republicans dropped many of the controversial aspects of their Medicare proposal that were opposed by the Democrats, such as increasing the eligibility age for Medicare from 65 to 67, making the Medicare Part B premium income related, and setting the Part B premium at 31.5 percent of Part B costs. And President Clinton announced that he would ensure the solvency of the Medicare Trust Fund for a period that was shorter than what the Republicans had been aiming for, thus requiring smaller savings. President Clinton favored postponing bankruptcy of the Medicare Trust Fund by reducing payments to hospitals and physicians.

The compromise BBA of 1997 made several short-term financial changes to Medicare, which moved its bankruptcy date 6 years into the future. No comprehensive changes were adopted that would have secured Medicare's future financial health. Instead, the only step Congress took toward resolving Medicare's long-term structural and financial problems was to create a Bipartisan Commission on the Future of Medicare to report its recommendations to the Congress in 1999.

The 1997 BBA solved Medicare's immediate financial problem by providing two short-term fixes. Home health care had been included in Medicare Part A and was the fastest-rising element of Medicare spending, thereby contributing to the Medicare Trust Fund's impending bankruptcy. It was shifted out of Part A into Part B, which is funded by general revenues. This had the immediate effect of reducing both the level and rate of increase in Medicare Part A spending. Second, $115 billion in projected Medicare Part A payments to healthcare providers, such as hospitals, were to be reduced over the next five years.

The political battle of how to change Medicare involved redistributive issues. Every attempt was made to impose as little additional cost as possible on the politically powerful aged. The aged received additional services. They were given seven new or expanded preventive services and their Medicare Part B premium was capped at 25 percent of the program's costs (lower than the 31.5 percent originally proposed by the Republicans).[15]

The only significant "cost" borne by the aged under the BBA was that the relatively small percent of seniors who join Medicare HMOs would no longer be able to switch back to traditional fee-for-service Medicare with only one month's notice. By 2003 they would have to wait almost a year before being able to switch plans.

The 1997 BBA managed to postpone Medicare's immediate problem: the expected 2001 bankruptcy of the Part A Medicare Trust Fund,

Consistent with the economic theory of legislation, given the inevitable bankruptcy of the Medicare Trust Fund, Congress will not undertake any politically difficult choice until there is an actual crisis. Second, by extending the solvency of the Medicare Trust Fund for several more years, the political problem is delayed for a future president and Congress to deal with it. And third, although the aged currently receive large subsidies under Medicare, short-term attempts to improve the Medicare Trust Fund's solvency do not stand in the way of providing the aged with still more subsidized benefits

State Children's Health Insurance Program

Two population groups considered worthy of government subsidies are the aged and children. The aged, because of the political support they (and their grown offspring) can offer politicians, have benefited greatly from subsidized medical care (Medicare) and pension benefits (Social Security). Subsidized medical care to children can be considered as a "charitable" redistributive program; it is not the children's fault that they cannot afford medical care. Subsidized medical care to the aged and children (using an income test for the latter group) are thus consistent with the economic theory of legislation.

Subsidies to these two population groups are also favored by those who ideologically favor universal coverage under a single-payer system. To include the entire population within a single-payer system, it makes sense to start with the aged, then include pregnant women and children (up to age 19 if possible), for reasons stated above, and then begin including the near-aged, then the parents of low-income children, and in this manner move from both ends of the age distribution until most of the population has been included in some government program. It then becomes politically possible to cover the few remaining population groups, such as those with employer-paid health insurance. Requiring employer-paid health insurance premiums to be included in a government pool (along with Medicare and Medicaid funds) would not be viewed as an additional employee tax by employees.

Single-payer advocates favor including additional population groups in Medicare, Medicaid, or employer-paid health insurance. These funds could then be aggregated to finance a single-payer system.

Opponents of a single-payer system are opposed to the existing (traditional) Medicare system, to allowing the near-aged to buy into Medicare, to expanding Medicaid, and to strengthening employer-paid health insurance because they want consumers to be directly affected if the government wants to include them in a single-payer system. Single-payer opponents favor choice of health plan and individual medical accounts, which would make it politically difficult for government to aggregate (by taxing) private accounts and force them into a different delivery system.

This conflict between single-payer advocates and their opponents who favor charitable redistribution programs manifests itself in the design of programs benefiting the aged and children.

Media accounts that growing numbers of uninsured children were failing to receive critical medical care for asthma, acute ear infections, strep throat, and other ailments, which could lead to serious heart and kidney problems, led to congressional proposals to alleviate this problem. About 90 percent of uninsured children live in a household where a parent or guardian has a full- or part-time job. About 7 million of the 10 million uninsured children have family incomes below 200 percent of the federal poverty level. These families no longer qualify for welfare, as the 1996 welfare reform bill resulted in many recipients moving into jobs (before they reached the five-year limit on cash assistance) thereby losing their free health coverage from Medicaid. The minimum wage that many former welfare recipients earn is insufficient to pay medical bills or buy insurance. States worry that when a child becomes sick, the parents will reapply for welfare so they can have Medicaid. Once back on welfare they become a burden to the state's budget.

The plight of America's children without health insurance and state concerns with former recipients returning to welfare led to a proposal—SCHIP—by Senators Orrin Hatch (R-UT) and Edward Kennedy (D-MA) for a block grant program to the states to extend health insurance to an estimated 5 million children. Funding for this initiative was based on an increased cigarette tax. States would receive funds to offer coverage to low-income children whose families are not poor enough to qualify for Medicaid. The federal government would pay 50 percent of the cost for the wealthiest states and up to 80 percent for the poorest states. The program was enacted as part of the 1997 BBA.[16]

The objective of SCHIP, helping uninsured children, had bipartisan support. However, the political parties in Congress differed on the design of the legislation, particularly over how much freedom to allow the states in designing their programs. President Clinton and the Democrats in Congress wanted the legislation to specify a set of comprehensive benefits that the states had to offer. Governors and the Republicans wanted to give the states flexibility in the design of benefits, claiming that too comprehensive a set of benefits would increase the program's cost and reduce the number of children a state could cover. The resulting compromise gave states a block grant and allowed them some flexibility in the benefits offered (states could choose from a list of possible benefit packages) as well as flexibility in how the states determined eligibility of children and how the money was to be spent. States could use traditional Medicaid, contract with private insurers to provide the benefits, or subsidize the employee's share of employer-paid health insurance.[17]

Overall, SCHIP illustrates the ideological divide between those desiring federally specified comprehensive benefits to be offered through government programs (Medicaid) versus those favoring flexibility in benefit design and offered through the private sector; the government as a contractor with private managed care plans rather than as a direct payer (using regulated prices) to individual providers.

The National Bipartisan Commission on the Future of Medicare

The 1997 BBA ensured the solvency of the Medicare Trust Fund only until 2007. Congress believed Medicare was in urgent need of reform, given the increasing number of aged (particularly after the baby boomers start retiring in 2011) and the relative decline in the number of workers paying payroll and income taxes. To examine how the Medicare Trust Fund's solvency could be extended for a longer period, the 1997 BBA created a bipartisan Commission that was to complete its report by March 1999. Members of Congress agreed that the Commission's recommendation had to be accepted by a "super majority," or 11 of its 17 members.

The Bipartisan Commission completed its work and could only agree, by a simple majority (10 votes), on its recommendations. The majority of the Commission favored allowing the aged to choose among different health plans. Medicare was to be modeled after the Federal Employee Health Benefits Program. Further, a "premium-support" plan was proposed that would have had the government provide a defined contribution toward the purchase of a health plan with a defined set of benefits. The government's contribution would have been based on the weighted average price of all the plans. The defined contribution would have paid the premium in full for the lowest-cost plans; plans that were more costly would require an extra payment by the aged. The defined contribution would have only paid 84 percent of the traditional fee-for-service Medicare premium, which would still be available for the aged. The reasoning behind the premium-support plan was to increase price competition among health plans as the aged would have to pay the full additional cost of more expensive plans.

Low-income aged (household income up to 135 percent of the federal poverty level) would have also received free drug benefits.[18]

The Commission also recommended increasing the Medicare eligibility age from 65 years to 67 years by 2025, similar to the phase-in of Social Security eligibility.

The conflict over the Commission's recommendations occurred over several issues: increasing the eligibility age, having the higher-income aged pay higher premiums, making the aged pay an additional premium for choosing the traditional Medicare plan, expanding the role of private managed care insurers in offering a choice of Medicare plans, and creating a new prescription drug benefit. Before the Commission completed its work, President Clinton undercut the Commission's recommendations by proposing to add a new prescription drug benefit, for all the aged, to the traditional Medicare system. Opponents of the president's proposal believed it would be a very expensive new benefit. More importantly, it would hinder efforts to reform Medicare. A stand-alone drug benefit would strengthen traditional Medicare and thus be a disincentive for the aged to choose managed care plans. (President Clinton also proposed allowing those between the ages of 55 to 64 years to buy into Medicare.)[19]

During this time period, federal budget forecasts had begun to change. Instead of years of federal deficits, huge budget surpluses were now being projected. Previous federal deficits had constrained government expenditures and limited the start of new programs. As the forecasted surpluses kept getting larger, President Clinton proposed using about $800 billion of these surpluses to extend the life of Medicare and pay for a new Medicare prescription drug program. This plan would commit massive general tax revenues to Medicare and forestall any urgency to reform the Medicare program.

The Commission failed to reach a super-majority consensus on reforming Medicare and ensuring its long-term solvency.

The 2000 Presidential Election

The Democrats once again hoped to use Medicare as an election issue. After President Clinton's proposal, Democratic presidential candidate Al Gore and Democrats campaigning for House and Senate seats proposed a new Medicare drug benefit for all the aged as part of the traditional Medicare plan. Once again, the Republicans perceived themselves to be on the defensive with Medicare during an election period. To counter the prescription drug plan of the Democrats, Republican presidential candidate George Bush and the Republicans proposed their own Medicare prescription drug benefit. Even though the Republican plan targeted low-income seniors, while the Democrat plan would have been available to all seniors, the competing proposals (particularly since the details were not clear to many) were sufficient to neutralize the Medicare drug benefit as a political issue.

Unless Medicare reform recommendations have bipartisan support, the political party proposing them is at a political disadvantage. The BBA of 1995 was vetoed and used in the election to the disadvantage of the Republicans. The BBA of 1997 was bipartisan; it achieved limited savings by shifting home health care from Medicare Part A to Part B and reducing provider payments, while providing the aged with additional Medicare benefits. The Bipartisan Commission could not achieve a super-majority because it proposed increasing some costs to the aged (raising the cost of the traditional Medicare plan) and treating low-income aged differently from high-income aged.

A new prescription drug benefit for all the aged raised the political stakes for both parties. To compete for the votes of the aged in the 2000 election, President Bush made a commitment to have a new prescription drug bill enacted during his first term.

Study Questions

1. The MCCA was enacted in 1988 and repealed in 1989. Use the competing theories of government to provide an explanation for these two events.
2. Why did healthcare reform become an important public policy issue in President Clinton's first term?
3. Which groups were in favor of an employer mandate and why?
4. Why was the employer required to pay 80 percent and the employee 20 percent of the employer mandate?
5. Why were the automobile companies and their union, the UAW, in favor of the Clinton healthcare reform plan?
6. Why did President Clinton's healthcare reform plan fail?
7. What were the main health insurance issues addressed by HIPAA?
8. How were the ideological conflicts compromised in SCHIP?
9. Why was the Commission on the Future of Medicare unable to develop a bipartisan consensus to reform Medicare?

10. Any proposals to reform Medicare will affect the aged, the working population, hospitals, physicians, and other healthcare providers. Which groups are most likely to be adversely affected by reform proposals that reduce the rate of increase in Medicare expenditures?

Notes

1. Julie Rovner, "Congress's 'Catastrophic' Attempt to Fix Medicare," in *How Congress Shapes Health Policy*, eds. Thomas Mann and Norman Ornstein (Washington, DC: The American Enterprise Institute and The Brookings Institution, 1995), 145–78. See also, Thomas Rice, Katherine Desmond, and Jon Gabel, "The Medicare Catastrophic Coverage Act: A Post-Mortem," *Health Affairs* 9, no. 3 (1990): 75–87.
2. William Recktenwald, "Insurance Forum Turns Catastrophic for Rostenkowski," *Chicago Tribune*, August 18, 1989, 1.
3. For an excellent discussion of the issues surrounding the Clinton plan, see Julie Rovner, "Congress and Health Care Reform 1993–94," in *How Congress Shapes Health Policy*, eds. Thomas Mann and Norman Ornstein (Washington, DC: The American Enterprise Institute and The Brookings Institution, 1995), 179–225.
4. Another redistributive mechanism within the employer mandate was to rely on "community rating," whereby employer and employee contributions for health insurance were not related to health risk factors. Older workers did not have to pay higher premiums than younger workers. The amount to be contributed on behalf of younger employees, who are less likely to vote, was expected to exceed their expected medical costs, thereby providing older employees with a subsidy.
5. For a discussion of interest groups and coalitions between such groups for and against healthcare reform, see Allen Schick, "How a Bill Did Not Become a Law," in *How Congress Shapes Health Policy*, eds. Thomas Mann and Norman Ornstein (Washington, DC: The American Enterprise Institute and The Brookings Institution, 1995), 227–72.
6. As the Clinton administration and the Democratic leadership tried to raise the necessary votes for reporting out a health bill from the various committees, legislators sold their votes for specific constituent benefits. For example, Senator Daniel Moynihan, whose state of New York includes a number of academic medical centers, inserted an amendment that would have provided all academic health centers with the funds generated by a 1.75 percent tax on all health insurance premiums; this benefit was valued at $75 billion

over 5 years. Chairman Dan Rostenkowski of the House Ways and Means Committee included an amendment that provided for a 3 percent interest-rate subsidy to Northwestern Memorial hospital for its $650 million construction program. The oil industry also received special tax breaks to ensure the votes of Senators John Breaux and Bennett Johnston, who are from oil-producing states.

7. Much has been written by others on the reasons for the defeat of President Clinton's health reform plan. See, for example, Daniel Yankelovich, "The Debate That Wasn't: The Public and the Clinton Plan," *Health Affairs* 14, no. 1 (1995): 7–23. See also in that same issue the "Perspectives" of several others, 24–36.

8. Len M. Nichols and Linda J. Blumberg, "A Different Kind of 'New Federalism'? The Health Insurance and Portability Act of 1996," *Health Affairs* 17, no. 3 (1998): 25–42.

9. The HIPAA also made a few changes in the tax laws that likely increased the demand for health insurance by self-insured persons. Previously, only employer-purchased health insurance was fully tax-exempt. This policy discriminated against those who were self-employed. The HIPAA attempted to rectify this by increasing the tax deductibility of health insurance premiums paid by self-insured persons. Also, HIPAA provided tax incentives for the purchase of long-term-care insurance.

10. An MSA works as follows: an employer may provide an employee with $3,000 in the employee's MSA account. The employee would have to purchase a catastrophic insurance policy costing, for example, $1,500 and having a $2,000 deductible. Thus, the employee has $1,500 remaining in the MSA account if he incurs no medical expenses. If he does become ill, he must pay up to $2,000 before his insurance policy becomes effective. If he does not spend the $1,500, the money accumulates in his account until he retires. The proponents of MSAs believe individuals will have a financial incentive not to be wasteful in using medical services.

11. "Medicare, Medicaid, 1997 Chronology," *CQ Almanac 1997*, (Washington, DC: CQ Press) retrieved from CQ Electronic Library, CQ Public Affairs Collection.

12. Surprisingly, the AMA, one of the provider groups targeted to suffer a reduction in physician payments under Medicare, came out in support of the House Republican plan (as did the American Society of Internal Medicine). In return for their support, which the Republicans considered to be very important to public acceptance of their plan, physicians received a number of concessions. For example, the reductions in payments to physicians would be smaller than

originally proposed; a limit would be placed on payment of damages ($250,000) to victims of medical malpractice; the aged would be permitted to set up MSAs, which would have no limits on the fees physicians could charge those patients; restrictions on physician self-referral laws to facilities in which they have a financial interest would be loosened; and, perhaps most important, a provision was included to make it easier for physicians to profit from their own managed care plans, known as provider service networks, by exempting them from the same capital requirements that HMOs and insurers have to meet. If these provider plans became bankrupt, the taxpayer is at risk for the losses. It is for this reason the National Association of Insurance Commissioners opposed this proposal.

Other healthcare groups were also provided with certain benefits to limit their opposition to the Republican's proposals. Christopher Georges, "House GOP Medicare Bill Wins Over Doctors with Hidden Enticements, Promise of Profits," *The Wall Street Journal*, October 12, 1995, A24.

13. David Wessel, "The Wall Street Journal/NBC News Poll: In Medicare Battle, Republicans Display Skill At Making Words Mean Just What They Choose," *Wall Street Journal*, September 22, 1995, A16.

14. Charles N. Kahn and Hanns Kuttner, "Budget Bills and Medicare Policy: The Politics of the BBA," *Health Affairs* 18, no. 1 (1999): 37–47.

15. The legislation also established a pilot program for MSAs, which allowed seniors to use tax-exempt accounts for qualified medical expenses. Seniors who selected this Medicare option, available to only 390,000 seniors, were also required to purchase a high-deductible insurance policy (up to a $6,000 deductible) to cover catastrophic illness. Medicare MSAs were very controversial; Republicans favored offering seniors more choice than traditional Medicare. The Democrats, led by Senator Kennedy, were opposed, believing the healthy aged would select MSAs, thereby worsening the Medicare risk pool. The pilot program was a compromise.

16. See the following for discussions on the development of the SCHIP legislation. David Hosansky, "Concern for Uninsured Children Has Not Led to Agreement," *CQ Weekly*, April 12, 1997, 850; Robert Pear, "GOP Leadership Agrees on a Plan to Cover Children," *New York Times*, July 24, 1997, 1; Peter T. Kilborn, "States to Give More Children Health Coverage," *New York Times*, Sept. 21, 1997, 1; G. Kenny and D. I. Chang, "The State Children's Health

Insurance Program: Successes, Shortcomings, and Challenges," *Health Affairs* 23, no. 5 (2004): 51–62.

17. Before enacting SCHIP, legislators were concerned that many uninsured children were in middle-class families and if a government program became available, parents would substitute public coverage for private coverage; subsidies would go to children whose parents might otherwise buy private insurance. (This phenomenon of substituting public for private coverage is referred to as "crowd out.") Crowd out occurred in 1986 when Medicaid eligibility for pregnant women and children was increased. Some of the working poor dropped their private health insurance and used the new Medicaid benefits. As a result Medicaid expenditures increased at a time when the government was attempting to limit rising costs. In an attempt to resolve the concern over crowd out and limit SCHIP funds, the federal law prohibits assistance under SCHIP to low-income children who are eligible for Medicaid.

18. For a discussion of the Commission's recommendations, see Mark McClellan, "Medicare Reform: Fundamental Problems, Incremental Steps," *Journal of Economic Perspectives*, 14, no. 2 (2000): 21–44. See also, Robert B. Helms, "Medicare Reform: Economics versus Politics," *The Independent Review*, 5 (2000): 209–18.

19. Mary Agnes Carey and Rebecca Adams, "Medicare Panel a Year Later: Deadlocked at Deadline," *CQ Weekly*, February 27, 1999, 481.

THE MEDICARE MODERNIZATION ACT OF 2003

After completing this chapter, the reader should be able to

- List the changes conservative Republicans wanted to include in the Medicare Modernization Act (MMA),
- Outline which ideological issues were important to liberal Democrats in the design of the MMA,
- Describe the "premium-support" concept,
- Identify AARP's condition for supporting the MMA,
- Discuss why President Bush was anxious to enact a Medicare drug benefit,
- List the benefits drug companies, hospitals, and physicians received as part of the MMA, and
- Explain why senators representing rural constituencies favored a stand-alone drug benefit.

In December 2003, President Bush signed into law the largest expansion of the Medicare program since it was enacted in 1965. Medicare was modeled after a standard private health insurance plan (a traditional Blue Cross–Blue Shield insurance policy), which did not include coverage for outpatient prescription drugs. The Medicare Prescription Drug, Improvement and Modernization Act of 2003 (referred to as the Medicare Modernization Act, or MMA) corrected that omission by adding outpatient prescription drug coverage for the elderly.

This chapter discusses why a new Medicare entitlement benefit was enacted at a time when federal budget deficits were rising and serious concerns existed regarding both the near-term and long-term financial solvency of Medicare. Further, to understand the complex design of the new Medicare outpatient prescription drug legislation, one has to be aware of the emerging ideological conflicts in health policy and the role played by concentrated interest groups.

The new Medicare prescription drug bill is a perfect illustration of how politics, ideology, and concentrated interests affect health policy.

Background on Medicare Prescription Drug Coverage

At the time Medicare was enacted, effective drug treatments for many chronic diseases affecting the aged did not exist. The cost of outpatient drugs was less of a concern to the elderly than the cost of hospital care, which could be a catastrophic medical expense. (Outpatient drugs that had to be administered by a physician were covered by Medicare to reduce the need for hospitalization.) Since 1965, many breakthrough drugs have been developed to treat conditions that were previously untreatable and to improve outcomes over previous treatment methods. The aged began to feel the financial burden of these costly drugs.

High out-of-pocket drug expenditures are a particular hardship for the elderly, who use prescription drugs more than any other age group. Many aged purchase supplementary health insurance to cover their Medicare hospital and physician out-of-pocket expenses and the cost of prescription drugs. Retiree health plans offered by large employers also provide such supplementary health coverage. In addition, those who join a Medicare managed care plan received prescription drug benefits. Before the enactment of the new Medicare prescription drug program, about 75 percent of the aged had some drug coverage.[1] As the cost of prescription drugs has risen over time, those without prescription drug coverage, typically the low-income aged, became particularly vulnerable to the financial hardship imposed by high prescription drug prices.

For a small percent of the aged, drug costs are a catastrophic expense; 25 percent of the aged account for 70 percent of total drug expenditures among the elderly.[2] The financial burden of outpatient drugs on some aged has been so great that they cannot afford to fill their prescriptions. The out-of-pocket cost of prescription drugs is a greater financial burden for the aged than open-heart surgery, which is covered by Medicare insurance.

A number of attempts have previously been made to include a drug benefit as part of Medicare.[3] The 1988 MCCA included an outpatient drug benefit (as discussed in Chapter 10), but Congress repealed the bill in 1989. Among the reasons for its repeal was the higher premium imposed on higher-income aged (because the bill had to be self-financed). The aged were required to enroll in the drug program (even though Medigap supplementary insurance provided a drug benefit for many), and although the aged were not going to receive their drug benefits for two years, they were required to start paying for those future benefits immediately.

After the failure of President Clinton's ambitious health reform program in 1994, Republicans achieved majority control of both houses of Congress in the 1994 elections. The new conservative Republican majority in the House, which was concerned with issues such as the rising federal budget deficit and the impending bankruptcy of the Medicare Trust Fund, engaged in a series of budget confrontations with the Clinton administration. The lack of agreement over the budget between the two sides led to a government shutdown. The Clinton administration prevailed as Republicans perceived they were losing public support for their position. The resulting BBA of 1997 included several changes to improve the short-term financial solvency of the Medicare Trust Fund and created the National Bipartisan Commission on the Future of Medicare. The commission was established at the behest of legislators who were concerned with the long-term financial solvency of Medicare, given that the baby boomers would start retiring in 2011, the number of employees per aged to finance Medicare was declining, and the cost of medical care continued to increase.

The goal of the majority of the members on the National Bipartisan Commission on the Future of Medicare was to restructure, or "reform," Medicare. They intended to achieve this reform by having the government provide each Medicare beneficiary with a subsidy (referred to as "premium support"), and the aged would then choose among different health plans, one of which would be traditional Medicare. If any plan, such as traditional Medicare, was more costly than the premium subsidy, the aged would have to pay the additional amount out of pocket. Opponents of premium support believed competition among health plans would lead to the eventual disappearance of traditional Medicare as healthier aged chose less expensive plans and the traditional plan serving the chronically ill became too costly to survive.

The proponents of competition needed a favorable vote by a super majority (11 out of 17) of the Commission's members to get their proposals recommended to Congress. As an inducement for Medicare beneficiaries to move from traditional Medicare into managed care plans, as well as to attract votes from more of the Commission's members, the proponents of competition included an outpatient prescription drug benefit in their recommendations. However, the proposals to reform Medicare did not receive the necessary super-majority vote.

While the Commission was debating its reform proposals, President Clinton, in his 1999 State of the Union address, proposed a "stand-alone" outpatient prescription drug benefit as part of the traditional Medicare program. Including a new drug benefit in traditional Medicare would have removed any incentive for Medicare beneficiaries to switch to a managed care plan to have access to a drug benefit.

Neither the proposal for Medicare reform with a drug benefit as recommended by a majority of the members of the Commission nor President Clinton's stand-alone drug benefit received sufficient support to make it through the closely divided Congress.

Republicans in the House, in anticipation of the 2000 elections, pushed through (over the objections of the Democrats) a Medicare prescription drug bill, knowing that it would not pass the closely divided Senate or be signed by President Clinton. It was seen as preventive medicine for House Republicans who controlled the House of Representatives by only a small (six-vote) majority. Democrats were viewed more favorably by the public on health issues, and the Republican leadership wanted to help vulnerable members in districts where Medicare drug coverage was an emerging issue. It was important for the Republicans to be able to negate this Democratic advantage by saying they had voted to provide the aged with a new Medicare drug benefit.

Both presidential candidates in the 2000 election also proposed differing Medicare drug benefit plans.

In mid-2001, Democrats gained control of the narrowly divided Senate.[4] Although there was little chance a drug bill would have passed the Senate before, once control shifted to the Democrats it was unlikely the Democratic-controlled Senate and the Republican-controlled House would be able to agree on a compromise bill.

In preparation for the 2002 congressional elections, the Democrats proposed a Medicare prescription drug benefit. They hoped to use this proposal to regain control of the House of Representatives and gain additional Senate seats. The Republicans hoped to deflect what was generally perceived as a Democratic advantage by proposing their own drug benefit. Republicans believed the differences between the two plans would not be as important as the fact that they were also proposing a drug benefit for seniors.[5]

Republicans improved their legislative positions in the 2002 election; they kept control of the House of Representatives and regained control of the Senate. The shift in control of the Senate was an opportunity for President Bush to fulfill his 2000 and 2002 campaign promises to enact a Medicare drug bill and thereby negate a Democratic advantage with seniors. President Bush believed that unless he could deliver on his election pledge, the public would lose trust in his promises and this would have negative consequences for him in the 2004 election.

Medicare reform was not only a top domestic priority for President Bush, but also for William Thomas (R-CA), the Chairman of the House Ways and Means Committee, and Senate Majority Leader William Frist (R-TN). (Chairman Thomas had cochaired the Bipartisan Commission and was strongly in favor of reforming Medicare.)

Similar to their proposals in the Bipartisan Commission, Republicans wanted to restructure Medicare by using a new drug benefit to induce Medicare beneficiaries to join private health plans.

The conflict over whether Medicare should have a stand-alone drug benefit or whether the drug benefit should be used as an inducement to introduce competition into Medicare was once again to be joined.

The Rise of Ideology in Health Policy

Previously, health policy was driven by groups having a concentrated interest, including health providers, health insurers, and even large employers with unfunded liabilities for their retirees' health benefits. Each sought legislative benefits to enhance their economic interests. For example, automobile companies, which are opposed to having government regulate their production of autos, are willing to have government intervene, through regulation and financing, to relieve them of their liabilities for retiree health benefits. Similarly, the aged and middle class seek redistributive legislation to shift the cost of their health benefits to the government, namely to taxpayers. Legislators have responded to these demands for legislative benefits in order to gain political support, campaign contributions, and the votes of the aged and middle class.

Constraining these demands was the Executive Branch, which bore the political cost of increased federal deficits and responsibility for the solvency of the Medicare Trust Fund. Increased regulation of Medicare hospital and physician payments occurred under both Democratic and Republican administrations. Politics took precedence over ideology when it came to an administration's responsibility for controlling Medicare expenditures.

However, primarily since the 1994 congressional elections, ideology has become a more important factor determining health policy. The Republicans gained 54 seats and took control of the House of Representatives for the first time in four decades.[6] The Republicans also took back control of the Senate. The leaders of the 1994 "Republican Revolution" that took control of the House of Representatives had campaigned on a document referred to as "A Contract with America," which promised to reduce the size and scope of government.

The rules under which the House of Representatives operates are such that when one party controls the House and its members are unified, bipartisan support is not necessary to pass a bill. The same is not true for the Senate, where it takes 60 votes to override a filibuster. Because Republicans did not have a 60-vote majority, and given that senators are more likely to vote independently of their party leadership, bipartisan compromise is necessary for a bill to emerge from the Senate.

The ideological battles over Medicare were mainly between conservative Republicans in the House and liberal Democrats in the Senate.[7] The ideological divisions between these two groups became pronounced when Republicans captured the House in 1994 and began to promote their viewpoint in legislation that passed the House but either failed in the Senate, was vetoed by President Clinton, or was, in greatly modified form, included in legislation that became law.

For a new Medicare prescription drug bill to be enacted in 2003, it would have had to receive the support of Republicans in the House while also receiving sufficient Democratic support for it to be accepted by the Senate. An ideological compromise would have been necessary for both sides to vote for the bill.[8]

Surprisingly, although there were strong differences on the comprehensiveness of the drug benefit—President Bush wanted to spend no more than $400 billion over ten years while Senate Democrats proposed spending upwards of $800 billion—*the difficult compromises involved ideological issues.*

Conservative Republicans considered the drug benefit as being secondary to reforming Medicare. They were opposed to adding a new entitlement to an existing entitlement that they believed was already out of control.

In designing the drug bill, the more important objective of conservative Republicans was slowing the growth in Medicare spending. They viewed Medicare as being unsustainable with its rapidly rising costs and an increased number of aged being guaranteed benefits under Medicare, which will become a huge financial burden on a working population that is declining (relative to the number of aged). In 2011, when the first of the baby boomers will become eligible for Medicare, the trust fund for Medicare Part A will be less than 20 years away from bankruptcy, and Part B expenditures, funded by general federal revenues, will consume an increasingly greater portion of the federal budget, necessitating tax increases or reductions in other politically popular programs. Huge tax increases will be needed to maintain the program into the future.

Medicare represents promises that cannot be kept. Modernization is needed to increase its efficiency, reduce the rate of increase in expenditures, and make Medicare financing more equitable. To achieve these goals, the aged need to be able to choose among competing health plans, and there has to be greater coordination of a patient's care. The market should determine the prices hospitals and physicians receive for treating Medicare patients in different regions of the country, rather than bureaucrats in Washington.

According to Medicare reform proponents, *the new drug benefit should serve as an inducement to the aged to join competing health plans.* Just adding a new, open-ended entitlement for all the aged would only make matters worse; it would be too expensive and would require even greater tax increases in future years. A drug benefit should only help those who need it and should only be used as an incentive to modernize Medicare.

Competition between traditional Medicare and private health plans was the basis of Medicare reform proposals. These plans would compete for Medicare beneficiaries on price and other attributes. The government would provide the aged with a health plan subsidy or voucher (the "premium-support" concept); those who choose a more expensive health plan would pay the additional out-of-pocket cost. Medicare beneficiaries would have more choice of health plans and a financial incentive to be concerned with their choice of plan. Medicare would be modeled after the Federal Employees Health Benefits Program. Conservative Republicans believed competition among health plans would result in enrollees receiving richer benefits and greater coordination of care, while saving Medicare money by encouraging innovation and better management of seniors' care.

Conservative Republicans in the House have different visions of the role of government and of Medicare than Democratic liberals in the Senate. They differ in the trust they place in private markets versus government decision making in the allocation of resources. The House Republicans believe the aged themselves, rather than the government, are better able to make decisions that are in their best interests and that to do so, the aged need to be able to choose among health plans that compete on price.

Democrats prefer the traditional approach to providing a new prescription drug benefit to the aged, namely, a uniform benefit administered by the government, offering generous coverage—over $800 billion over ten years—and direct negotiation by government with the drug companies to lower the cost of the new benefit. (This would have the effect of imposing drug price controls, similar to price controls on hospital and physician payments under Medicare.)

Liberal Democrats want to protect Medicare's traditional fee-for-service system and its principle of providing equal benefits for *all* the aged and providing the same subsidy regardless of income (even though this means benefits are more affordable to seniors with higher incomes). They believe Medicare can and should be sustained as it currently exists and that President Bush's tax cuts should be repealed and the funds used to support Medicare.

Liberals are opposed to changing Medicare's basic design and structure. They view Medicare as a very successful program, an example of how government can assist the aged. Further, liberals believe the private market and competition have failed to meet the needs of the poor and the aged, and they are concerned about the ability of consumers in these groups and others to make informed decisions in a competitive market.

In line with their philosophy, liberals wanted a new, stand-alone Medicare drug benefit. They contended that the aged should not have to leave traditional Medicare to receive a drug benefit, and Medicare should not have to compete with private health plans.

Given the different philosophies regarding Medicare, it is not surprising that the most controversial provision of the bill was the requirement that the traditional Medicare plan compete directly with private health plans (the "premium-support" concept). If traditional Medicare had higher costs than the private plans, beneficiaries would have to pay higher premiums to remain in Medicare. Fewer beneficiaries would be able to afford the higher premiums, the healthy aged would shift to lower-priced private plans, and this would eventually lead to the demise of traditional Medicare.

Those opposed to forcing traditional Medicare to compete with private health plans included Minority Leader Tom Daschle (D-SD), who claimed, "This is about the future of Medicare and whether it survives."[9] Senator Edward Kennedy (D-MA) warned that one particular provision in the House bill was unacceptable, that is, setting up direct competition between private plans and traditional Medicare.[10]

Given these strong ideological differences, how was it possible that a new Medicare prescription drug benefit was enacted?

The Role of Concentrated Interest Groups

Organizations that perceived significant economic benefits accruing to their members were important advocates for a new Medicare prescription drug bill. By providing benefits to these organizations, legislative proponents were able to build support for the bill. Lobbyists for these organizations played a significant role in persuading wavering legislators to vote in favor of the bill.[11]

Fred Graefe, a healthcare lobbyist representing hospitals and manufacturers, stated, "Members (Congressmen) should view Medicare as pork—it's just as important as a highway or an appropriations bill. It's important for members to show that in an era of surplus they can return Medicare dollars to their districts, which benefits both beneficiaries and providers."[12]

Following are some of the more important interest groups that strongly lobbied in favor of the bill and the benefits they received. (They were opposed by the AFL-CIO and the Consumers Union.)

The Pharmaceutical Companies

Any legislation affecting pharmaceutical products affects the profitability of pharmaceutical companies. Therefore, they have a concentrated interest in the design of that legislation.

The aged, whose use of prescriptions per capita is greater than that of any other group, will, as a result of the new drug benefit, receive a subsidy that will further increase their demand for prescription drugs. A new drug benefit would greatly increase the demand for drugs, hence increase drug firm profits. As discussed earlier (Chapter 4: The Demand for Legislation by Health Associations), no industry wants to be paid directly by government because the government, to reduce its expenditures, will eventually regulate the industry's prices. (The precedent for the government's controlling medical prices to reduce Medicare spending was controls on hospital and physician payments.)

Democrats claimed that, given its potential purchasing power for prescription drugs, the government could reduce the cost of the drug benefit by negotiating prices directly with the drug companies.

The drug manufacturers' major objective was to be paid by private payers, not the government.

Pharmaceutical companies were adamantly opposed to having to negotiate with the government, which they believed would have led to price controls.[13] The pharmaceutical companies, over the objection of Democrats, were successful in having the legislation include a prohibition against Medicare's using its purchasing power to negotiate with drug companies.[14]

A second priority of the drug companies, in which they were again successful, was to prohibit unlimited reimportation of drugs to the United States. If Americans could use the Internet to buy drugs overseas at lower prices, U.S. pharmaceutical company profits would be reduced. The proponents of drug reimportation were legislators from states bordering Canada, irrespective of political party. They favored allowing Americans to reimport drugs from Canada and other countries where drug companies sold the same drug at greatly reduced prices. Some legislators even wanted to require drug companies to sell unlimited amounts of their drugs to Canada so that they could be reimported back to the United States.

Reimportation legislation was previously enacted, but it was contingent upon the Secretary of Health and Human Services certifying that reimported drugs would be safe (not counterfeit). Under both the Clinton and Bush Administrations, the secretaries of Health and Human Services did not permit reimportation because they could not guarantee safety. Proponents of reimportation wanted the MMA to remove the secretary's discretion to certify that reimported drugs would be safe. Reimportation proponents were unsuccessful in having the law changed.[15]

American Association of Retired Persons

The AARP has a concentrated interest in all issues affecting the elderly. Its objective is to promote an intergenerational transfer of wealth, from the working-age population to those who are retired. The AARP's support for the new drug benefit should be understood within this perspective. The new drug benefit subsidized the elderly at the expense of taxpayers. Although the new benefit was not as generous as the AARP leaders preferred, they believed it was a foot in the door and could be expanded at a future time.

As a lobby organization for seniors, the AARP has been very effective in mobilizing the elderly to contact their legislators and to provide their "Good Housekeeping Seal" to legislation (as well as to products and services offered to seniors).

Given the rising deficits, the $400 billion set aside by the congressional resolution, and the upcoming 2004 election, the chief executive officer of the AARP, William Novelli, believed this was a window of opportunity to enact a drug benefit that could later be made more comprehensive. As the AARP's chief lobbyist, John Rother, stated, "Well, we represent a constituency that doesn't have that much time to wait. There was no prospect in the short term that we were going to get a better bill, and there was a real risk that we could end up with a worse bill."[16]

The AARP's endorsement was a huge victory for the Republicans and substantially increased the chances that the House and Senate conference committee's bill would be approved in the Senate. The AARP's endorsement angered its usual allies in the Democratic Party and the labor unions. Liberal Democrats accused AARP of a conflict of interest for trying to profit from its commercial interests.[17] AARP's brand name has a great deal of market power among seniors. In addition to offering, through other companies, life, health, auto, and homeowners insurance; investment services; and travel services, AARP also offers pharmacy services through United HealthCare. Under the new Medicare drug bill, AARP stands to earn hundreds of millions of dollars more under its drug royalty agreements. In response to these criticisms of financial conflict, William Novelli claimed that the business side of AARP has no influence on its policy side.[18]

As the price for AARP's support of the Medicare drug bill, Novelli insisted on three conditions, all of which were met by the Republican leadership. First, the proposal for competition of private plans with traditional Medicare had to be experimental, not permanent. (This meant that House Republicans' proposal for competition between private plans and traditional Medicare had to become a demonstration project and not be implemented before 2010, if ever.) Second, employers had to be given an incentive to maintain retiree prescription drug benefits. Third, the drug benefit must be free for low-income seniors.[19]

Rural Constituents, Including Rural Hospitals and Physicians

Senator Chuck Grassley (R-IA), chairman of the Senate Finance Committee, had the responsibility of passing the drug bill through the finance committee and then having it approved by the Senate. In addition to ensuring that the bill contained sufficient ideological compromises and benefits for the constituents of other senators (Democrats as well as conservative Republicans) so that the bill could withstand a possible filibuster by opponents, Senator Grassley, who represented a rural area, was running for reelection in 2004 and wanted to make certain that his constituents were well taken care of. Senator Grassley, however, was not the only senator on the committee representing rural interests; many other senators on the committee from both parties had similar interests, and their votes were needed.

Looking out for the interests of elderly Medicare beneficiaries living in rural areas, who are overwhelmingly dependent on traditional Medicare and therefore less likely to have access to a private health plan, was a top priority of Senator Grassley. The Bush administration's initial intent was to use the drug benefit as an incentive to entice seniors into private health plans. However, senators representing rural constituents wanted the elderly to be able to remain with traditional Medicare and receive the drug benefit. To achieve this goal, the drug benefit would have to be a stand-alone benefit.[20]

Senator Grassley's second priority was to ensure that rural hospitals and physicians would remain in rural areas; therefore, he wanted them to receive additional monies as part of the MMA. The *Des Moines Register*, the state's largest newspaper, published many editorials advocating an increase in Medicare payments to rural hospitals.[21] It was in Senator Grassley's political interest to make sure these additional funds were included in the MMA.

The MMA included $25 billion in additional payments to rural healthcare providers over the next ten years. The payments included providing hospitals in rural and small urban areas with a permanent 1.6 percent increase in payment for caring for Medicare patients. Hospitals in low-wage areas would receive more money to help them compete for workers by paying higher wages. Medicare payments to physicians working in rural areas would be increased by an additional 5 percent. And home health care providers caring for Medicare patients in rural areas would be provided with bonus payments.

Hospitals

Hospital association lobbyists were successful in including in the senate bill anticompetitive language prohibiting physicians from referring patients to hospitals in which they have an ownership interest. Community hospitals claimed that specialty hospitals that treat one type of patient, such as orthopedic cases, take the more profitable patients and leave community hospitals with the less profitable patients. An 18-month moratorium was placed on physician referrals for Medicare patients to new specialty hospitals in which they have an investment interest.

Hospitals also received additional benefits, such as increased Medicare payments in 2004 by the full rate of change in cost for a "market basket" of items hospitals use. By reclassifying the Medicare hospital wage index, hospitals received an additional $900 million over five years and teaching hospitals received an additional $400 million over ten years. Further, hospitals that serve a large number of uninsured patients and Medicaid patients, known as disproportionate-share hospitals, received more federal money to compensate them for that care. And for teaching hospitals, the Indirect Medical Education adjustment factor was increased for the next four years.

Physicians

Since 1997, Medicare has based the amount by which it annually increases Medicare physician expenditures on the sustainable growth rate. One component of the sustainable growth rate is the percentage increase in real gross domestic product per capita. Thus, when the economy is doing well, physicians' Medicare payments increase. However, in 2000 the economy entered a recession, and the consequence was that physician payments decreased by 5.4 percent in 2002.

A high priority of the AMA was to prevent further scheduled decreases in physicians' Medicare payments. The MMA blocked a scheduled 4.5 percent reduction in physician Medicare payments in 2004 and 2005. Instead, physicians received a 1.5 percent increase in each of those years.

Further, the sustainable growth rate, which determines how much Medicare pays physicians (and which has been the reason for the proposed cuts in physician payments—which Congress overturned), will be modified under the new law.

Physicians will also receive additional payments for drug administration services.

Health Insurers

Previously, as part of Medicare Part C (called Medicare+Choice), private health plans were able to enroll Medicare beneficiaries. The Bush administration wanted to promote the use of private health plans for Medicare beneficiaries. As part of the new drug legislation, Medicare+Choice was renamed Medicare Advantage. The new drug benefit can be provided by stand-alone prescription drug plans as part of traditional Medicare or as part of Medicare Part C, in which Medicare Advantage health plans integrate (and enhance) Part A and Part B benefits.

The Republicans wanted the Medicare Advantage plans to serve more Medicare seniors, and eventually, to compete with traditional Medicare. Government payments to Medicare Advantage plans were increased under the new drug bill. By strengthening (subsidizing) these plans and having them increase their proportion of Medicare seniors (to 35 percent), the Republicans and health insurers believed the Medicare Advantage plans would have greater political power relative to traditional Medicare in the annual struggle for funds.

Health insurers were strongly in favor of the MMA provisions to inject market forces and competition in the delivery of Medicare services.[22]

Under the MMA, Medicare would sign contracts with preferred provider plans in each region of the country starting in 2006. These plans would provide drug benefits, along with a full range of medical services.[23] Medicare may designate 10 to 50 regions to cover the United States. Health insurers were concerned that a contract for a region would include both urban and rural areas. In the past, health insurers withdrew from many rural markets because they claimed Medicare payments were insufficient for serving those areas. Insurers have been able to establish preferred provider networks of physicians and hospitals in urban areas. However, in rural areas, because there are so few hospitals and physicians, these providers have market power and can charge very high prices to participate in an insurer's network, much more than they are paid by traditional Medicare. Insurers were concerned that unless they were provided with additional subsidies, they would be unable to compete with traditional Medicare in rural areas.[24]

As part of the MMA, HMOs (and other managed care plans) received a subsidy of $500 million for 2004 and $14.2 billion over ten years.

Other Providers

Other provider groups also benefited from the MMA. For example, to benefit the trade association of pharmacies, insurers would be required to accept any pharmacies willing to agree to the health plan's terms and conditions. (This is similar to anticompetitive any willing provider laws.) Dentists, podiatrists, and optometrists would be able to privately contract with Medicare beneficiaries. Per diem payments to skilled nursing facilities that treat AIDS patients would rise by 128 percent. And healthcare providers providing emergency services to undocumented immigrants would also receive additional funds.

The Country's Largest Employers

The MMA enabled these companies to shift part of their retirees' soaring prescription drug costs to the government. These "old-line" companies with a large number of retirees were committed to providing their employees and their retirees with generous health benefits, including prescription drugs. These companies, however, did not prefund their healthcare liabilities. As the costs of healthcare have risen, these companies' unfunded liabilities for retiree healthcare costs have also risen rapidly. For example, GM has an unfunded healthcare liability of $70 billion for its current and future retirees.

Under the Financial Accounting Standard 106, an accounting rule established by the Financial Accounting Standards Board in 1991, unfunded retiree (and future retiree) healthcare liabilities must be recognized on the financial statements of these companies. This accounting rule requires companies to expense a portion of their liability each year, thereby reducing their profits. As a result, the profits of these companies are reduced each year by hundreds of millions of dollars.

A major legislative objective of these companies was to shift their burden for retiree health benefits to the government, hence taxpayers.

Under the MMA, employers who provide retiree drug coverage with actuarially equivalent drug benefits as provided in Part D will receive a government subsidy equal to 28 percent of those costs above $250 but not greater than $5,000 (in 2006) per Medicare beneficiary. This amount would be adjusted annually by the percentage increase in Medicare per capita prescription drug costs.

As a result of the MMA, Ford Motor Company, which has an unfunded healthcare liability of $30 billion, is expected to save $50 million or more of its current spending for retirees' drug costs—in addition to a $40 million reduction in its annual accounting estimate of future spending for retirees.[25]

Under the MMA, these tax-free subsidies to employers who maintain drug coverage for retirees was estimated to be worth $70 billion over ten years.[26]

The funds allocated for the prescription drug bill, $400 billion over a ten-year period, were not just for federal subsidies for seniors' drug expenditures. A significant portion of the $400 billion went to benefit concentrated interests, such as health plans, large employers providing a retiree drug benefit, hospitals, physicians, other providers, and rural areas.

Economic interests outweigh ideological interests for groups that have a concentrated interest. Such groups typically oppose government regulation, except when it is in their own economic interest.

The Politics Underlying a New Medicare Prescription Drug Bill

Legislative proposals are driven by political considerations. The year 2004 was a presidential election year, and the two political parties expected the election to be very close. The aged are an important demographic group in Florida, a state that determined the 2000 presidential election and that President Bush won by fewer than 600 votes. Opinion polls showed that on health issues, the public trusted Democrats more than Republicans, and the Democrats had been proposing a new drug benefit for the aged.

President Bush wanted to enact a drug benefit for the aged to remove it as a campaign issue; he wanted to neutralize the Democrats' political advantage with the elderly. President Bush had previously talked about a Medicare drug benefit in the 2000 election campaign. The Republicans and President Bush made a Medicare prescription drug bill their number one domestic priority and believed they had to enact such a bill before the 2004 elections. President Bush raised the visibility of a Medicare drug benefit by including it in his 2003 State of the Union address. If he succeeded in enacting such a bill, the president would be able to take credit for an issue important to the aged and an issue where the Democrats have been viewed more favorably by voters than Republicans.

President Bush, who was politically responsible for the rapidly rising federal budget deficit, proposed a drug plan costing $400 billion over ten years. Although the Democrats tried to outbid the president for the votes of the aged by proposing prescription drug legislation that would cost the federal government about $800 billion over ten years, the Congressional Budget Resolution for Fiscal Year 2004 allocated $400 billion over ten years for a new Medicare prescription drug benefit, which represented only about 20 percent of seniors' total drug expenditures.

Given the large projected federal deficits, Democrats and Republicans realized that $400 billion might not be available to provide the aged with a new drug benefit for many years. Although the $400 billion was much less than Democrats and the AARP wanted, it was still a significant amount of money allocated to a drug benefit at a time when the war in Iraq was consuming a lot of money. The baby boomers would soon begin to retire and greatly increase Medicare spending still further, and under these circumstances, they did not think a drug benefit would be proposed again for some time.

The MMA's design was very complex because it was affected by the spending cap of $400 billion over ten years and by political considerations.

The spending cap meant that compromises had to be made in coverage. The greatest financial hardships occur from unexpected catastrophic expenses. Individuals are able to afford small expenses. Thus, any form of insurance, whether it is medical, auto, or home insurance, should primarily cover catastrophic expenses. It would be expected that an important part of the new drug benefit would be to cover catastrophic drug expenditures; that is, those drug expenses that exceed a large dollar amount, such as $5,000 per year per beneficiary. And because a lower expenditure limit could also represent a financial hardship to low-income aged, additional subsidies would have to be provided for them.

The political difficulty of allocating limited federal dollars just for catastrophic drug expenses and for subsidies to low-income aged is that most (particularly middle- and high-income) aged would not receive any benefit from the new legislation.

The political objective of subsidizing the aged is to receive their appreciation and votes, therefore, legislators had to design the legislation so *all* aged would receive some benefit. Consequently, small drug expenses were also subsidized. The cost of a catastrophic drug plan is relatively small; however, once small expenses are also included, the cost of the government plan greatly increases. To limit the cost of the plan, a very large deductible was inserted *between* the small drug expenses and the catastrophic coverage.

Consequently, the drug benefit consists of a deductible of $250, which will increase annually based on the growth in per capita Part D drug spending; it is estimated to be $445 by 2013.

The beneficiary would then have to pay 25 percent of drug costs from $251 to $2,250 in 2006 (which then increases to an estimated $4,000 in 2013). *Then patients have to pay 100 percent of their prescription drug expenditures between $2,250 and $5,100 in 2006, rising to $9,066 in 2013.* (This gap in drug coverage has been referred to as the "doughnut hole.") Once the patient reaches that threshold, there is "stop-loss" coverage; the patient only has to pay $2 for generic drugs or $5 for branded drugs (which are indexed to increase over time by the rise in per capita Part D drug spending) or a 5 percent coinsurance, whichever is greater. (However, a formulary would be used and drugs bought that are not on the formulary would not count toward the beneficiary's out-of-pocket limit.)

The "doughnut hole" was created to save money as all the aged benefit when they are provided with coverage up to $2,250. Such a design is rare in private insurance. Designing the drug benefit with a big gap only makes sense in terms of politics, not insurance. The idea was to give everyone some benefit, but also to limit total costs of the program. (Once the aged discover this big gap, it is likely they will clamor for more, and this will increase the cost of the bill.)

The first stage of the legislative battle over the Medicare drug benefit occurred when the Senate and House had to pass their respective drug bills.

In June 2003, the Senate, without a great deal of controversy, passed its version of the MMA, which then went to conference to be reconciled with the House version of a prescription drug bill. To have a Medicare drug bill pass the Senate, its proponents, primarily the Bush administration, had to accept a great many changes to what they originally proposed. Thus, the drug bill passed by the Senate in 2003 was very different than the one passed by the House, which meant that the two bills would have to be resolved through a conference committee.

Although the drug benefit in the Senate bill was not nearly as comprehensive as Senate Democrats wanted, given the size of the federal deficit and the additional funding required for the war in Iraq, many Democrats believed another $400 billion would not be available for a long time if they did not get a drug bill this time. Senator Edward Kennedy (D-MA), a liberal in favor of providing the aged with a comprehensive drug benefit as part of traditional Medicare, endorsed the initial bipartisan drug bill that passed the Senate. Without his support, the Senate would not have been able to pass the bill.

Once enacted, Democrats would be able to propose a more comprehensive drug benefit. In this way, the Democrats would be able to keep the drug benefit alive as an election issue to help win seniors' votes.[27]

In previous years, House Republicans were able to push drug legislation through the Republican-controlled House (with mostly Republican votes) with the knowledge that the legislation, which included proposals that were anathema to Democrats, would fail in the closely divided Senate. House Republicans could then claim at election time that they had voted for a Medicare drug benefit.

In June 2003, realizing that the enactment of a Medicare drug bill was a real possibility, the Republican-controlled House of Representatives narrowly passed its bill—by just one vote. In the closely divided House of Representatives, with House Democrats nearly unanimous in their opposition to the bill, the Republican leadership needed the support of conservative Republicans, who were concerned about enacting a new, costly Medicare drug entitlement when there was already doubt about Medicare's long-term solvency. The new bill, they argued, had to restructure Medicare, which meant requiring traditional Medicare to compete against private health plans. In June 2003, a group of 42 House Republicans notified the Speaker of the House, Dennis Hastert (R-IL), that they would not support any compromise bill unless the bill promoted competition with private health plans.[28]

The bill passed by the House in June 2003 included a number of proposals previously included in House bills that the Senate had rejected and therefore had not become law. In the past, Congress had permitted managed care plans to serve Medicare beneficiaries as an alternative to traditional Medicare. The aged could voluntarily join these plans and return to traditional Medicare with 30 days' notice. However, this form of competition was very different than what Republicans desired. Republicans wanted "premium support," which would have turned Medicare into more of a voucher system, from a defined benefit to a defined contribution.

Conservative Republicans in the House were adamant about having traditional Medicare compete against private plans, while both House and Senate Democrats were equally vigorous in opposing such competition.

Competition between private health plans and traditional Medicare became the most contentious issue holding up agreement on the prescription drug act.

The bill passed by the House in June 2003 (by a one-vote majority) was intended to reform Medicare in anticipation of the retirement of the baby boomers and rapidly increasing Medicare expenditures. There were significant ideological differences in the bills passed by the House and Senate. Consequently, a conference committee to reconcile these differences was started in July 2003. The conference committee bill would have to be brought back to each chamber for a vote before going to the president.

The conference committee had to construct a bill that would attract some Democratic support in the Senate while also enabling House conservatives to vote for the bill, as almost all Democratic House members were expected to vote against it. To attract the necessary votes from some legislators, the bill included benefits for various interest groups. (In fact, the Bush Administration asked many lobbyists to campaign hard with legislators for their vote in favor of the final bill.) However, the greater the benefits given to interest groups, the higher the cost, and the bill had to be within the $400 billion Congressional resolution. The conference bill had to weigh these many trade-offs.

The Republicans, who controlled both houses of Congress, also controlled the conference committee. Senate Republicans decided to exclude Senate Democrats from the conference committee's discussions, except for two senators who were crucial to the bill's success, Max Bauchus (D-MT) and John Breaux (D-LA), who were considered the only two Democrats willing to compromise with the Republicans. House Republicans excluded House Democrats, because they had opposed the House bill and were expected to oppose the conference bill.[29]

The Compromise Bill

The resulting conference committee bill compromised on many issues, including ideological conflicts. The design of the drug benefit was itself a compromise between those who wanted a more comprehensive benefit for all aged versus those who wanted a catastrophic drug benefit for just those aged who incurred such costs. Hence the inclusion of the "doughnut" concept; the aged would have to pay a large deductible after having received some drug benefits.

The MMA provides for a voluntary outpatient prescription drug benefit under Medicare Part D. Seniors can obtain prescription drug coverage in two main ways: by joining a managed care plan or by remaining in traditional Medicare and buying a separate drug-only insurance plan, which did not previously exist. The new drug benefit becomes effective January 2006. For the two years before the start of the new benefit (2004 to 2005), a subsidized drug discount-card program for low-income elderly without other drug coverage became available.

Medicare Part D subsidies will be financed by general federal revenues (and by maintaining effort payments by state Medicaid programs). The federal subsidy for Part D is 74.5 percent, provided through direct premium subsidies and reinsurance. The federal government will provide premium subsidies for low-income Medicare beneficiaries.[30]

Further, Medicare beneficiaries enrolled in the new drug plans are not permitted to buy Medigap (supplementary) policies that would cover out-of-pocket expenses. The reason is that lowering the beneficiary's out-of-pocket costs, thereby insulating them from any costs, would encourage them to overuse the drug benefit and increase total government drug expenditures.[31]

The benefit design of the drug bill was less contentious than other aspects because the Democrats believed that once the legislation was enacted, they would be able to propose enhancing the benefits and place Republicans in the position of opposing increased drug benefits for the aged.

Compromises were also reached on ideological issues. House Republicans had to give up a great deal for the bill to win the support of moderate Senate Democrats (and Republicans). House Republicans wanted a more far-reaching bill that would reform Medicare ("premium support") and limit Medicare spending. Instead, all they received was a (face-saving) limited demonstration project for competition between traditional Medicare and private health plans that would not occur until 2010.[32]

The conference committee bill infuriated conservative House Republicans. The bill did not go far enough in restructuring Medicare to provide incentives for seniors to switch into private plans; their desire for subjecting traditional Medicare to competition with private plans was relegated to a demonstration project to begin years later.

To compensate conservative Republicans for their loss of Medicare reform, the legislation established tax-free HSAs for persons under the age of 65 years who have high-deductible policies.[33] The plan must have an annual deductible of at least $1,000 for individual coverage and $2,000 for family coverage. Out-of-pocket expenses must be no more than $5,000 for individual coverage and $10,000 for family coverage. The maximum aggregate annual contribution that can be made to an HSA is the lesser of 100 percent of the annual deductible under the high-deductible plan. Contributions to such accounts are tax free. These accounts are owned by the individual, but when the individual dies, HSA ownership can be transferred tax free to the person's spouse.[34]

To further mollify conservative Republicans who were concerned with the cost of a new entitlement, two significant cost-containment measures were included in the compromise bill.

A trigger mechanism was included that requires the president and Congress to act if expenditures increase to a much greater extent than forecast. If Medicare's trustees forecast for two consecutive years that within the next seven years general government revenues will exceed 45 percent or more of total Medicare expenditures, the president has to submit "corrective" legislation to Congress. The House of Representatives would be required to act under a fast-track procedure; however, in the Senate filibustering rules would still apply. This cost-containment mechanism does not ensure that corrective legislation will be enacted, but the president and Congress would be forced to acknowledge the problem and examine possible solutions.

The first of two warnings could occur in 2006, the second in 2007. After two consecutive such reports are issued, the president is required (15 days after he submits his next budget, which would be in February 2008) to submit legislation to correct this deficiency. Congress then has to deal with it in an expedited fashion in June of the same year, 2008.[35] However, 2008 is a presidential election year. It is highly unlikely that competing presidential candidates or legislators up for election in 2008 will propose solutions that would impose a burden on any voting group, particularly the aged, who have the highest voting-participation rate.

Relating the Medicare Part B premium to income was another measure to keep the cost of the bill within the $400 billion estimate. Beginning in 2007, higher-income beneficiaries will pay a higher Part B premium. The government subsidy for the Part B premium will decrease by different percentages for different income levels, from a 65 percent subsidy for those in the $80,000 to $100,000 income bracket to as low as a 20 percent government subsidy for those enrollees making more than $200,000 a year. Estimates are that only 3 percent of Part B enrollees will be affected by the income-related premium in 2007, increasing to 6 percent in 2013.

The Republican leadership had difficulty gaining support for the drug plan from their own legislators, who believed it provided for an expensive new entitlement they already thought was "unsustainable," poorly designed, inequitable (all the aged, regardless of income, would receive a large subsidy), and diminished the chances of ever having competition between Medicare and private plans occur.

The conference bill, when voted on by the House of Representatives, was very close; House Republican leaders had to keep the vote open for an unusually long period, three hours, and engaged in strong lobbying to get conservative Republicans to vote for the bill. The final vote was 220-215.

Although the Republican leadership had to cajole conservative Republicans to vote for the conference committee bill when it was voted on in the House, in the Senate it was the liberals who were opposed to it.

Senator Edward Kennedy (D-MA), an influential Democrat, particularly on health issues, initially gave his approval for a Medicare drug benefit, which made it acceptable for other Democrats to vote for the Senate bill in June 2003. Senator Kennedy wanted to expand Medicare benefits and extend Medicare to population groups other than the aged. By enacting a new Medicare drug benefit, he believed it would just be a matter of time before political pressures by the aged, stimulated by Democrats, would make the new drug benefit more comprehensive.

Subsequently, Senator Kennedy withdrew his support and opposed the conference committee bill because it included a demonstration project on competition ("premium support") and increased premiums for higher-income aged. Senator Kennedy and other Democrats claimed that the competition demonstration would result in privatizing Medicare and that relating Part B premiums to income would change the political support for the program. Medicare would become like Medicaid, a welfare program. Instead of being a middle-class entitlement, higher-income aged would drop their support and it would become less politically popular and vulnerable to future budget cuts, like Medicaid.

Senate Democrats also criticized the bill for prohibiting the government from negotiating drug prices directly with the drug companies and for not permitting drug reimportation from Canada. (In the bill, the Secretary of Health and Human Services had to approve reimportation).

However, by the time the conference committee bill reached the Senate, the bill had enough votes to pass. The Senate, with help from Democrats, ended a filibuster led by Senator Kennedy and others.

AARP's endorsement of the bill in November 2003 was seen as a turning point. It provided the Republicans with political cover from Democrat charges that the bill was not in the best interests of the aged and that Republicans were trying to destroy Medicare as we know it. It also helped Republicans counter Democratic charges that the bill did not provide enough benefits.

Enough Democrats voted for the bill to overcome a filibuster; they were concerned that if they did not support the bill, they would be seen as obstructionists preventing seniors from having a drug benefit and this would give the Republicans an advantage going into the 2004 election.

Summing Up

As a Republican committed to lessening the role of the federal government, President Bush proposed an enormous increase in federal expenditures and, over time, as pressure built to reduce prescription drug expenditures, likely federal regulation of drug prices. Political considerations overrode ideology.

In addition to concentrated economic interest groups, ideology and politics are used to explain the passage of the MMA. The use of ideology and politics enhances the explanatory power of the economic theory of regulation. Both politics and ideology represent opposing group's economic preferences regarding redistribution.

Ideology can be defined in terms of conflict over economic redistribution. Liberals are for greater income redistribution, as indicated by their support for higher taxes, increased size of government, and greater equality of income. Conversely, conservatives have a greater acceptance of inequality of incomes. Thus, ideology represents voters favoring different tax, expenditure, and redistribution policies.[36]

Similarly, politics can be considered to represent economic redistribution, as the MMA caters to the economic interest of the aged, a politically important voting bloc, particularly in Florida. Although a conservative, President Bush favored the MMA on political grounds, believing he would need the MMA for reelection. To ideological conservatives, the MMA represented a large increase in the role of government, together with a substantial increase in the federal deficit. Presidential politics and the conservative ideology of House Republicans resulted in significant conflict between the president and his own party in enacting the MMA. Liberals favored a vast new redistributive program, a comprehensive benefit for all the aged, while conservatives favored a more limited benefit and wanted it to be income related.

Both Republicans and Democrats compromised on ideological issues. Republicans lost their major objective, which was to restructure Medicare by having traditional Medicare compete with private health plans ("premium support"). Instead, they received a demonstration project that few expect to occur.

However, to secure the political support of conservative Republicans, the bill added features unrelated to prescription drugs, such as allowing tax-deductible HSAs for those younger than 65 years, prohibiting the government from directly negotiating with drug companies, and providing a new mechanism to force the president and Congress to take action if federal tax revenues exceeded 45 percent of Medicare spending.[37]

Eventually, the rising costs of the drug benefit (and the 45 percent limit) will cause the federal government to have a concentrated interest in holding down total Medicare drug expenditures. At that time, federal regulation of drug prices may occur, in which case the Republicans will have lost another ideological battle.

The Democrats (with the help of Republican senators representing rural constituencies) achieved two of their major ideological priorities, namely, a stand-alone Medicare drug benefit so seniors would not have to leave traditional Medicare to have a drug benefit, and second, an end to Republican hopes of having traditional Medicare compete with private health plans. They were able to postpone the tough decisions that Medicare reform would require, namely, reducing Medicare benefits and increasing payroll taxes, until later.

Democrats, however, lost on an important ideological issue. For the first time, Medicare premiums became income related. Seniors with higher incomes will have to pay higher premiums. Since Medicare's inception, all beneficiaries have received the same benefits at the same price. Although few aged will be affected initially, symbolically this is an important change. Democrats also lost on several other issues: reimportation drugs, prohibiting the government from negotiating drug prices directly with drug companies, HSAs for those under the age of 65 years, and a potential limit (45 percent) on the use of tax revenues to finance Medicare. Democrats are concerned this limit will be used to reduce Medicare benefits and increase Medicare premiums.

Incremental changes will likely be made to the MMA in coming years. The Democrats will press for expanding the drug benefit, and projections of the cost of the drug benefit will require whichever administration is in office to take steps to limit increases in Medicare drug expenditures.[38] The political and ideological fights over the drug benefit have only temporarily ceased.

Looking Ahead

Medicare is unsustainable. The 2004 Medicare and Social Security Trustees' Report calculated the present value of the difference between federal Medicare expenses and revenues. The present value of the additional revenues required by Medicare is $62 trillion dollars. This estimate is five times greater than the projected deficit for Social Security, which is $12 trillion. (The recently enacted Medicare prescription drug benefit will require an additional $17 trillion.) This $74 trillion revenue shortfall requires that this amount of money be invested and earn interest to be able to meet commitments made to the aged. Each year, this tremendous shortfall increases by $2 trillion.

The surpluses of the Medicare and Social Security Trust Funds have been spent to fund current government programs; nothing has been saved—there is no cash in those trust funds. In return for the use of these funds, the government has given an IOU to the respective trust funds. When expenditures under these programs exceed each fund's payroll tax revenues, the U.S. Treasury cannot use the surplus that was generated in these funds, because the money has already been spent. Instead, to pay the Medicare and Social Security commitments made to the aged, the government will either have to borrow money, increase taxes, or reduce spending on other government programs.

The Medicare and Social Security Trust Funds are currently generating a small surplus and are not expected to be technically bankrupt for about 12 to 15 years. However, in 2005, for the first time, the federal government will spend on Medicare and Social Security all the payroll taxes that are collected and will have to use $4 billion of general revenues to cover the excess of spending over revenues for these entitlement programs. (The government will be paying back the IOUs by using general revenue funds.) Funding problems will become even more severe when the baby boomers start retiring in 2011. The federal government will then be spending about 15 percent of all income- tax revenues, in addition to the payroll taxes collected, on these aged entitlements. The Social Security Fund is estimated to become technically exhausted by 2017 and the Medicare Trust Fund by 2019. By then, 25 percent of all federal income-tax dollars will have to be used to pay entitlement benefits to the aged. That amount of money will necessitate a drastic reduction in all other federal programs unless changes are made.[39]

The aged and near-aged will receive large intergenerational transfers. Delaying the time when Medicare's financing is reformed only increases the tax burden on the younger generation.

Previously, when the Medicare trustees claimed that Medicare expenditures were expected to exceed the funds provided by Medicare payroll taxes, Medicare payroll taxes were increased, as was the wage base, and (the annual update) payments to hospitals were reduced. These approaches for delaying bankruptcy of the Medicare Trust Fund will no longer be possible. After the first of the baby boomers begin to retire in 2011, estimated Medicare expenditures will start exceeding Medicare taxes by larger and larger amounts in succeeding years. Reducing hospital payments and increasing the Medicare payroll tax to cover the shortfall will reduce hospital access and quality; much higher payroll taxes will create political opposition. Medicare will have to be reformed.

Medicare expenditures will continue to rise sharply as the baby boomers retire, life expectancy of the aged increases, medical technology expands what can be done for patients, and the cost of producing medical services (wages) continues to increase. How will these expenditures be financed? Which population groups will bear this burden?

There are no simple solutions to the impending Medicare financial catastrophe. Medicare reform will occur when the tax burden placed on the working population for providing medical benefits to the aged rapidly increases. As this occurs, future generations will have an incentive to try and reduce these costs. The previously diffuse cost of aged health and retirement benefits will become a concentrated cost to the working population.

To make Medicare financially secure over the long term, costs would have to be imposed on politically important constituencies. Medicare reform will require future retirees, healthcare providers, the working population, and the current aged to bear some of the cost of forestalling Medicare's bankruptcy. Legislators are unlikely to vote on an issue that will antagonize important constituencies. Reform carries too great a political cost and therefore has been deferred to a future Congress and president.

Study Questions

1. What changes did conservative Republicans want to include in the MMA?
2. What ideological issues were important to liberal Democrats in the design of the MMA?
3. Describe the "premium-support" concept and how its proponents expect it to modernize Medicare.
4. What were the AARP's conditions for supporting the MMA?
5. Why was President Bush anxious to enact a Medicare drug benefit?

6. What benefits did the following concentrated interest groups receive as part of the MMA: drug companies, hospitals, and physicians?
7. Why did senators representing rural constituencies favor a stand-alone drug benefit?

Notes

1. John A. Poisal and Lauren Murray, "Growing Differences Between Medicare Beneficiaries With and Without Drug Coverage," *Health Affairs* 20, no. 2 (2001): 74–85.
2. Congressional Budget Office, *Prescription Drugs: Expanding Access to Federal Prices Could Cause Other Price Changes*, GAO/HEHS-00-118 (Washington, DC: U.S. Government Printing Office, 2000).
3. For a historical perspective on proposals for a Medicare outpatient prescription drug benefit, see Thomas R. Oliver, Philip R. Lee, and Helene L. Lipton, "A Political History of Medicare and Prescription Drug Coverage," *The Milbank Quarterly* 82 (2004): 283–354.
4. Senator James Jeffords (R-VT) left the Republican party to become an independent and vote for Democratic control of the Senate.
5. Robert Pear, "Drug Plans For Elderly Are Unveiled By 2 Parties," *New York Times*, May 2, 2002, A21.
6. Using Americans for Democratic Action scores as the measure of ideology, Grofman, et. al., examine the change in the location of the median and mean voter in the House of Representatives during different time periods. They conclude that the shift in the median House voter from 1993–1994 to 1994–1995 was the single greatest shift in ideology in the modern era. The median voter's Americans for Democratic Action score shifted from nearly 50 in the previous five congresses to only 24, which, after one election, was a shift in the House median of more than 25 points; such a shift in the median could certainly be characterized as revolutionary. After the 1994 elections there was a 79-point difference in the Americans for Democratic Action score between the median House Republicans and the House Democrats, a huge ideological difference between the two political parties. Bernard Grofman, et. al., "Changes in the Location of the Median Voter in the U.S. House of Representatives, 1963–1996," *Public Choice* 106 (2001): 221–232.

    Consequently, ". . . a small shift in the average ideology of the legislature can lead to a large shift in the particular policy chosen as the outcome of voting if the small shift moves from a liberal majority to a conservative majority." (392); James B. Kau and Paul H. Rubin, "The Growth of Government: Sources and Limits," *Public Choice* 113 (2002): 389–402.

7. The term "conservative" usually represents a person who favors the status quo, while a liberal favors change. In politics the term has taken on its opposite meaning, whereby conservatives favor changing Medicare while liberals favor the status quo.

8. Robin Toner, "Medicare: Battleground for a Bigger Struggle," *New York Times*, July 20, 2003, 4.1.

9. Deborah Barfield Berry, "The New Deal on Medicare," *Newsday*, November 25, 2003.

10. Robert Pear and Robin Toner, "House Committee Approves Drug Benefits for Medicare," *New York Times*, June 18, 2003, A19.

11. Attached to complex legislation are targeted provisions meant to benefit specific institutions or small groups of individuals. These benefits would never be enacted separately. For example, Senator Grassley (R-IA), the lead Senate negotiator of the Medicare bill and whose state is home to a large chiropractic college, included pilot programs to determine whether Medicare should pay for more chiropractic services. Senator Ted Stevens (R-AK), chairman of the powerful Senate Appropriations Committee, included a provision for Medicare to pay more to physicians working in Alaska, which has the smallest percentage of Medicare beneficiaries than any other state. Christopher Lee, "Medicare Bill Partly a Special Interest Care Package," *Washington Post*, November 23, 2003, A11.

12. Mary Agnes Carey, "GOP's Prescription Drug Bill: A 'Political Imperative'?", *Congressional Quarterly Weekly*, June 17, 2000. Also, "Medicare has become pork barrel. It plays to retirees' desires and raises their discretionary income. The question of generational justice is nearly absent. Who cares about the long-term budget outlook or about clueless younger workers?" Further, "The new drug benefit will make a national problem—paying the baby boom's retirement benefits—worse. In its first decade, costs are expected at about $400 billion. . . . But if a new "blockbuster" drug appears, forget the $400 billion estimate. Spending will explode anyway as baby boomers retire and drug use rises. (The) director of the Congressional Budget Office (the agency responsible for costing out proposed legislation) puts the second decade's costs between $1.3 trillion and $2 trillion." Robert Samuelson, "Medicare as Pork Barrel," *Washington Post*, November 24, 2003, A21.

13. The drug companies, as would any company, prefer to negotiate with many private buyers for their products rather than a single (monopsonist) buyer.

14. Robert Pear, "Medicare Law's Costs and Benefits Are Elusive," *New York Times*, December 9, 2003, A1.

15. The pharmaceutical companies, however, did not get all that they wanted. As part of the cost-containment measures to reduce the cost of the drug benefit, Congress limited drug manufacturer's ability to delay the introduction of generic drugs, which are low-cost substitutes. The new law contains provisions to speed less expensive generic versions of drugs to market by limiting brand name manufacturers to a single 30-month stay of approval. Previously, brand name drug manufacturers were able to accumulate multiple 30-month stays and delay approval of generic substitutes.

16. Sheryl Gay Stolberg, "An 800-Pound Gorilla Changes Partners Over Medicare," *New York Times*, Nov. 23, 2003, 4.5.

17. The AARP has a tax-paying entity called AARP Services Inc., which generates several hundred million dollars a year in the form of royalties from insurance, financial services, and other companies that market their products to AARP members. Almost all of these revenues are returned to AARP to be used for lobbying, research, publications, and other member programs.

18. Bara Vaida, "Lobbying—AARP's Big Bet," *National Journal*, March 13, 2004.

19. David Broder and Amy Goldstein, "AARP Decision Followed a Long GOP Courtship," *Washington Post*, A1.

20. Robin Toner, "Reshaping Medicare, Rural Roots in Mind," *New York Times*, June 2, 2003, A14.

21. Robert Pear, "Bill on Medicare Drug Benefit Is Stalled by House-Senate Republican Antagonism," *New York Times*, August 27, 2003, A15.

22. The prescription drug benefits will be provided by private, risk-bearing plans. There must be a minimum of two plan options in each area; otherwise, the government will contract with private plans to serve as a "fallback" option. Private plans are paid by a combination of enrollee premiums and government contribution. The government also shares risk with the private plans through reinsurance; the government pays 80 percent of allowable drug costs exceeding the stop-loss threshold.

    The private plans may use a formulary, as long as the formulary meets certain standards. Further, before removing a drug from the formulary or changing its tier status, enrollees must be notified. Patients may appeal for coverage of a nonformulary drug if the prescribing physician believes a formulary drug would not be as effective for the patient or have significant adverse effects.

    The private plans would negotiate prices with both the manufacturers and suppliers of the drugs and pharmacies.

Prescription Drug Coverage for Medicare Beneficiaries: A Summary of the Medicare Prescription Drug, Improvement, and Modernization Act of 2003 (The Henry J. Kaiser Family Foundation, 2003).

23. These preferred provider plans must offer a single deductible for Part A and Part B benefits and catastrophic out-of-pocket limits for in-network services. Beginning in 2006, plans in each region will be paid on the basis of the bids in relation to a benchmark price. Plan bids above the benchmark price will be paid the benchmark price by the government and will be paid the additional amounts by enrollee premiums. Plans whose bids are below the benchmark price must provide enrollees with additional benefits worth 75 percent of the difference between their bid and the benchmark price they receive; the remaining 25 percent is to be returned to the government.

    Beginning in 2010, a six-year demonstration project will be started in up to six metropolitan areas to test competition between Medicare Advantage (MA) plans and traditional Medicare. The demonstration cannot be extended or expanded without congressional action.

24. Robert Pear, "Private Health Insurers Begin Lobbying for Changes in Medicare Drug Legislation," *New York Times*, July 1, 2003, A20.

25. Milt Freudenheim, "Employers Seek To Shift Cost of Drugs to U.S.," *New York Times*, July 2, 2003, A1.

26. Robert Pear and Carl Hulse, "Senate Removes Two Roadblocks to Drug Benefit," *New York Times*, November 25, 2003, A1.

27. Adriel Bettleheim, "Medicare Reform: Will Policymakers Agree on Prescription Drug Benefits," *The CQ Researcher Online*, August 22, 2003, Volume 13, Number 28, file://C:\EMP\cqresrre 2003082200.htm, p. 5 (673–696).

28. Ibid, p. 27.

29. A conflict soon developed between the two chairmen of the Senate and House committees responsible for negotiating a compromise bill: Senator Grassley (R-IA), chairman of the Senate Finance Committee, and Representative William Thomas (R-CA), chairman of the House Ways and Means Committee. Representative Thomas, representing the more conservative Republicans in the House, wanted to slow the growth in Medicare spending for hospital care. Senator Grassley wanted to increase funding for rural hospitals. This particular conflict delayed a final compromise bill until November, 2003.

30. The additional monthly premium for Part D was estimated by the Congressional Budget Office to be $35 a month, rising to $58 a month by 2013. As the new drug benefit is voluntary, and those enrolling at a date later than when they first become eligible will be

charged an additional (penalty) amount each month. (To limit adverse selection—only those enrollees with high drug costs join the program—the additional premium for joining late is meant to encourage a greater number of enrollees, particularly those with little or no drug costs, to enroll when they first become eligible, thereby spreading the drug costs over a larger number of enrollees.)

31. Robert Pear, "New Medicare Plan for Drug Benefits Prohibits Insurance," *New York Times*, December 7, 2003, 1.1.

32. Many believe the demonstration tests will never take place, as previous pilot programs authorized by Congress in Baltimore (1996) and Denver (1997) were stopped by local opposition. Also, few, if any, senators or legislators will want their state to be one of the demonstration sites for traditional Medicare to compete against private plans.

33. The concept of HSAs, allowing individuals to have greater control and choice in their healthcare decisions, was previously included by the Republican-controlled House of Representatives in a 1995 bill (as MSAs) that President Clinton vetoed. It was resurrected and included in HIPPA, which was enacted in 1996, and also in the 1997 BBA. These previous attempts by Republicans to change the financing and delivery of medical services by nonaged culminated in the 2003 MMA, which greatly expanded the concept and renamed it HSAs.

34. Mary Agnes Carey, "Provisions of the Medicare Bill," *Congressional Quarterly Weekly*, January 24, 2004.

35. Marilyn Weber Serafini, "Health Care—The Real Medicare Crisis Ahead," *National Journal*, June 4, 2004. http://www.ncpa.org/prs/rel/2004/20040604bnr.htm.

36. James B. Kau and Paul H. Rubin, "The Growth of Government: Sources and Limits," *Public Choice* 113 (2002): 389–402 (especially 392). See also, Claudio A. Bonilla, "A Model of Political Competition in the Underlying Space of Ideology," *Public Choice* 121 (2004): 51–67.

37. Robert Pear and Robin Toner, "Counting Votes and Attacks in Final Push for Medicare Bill," *New York Times*, November 20, 2003, A25.

38. Less than two months after the drug bill was enacted, the Bush administration announced that the ten-year cost of the bill was expected to be at least $530 billion instead of the original $400 billion estimate, an increase of one-third, before the program has even started.

Many conservative Republicans in the House were upset because the administration assured them that the ten-year cost of the bill would not exceed $400 billion. They reluctantly voted for the bill and would have opposed it if they had thought the cost was more than $400 billion. At the same time, the Democrats intro-duced legislation to expand what they believe is a meager drug ben-efit and to save money by having the government negotiate directly with drug companies.

Robert Pear, "Bush's Aides Put Higher Price Tag on Medicare Law," *New York Times*, January 30, 2004, A1.

39. Andrew Rettenmaier and Thomas Saving, "The 2004 Medicare and Social Security Trustee Reports," *National Center for Health Policy Analysis*, June 4, 2004. http://www.ncpa.org/pub/st/st266/.

NATIONAL HEALTH INSURANCE: HAS ITS TIME COME AND GONE?

After completing this chapter, the reader should be able to
- list the objectives of national health insurance according to the public interest and economic theories,
- explain why large employers have a concentrated interest in lowering rising healthcare costs,
- identify what objective different concentrated interests would like to achieve though national health insurance, and
- outline the competing theories of government and discuss the prospects for universal coverage based on an equitable financing mechanism.

National health insurance means different things to different groups. Traditionally, it has meant increased access to care, particularly by the uninsured and those with low incomes. Some also propose national health insurance as a means of controlling the rapid rise in medical expenditures. These are conflicting objectives. However, these differing objectives go to the heart of the debate over national health insurance. The divergent objectives also illustrate the difference between the public and self-interest theories of government.

The Objectives of National Health Insurance

To understand why this country has not had national health insurance it is necessary to understand the actual rather than the stated objective behind such a visible redistributive goal. Further, the debate over the structure and financing of national health insurance actually represents the controversy over the underlying objective to be achieved. Discussing the possible goals of national health insurance therefore clarifies the design features of different national health insurance proposals and provides insights into why this country has not had national health insurance.

The public and self-interest theories provide competing explanations regarding the objectives underlying national health insurance and the difficulty of enacting legislation to assist the uninsured and working poor.

Universal Coverage

According to the public interest theory, the motivation underlying national health insurance is to increase access to medical care by the uninsured and those with low incomes. The poor either have no health insurance and must fall back on Medicaid if they become ill, or their insurance is less comprehensive than the insurance purchased by (or on behalf) of those with higher incomes. In support of the goal of universal access are the numerous studies that document the size of the uninsured population (approximately 15.6 percent or 45 million people) and the problems encountered by those with low incomes who are seeking medical care.[1]

The financing mechanism consistent with a goal of increasing access to those with low incomes would be income taxes and an income-related premium. The funds to finance universal access would have to come from those with higher incomes. Thus, the public interest theory would predict that national health insurance would be redistributive, that the main beneficiaries would be those with low incomes, and that the costs would be financed by higher-income groups.

According to the self-interest theory, although many people support increased services to the poor, this is not, nor has it ever been, the driving force behind national health insurance. Those with low incomes already have national health insurance; *Medicaid is national health insurance for the poor.* Medicaid is generally acknowledged to be an inadequate program. Because it is administered by the states, Medicaid eligibility rules vary from state to state; those states with the lowest per-capita incomes also tend to have the lowest percentage of their population, as a percentage of the federal poverty level, covered. In aggregate, according to 2003 data, only about 42 percent of those below the federal poverty level are eligible for Medicaid.[2]

There is also a sharp cutoff from eligibility if a person's income increases. A disincentive exists for a Medicaid-eligible low-income person to earn additional income because their loss of medical and other benefits would exceed the additional wages earned.

Medicaid also pays providers lower fees than either Medicare or private insurers. Thus, many providers refuse to care for Medicaid patients. Even though a person may be eligible, she may have difficulty finding a provider who will treat her.

The inadequacy of Medicaid, however, is neither the result of malevolent bureaucrats nor a lack of will on the part of legislators or the administration to improve it. Instead, the funding provided for Medicaid, and its eligibility, reflect the preferences of the nonpoor, who provide the political support for programs to those with low incomes. Eligibility levels and medical benefits provided to Medicaid recipients reflect how much the nonpoor are willing to tax themselves to provide benefits to those who are poor.[3]

If the motivation for national health insurance were to increase access to care by those with low incomes, Medicaid could be improved. Eligibility could be increased, up to and beyond the federal poverty level; a gradual cutoff of eligibility could be instituted as wages increased; benefits could be enhanced; and more generous payments could be made to providers to increase their willingness to see Medicaid patients. It would not be necessary to enact a separate national health insurance program to achieve this.

The middle class, however, is unwilling to fund such an increase in Medicaid eligibility and benefits. *If the middle class is unwilling to improve Medicaid, why would middle-class people be willing to tax themselves to enact national health insurance for the poor?* Therefore, one must conclude that the main objective of national health insurance is not to help those with low incomes by increasing taxes on those who have higher incomes.

Using the Power of Government to Benefit Politically Powerful Groups

An alternative goal of national health insurance is one that is consistent with the self-interest theory, namely, to use the power of government to benefit politically powerful groups. Groups are politically powerful when they are able to provide legislators with political support, that is, votes, money, or volunteer campaign time. Politically powerful groups attempt, through the legislative process, to redistribute wealth by receiving benefits in excess of their costs.

Previous visible redistributive programs, such as Social Security and Medicare, provided the aged with benefits in excess of their contributions to such programs. (With regard to Medicare, other politically important groups also benefited, such as the AFL-CIO unions, hospitals, and physicians.) Regressive taxes (a payroll tax up to a certain wage level) were used to finance these programs, which were borne by the nonaged. The size of the payroll tax was hidden, and made more diffuse, by imposing half of the tax on the employer and the other half on the employee. A regressive financing mechanism was necessary if the aged and the retirees from the AFL-CIO unions were to be eligible to receive benefits in excess of their costs.

The reason health policies change over time is that groups who have borne a diffuse cost find that the cost has increased to where the group develops a concentrated interest in reducing it. Once a diffuse cost develops into a concentrated interest, the group has an incentive to represent its interests in hopes of reducing that cost.

To understand the pressures for health reform, it becomes necessary to understand the objectives of those groups having a concentrated interest.

Major Groups with a Concentrated Interest in Health Reform

Federal and State Governments

Federal expenditures under Medicare and Medicaid have been rising rapidly. The Medicare Trust Fund, which collects payroll taxes to pay for Medicare Part A, is expected to be bankrupt in the relatively near future. To forestall bankruptcy of the trust fund, the government will have to increase the Medicare portion of the Social Security tax, which is already 2.9 percent on all earned income; pay physicians and hospitals less; and/or reduce Medicare benefits to future and/or current aged.

Because it is politically difficult to reduce benefits to current aged, previous impending bankruptcies of the trust fund were resolved by increasing both the Medicare tax and the wage base to which it applied and by paying hospitals and physicians less. Both of these choices are becoming more difficult. Although the Medicare payroll tax is now a proportional tax on all earned income, increasing it further raises its visibility and opposition. To continue reducing Medicare payments for physicians and hospitals will result in fewer services being provided to the aged and/or decreased access to care. Thus, the government must explore other approaches for reducing the rise in Medicare Part A payments.

Similarly, Medicaid and Medicare Part B (which pays for nonhospital services) and Part C (the newly enacted prescription drug benefit) contribute to the federal deficit. These programs are subsidized from general tax revenues. Controlling the federal deficit is a goal that has a large amount of political support. If expenditures under these programs continue their rapid rise, other politically popular programs will have to be sharply reduced, or taxes increased, if the deficit is not to be increased further. Increasing taxes and/or reducing benefits under Medicare Parts B and C would be politically unpopular.

The states have also seen their expenditures under Medicaid rise rapidly. Because the states' portion of Medicaid is funded from general tax revenues, and states, unlike the federal government, are required to balance their budgets each year, rising Medicaid expenditures leave the states with few options. States could reduce expenditures on other politically popular programs, such as prisons and education; taxes could be increased; Medicaid eligibility could be limited; or payments to providers, hospitals, physicians, and nursing homes could be reduced. To minimize their loss of political support, legislators have previously chosen to limit Medicaid eligibility and reduce provider payments.

Continued rapid increases in Medicaid expenditures will force states to consider these difficult choices.

Thus, both the federal and state governments have developed a concentrated interest in reducing the rise in Medicare and Medicaid expenditures. Legislators at both the federal and state level are likely to oppose healthcare reform proposals that place an even greater financial commitment on the federal and state governments. Instead, such legislators view health reform as a means of reducing and/or shifting governments' health expenditures.

Employers and Unions

As health insurance premiums have rapidly increased over time, the cost of healthcare to employers and unions has changed from a diffuse to a concentrated cost. As such, both have attempted to reduce these costs through legislative action.

The 1993 requirement by the Financial Accounting Standards Board required employers to accrue the costs of providing retiree medical benefits over the working careers of their employees, in the same way corporations account for retirement plans. Companies had to list such benefits on their balance sheet and annually expense their (current and future) retiree medical obligations. This ruling (FASB 106) caused many large firms that provide retiree medical benefits, particularly those located in the Midwest and Northeast, to reduce their net worth and earnings per share. GM, which provides health insurance for 1.1 million active and retired workers and their families in the United States, has unfunded retiree medical liabilities of $77 billion. Any reduction in the rate of increase in medical expenditures reduces these company's retiree medical liabilities.[4]

Many large unions, such as the UAW, have very generous medical benefits. (UAW members pay, on average, only 7 percent of their healthcare costs compared to salaried employees at GM, who pay 27 percent of their costs.) As the cost of medical care has risen, these unions have had to accept smaller wage increases to maintain their comprehensive medical benefits. GM will spend $5.6 billion in 2005 (up $800 million from 2003) on medical expenses for its employees, retirees, and dependents. When calculated per employee, GM spends $14,000 annually on healthcare, which would otherwise be used to increase employee wages if these costs were to be shifted to the taxpayer.[5] The unions' legislative objective has been to maintain benefits without having to pay the required cost.

To achieve the employers' goal of reducing their unfunded retirees' medical liabilities, and the union's goal of reducing the employees' cost of rising medical costs, these costs have to be shifted to others. Automobile firms and their unions favor a government financing mechanism that requires union members to pay less than their full costs by shifting part of the cost to taxpayers. For example, they have favored an employer mandate that limits the percent of payroll that goes for medical care (such as the 12 percent proposed in the Clinton health reform plan), as that amount for auto workers greatly exceed the national average (it is close to 18 percent).[6]

Large employers and unions hope to achieve through national health insurance a reduction in the rise of (and their obligation for) their medical expenditures. In this regard, it should come as no surprise if the auto companies and their unions were to support a regulatory system that limits overall expenditure and/or premium increases, similar in its effects to a single-payer system, such as the Canadian healthcare system.

Physician and Hospital Associations

The growth of additional groups that have a concentrated interest in healthcare has resulted in a decline in the relative political influence of physician and hospital associations. For example, provider organizations, such as chiropractors, psychologists, and podiatrists, have sought to compete with physicians by becoming eligible for reimbursement by insurance companies and Medicare and Medicaid. The HMOs and insurers have opposed medical societies in their attempt to enact restrictive legislation, such as any willing provider laws and patient's rights laws that would increase costs for HMOs. And the federal government has a concentrated interest in reducing the rate of increase in Medicare expenditures by placing reimbursement limits on physicians and hospitals.

The fact that both the AMA and the AHA have a diverse membership also decreases their political influence. Within the AMA there are many different specialty groups of physicians. Similarly, within the AHA, there are separate groups of hospitals, such as the urban, rural, teaching, and state hospital associations, that have a concentrated interest in increasing federal funds to their own constituencies at the expense of other constituencies, within a budget-neutral environment.

When the federal government phased in (over a five-year period) the new Medicare hospital payment system in 1983, it was determined that it would be "budget-neutral," that is, although the payment method changed to DRGs, the total amount to be spent on hospitals would be the same. Thus, any gains to one group of hospitals had to be offset by losses to other groups of hospitals. The effect of budget-neutrality was to lessen the political influence of the AHA, because the AHA could only favor revenue increases to all hospitals—not to specific groups of hospitals. Each group of hospitals then developed their own lobbying organization to try and receive more Medicare funding and to protect themselves against the lobbying efforts of other hospital associations. Hospitals no longer spoke to legislators with one voice.

The Medicare physician payment system (using the RBRV) introduced in the 1990s was also based on budget-neutrality. One of its objectives was to redistribute income away from procedure-oriented specialists toward family physicians. Each medical specialty association engaged in the political process, both to receive higher reimbursement and to protect the interests of its own members. Although a majority of its membership is specialists, the AMA could not favor one medical group over another for fear of losing the membership of these large medical associations. These medical societies were also very active during the debate over President Clinton's health reform proposal; for example, the American College of Surgeons (52,000 members) and the American College of Physicians (70,000 internists) supported an overall budget limit and fee controls, which the AMA and other medical societies opposed.

The existence of multiple hospital and medical associations, each with its own concentrated interest and representing those interests, has politically weakened the umbrella organizations, the AMA and the AHA.

The AMA and AHA have attempted to represent the interests of all of their members by lobbying for more federal funding and against any further reductions in Medicare payments. The membership of both organizations was significantly rewarded by the Bush administration by helping the administration lobby wavering legislators to vote in favor of the MMA.

Given the limited funds available at the federal and state level for assisting the uninsured and expanding Medicaid, the AMA and the AHA have favored health reform proposals that increase the demand for medical services in the private sector, such as an employer mandate and HSAs, while opposing further reductions in Medicare and Medicaid provider payments.

Health Insurers

Health insurers want to ensure that any health reform program retains the private health insurance industry and, second, that there is an increase in the demand for private insurance.

The health insurance industry, however, is split between large and small insurers. Large insurers would like to see small insurers exit the industry. Large insurers are in favor of managed care and HMOs because they believe they can develop such organizations and can use their marketing systems to increase their market share. Smaller insurance companies would prefer to sell traditional indemnity and catastrophic insurance, that is, continue to manage risk rather than manage care, as large insurers are slowly attempting to do. (Under the Clinton health plan, smaller insurers opposed larger insurers, believing they would no longer have a role if the large purchasing pools, referred to as health alliances, chose participating insurers and HMOs.) The difference in economic interests between insurers also explains why large insurers favor health insurance reform regulations, such as guaranteed renewability and portability (permitting an employee to keep his insurance when changing employers), because large insurers will be better able than small insurers to bear these costs, thereby giving them a competitive advantage over small insurers.

An issue health insurers (and HMOs) would like resolved in any national health insurance plan is which medical treatments are considered experimental and do not have to be covered in their benefit package. Denying medical treatments that are considered experimental or that have very low probabilities of success for certain patients leaves the insurer liable for large damage awards. It is difficult for insurers to calculate a premium if it is not known which new medical treatments will be part of their enrollees' benefits. Insurers would prefer that the federal government establish technology assessment panels that would undertake cost-effectiveness studies of new technology and presumably limit access to expensive medical treatments. Opposing insurers on this issue are pharmaceutical and medical technology companies whose revenues and profitability would be decreased.

Health insurers would also like to limit lawsuits over denial of care by relying on outside review panels for deciding such issues. Opposed to any limits on patient lawsuits over denial of care have been trial lawyer associations. The issue of lawsuits has been an important stumbling block to reaching any compromise between these two organizations on enacting federal patient rights legislation.

The Aged

The aged already have national health insurance for acute care: Medicare. The aged, however, still spend a significant portion of their medical expenses out-of-pocket, approximately 17 percent.[7] They would like lower out-of-pocket payments for their medical expenses, particularly for outpatient prescription drugs. Given the high voting-participation rate of the aged, the closeness of the 2000 presidential election, and the electoral significance of Florida with its many elderly voters, both political parties competed to provide the aged with a prescription drug benefit. In 2003 the aged received a very expensive prescription drug benefit. However, the drug bill is complex, difficult to understand, and contains large copayments and deductibles. Despite the drug bill's impact on the deficit, there will be political pressure by the aged to make the drug benefit more comprehensive.

In coming debates over reducing the federal deficit, healthcare reform, and ensuring Medicare's financial solvency, the aged will lobby for maintaining their existing Medicare benefits, that is, traditional Medicare, while pressuring legislators for enhancing the drug benefit.

If the federal deficit were not a political problem, the aged would next like to have financial protection against the high costs of long-term care. Low-income aged must rely on Medicaid for their long-term-care needs. Middle- and high-income aged do not want to spend down their assets to qualify for Medicaid if they incur large long-term-care expenses. Rather than purchase asset protection (long-term-care insurance) through the private market, middle- and high-income aged would prefer government long-term-care insurance so that their cost can be shifted to others.

The approach presidents and legislators have used to receive the political support of the aged has been to gradually increase their health coverage, for example, by expanding Medicare to include home health care, additional preventive services, respite care, prescription drugs, and even lifestyle drugs (e.g., Viagra). The aged have not paid the full cost of those benefits. Consistent with the self-interest theory are the large subsidies provided to the current aged, regardless of their incomes, by imposing a large financial burden on future generations, at a time of large federal deficits and impending Medicare insolvency.

The Middle Class

Visible redistributive issues, such as national health insurance, require the political support of the middle class. The middle class has a disproportionate amount of political power because political parties cannot form a majority without those in the middle. Legislators would respond and enact national health insurance if a national health insurance proposal had widespread support from the middle class. Therefore, it becomes important to determine the objectives of the middle class with regard to national health insurance.

Until the mid-1980s, the middle class was insulated from the rising costs of medical care. Employers paid the employee's health insurance premium for a traditional indemnity health plan, which permitted the employee and the employee's family to go to any fee-for-service provider and pay very little out-of-pocket costs.

Employer health insurance contributions on behalf of the employee are not considered part of the employee's taxable income. The beneficiaries of employer-paid health insurance are primarily those who are in higher marginal income-tax brackets, namely, those with higher incomes. If the employer increased the employee's wage by $10,000, the employee would have to pay federal, state, and Social Security taxes on that additional $10,000. The employee would be left with approximately $5,500. (Assuming the employee is in a 31 percent federal tax bracket, pays 7 percent state income tax, and 7.5 percent Social Security tax.) These tax savings are greatest for employees in the highest income-tax brackets. If, instead of giving the employee a raise of $10,000, the employer purchased, on behalf of the employee, $10,000 worth of health insurance (with before-tax dollars), the higher-income employee can receive almost twice as many medical services and reduce their out-of-pocket expenses.

Employer-purchased health insurance has been a form of subsidized national health insurance for middle- and high-income groups. Thus, medical care costs did not represent a serious financial risk to the middle class. They were at greater financial risk for the long-term-care needs of their parents. The lost federal tax revenue (foregone federal and Social Security taxes) from employer-purchased health insurance was about $188.5 billion in 2004.[8] These lost taxes could more than pay for subsidies to cover the uninsured. (Yet neither political party proposes limiting these tax subsidies as a means of financing national health insurance for the poor. In addition to middle- and high-income groups, unions, health insurers, and health-care providers are all strongly opposed to a tax cap on employer-paid health insurance.)

President Clinton viewed the 1992 election as a mandate to introduce comprehensive healthcare reform. According to various polls, the middle class expressed a great deal of dissatisfaction with the current health-care system at that time; however, the polls did not indicate any consensus on what type of reform the middle class favored. Middle- and high-income groups already had subsidized national health insurance. "Half of the voters . . . said they were willing to pay an additional $20 a month to support a national plan that would provide insurance coverage to all Americans, but only 24% were willing to pay an additional $50 per month."[9] Willingness to pay higher taxes also varied by the type of tax. Sin taxes being preferred over income taxes (consequently President Clinton proposed an increase in the cigarette tax).

The public was clearly unwilling to tax themselves sufficiently to provide comprehensive health insurance for everyone. The middle class was more concerned with their own rising insurance premiums (which meant lower take-home wages), the fear that they would lose their insurance if they became ill or changed jobs, and the greater restrictions placed on their choice of provider by managed care organizations. The middle class basically wanted what they previously had—traditional indemnity insurance with free choice of provider—but at a lower cost.

The only way for the middle class to have unlimited access to care and to the latest medical technology at subsidized premiums is to shift the rising cost of care to others; however, that is just not possible. Paying hospitals and physicians less limits their willingness and ability to absorb rising costs. Shifting costs to other population groups is also difficult; those with low incomes could not afford to pay the increased taxes to subsidize the large middle class and their medical costs. It is unrealistic to expect the small percentage of the population with very large incomes to bear the enormous medical costs of the entire middle class. Thus, it is not possible for the middle class to achieve its goals by shifting its costs to other groups.

The inability of the middle class to achieve unlimited access at a reduced cost, however, has not prevented some politicians from claiming it can be done. Single-payer advocates claim that reducing administrative costs and removing profit from healthcare will save sufficient funds to provide universal healthcare to all, free access to all healthcare providers, and at no additional cost.

The Prospects for National Health Insurance

National health insurance (universal coverage) is unlikely to be enacted in the foreseeable future. Although the public, the media, and legislators decry the number of uninsured (and underinsured), given the size of the federal deficit and the additional burden on federal tax revenues of the Medicare prescription drug benefit, additional federal funds will not be available to fund expensive new programs for the uninsured. Further, the middle class is unwilling to tax themselves to provide the necessary funds to either expand coverage to the uninsured or to enhance Medicaid.

The pressures forcing Congress to consider health reform are middle-class concerns, and that is the group that provides the political support for such visible redistributive legislation. For this reason health insurance reform (HIPAA) was enacted. These reforms were not enacted to provide insurance for those unable to afford such insurance, but instead to relieve middle-class anxieties about being denied coverage or losing their coverage if they changed jobs. Similarly, minimum length of hospital stays for maternity patients was a response to anecdotes regarding early hospital discharge after a normal delivery, although there were no definitive studies indicating that early hospital discharge had an adverse effect on quality.[10] Proposals to enact patient rights legislation and to remove restrictions imposed by managed care companies that limit the patient's choice of provider are additional attempts by legislators to curry favor amongst the voting public.

Congress provides these regulatory benefits to the public without imposing any visible cost. Insurance companies and HMOs are simply required to provide them. The public is pleased by seemingly receiving something for nothing. Although the costs of these regulations are apparently borne by the insurers and HMOs, in reality those (diffuse) costs are shifted toward purchasers in the form of higher insurance premiums.

Limiting rising healthcare costs is likely to be the major redistributive issue in coming years. The increasing burden on federal revenues caused by the new Medicare prescription drug benefit will pressure the administration to hold down prescription drug costs. Concern over the insolvency of the Medicare Trust Fund and rising Part B expenditures will place the administration in conflict with hospital and physician associations. As insurance premiums increase, the number of uninsured will increase, placing greater pressure on state Medicaid budgets. Large employers and their unions, facing large unfunded retiree health obligations and lower take-home pay, will press for regulatory action to reduce rising medical costs. And market pressures are forcing the middle class to make the trade-offs that politicians are reluctant to propose for Medicare.

To reduce their insurance premiums, the middle class is accepting higher deductibles and copayments. Some of the more popular insurance products on the market are high-deductible insurance plans, such as HSAs. As an alternative to these "consumer-directed" insurance products for lowering insurance premiums, managed care products relying on limited provider networks are returning.

The growth in these new insurance products reflects the public's willingness to choose lower premiums in return for larger out-of-pocket payments and restrictions on their choice of provider. Market competition has previously lowered the rate of increase in medical expenditures and is being relied on to do it again. As in other markets, the competitive healthcare market offers different tiers of medical care for those who are willing to pay different amounts.

Sharp ideological differences between the political parties have made it difficult to provide these different choices to Medicare beneficiaries. In Medicare, fewer restrictions on choice of provider mean higher Medicare expenditures. Many politicians, however, have been reluctant to publicly promote multiple tiers of medical care within Medicare, such as proposed by advocates of "Medicare reform," even though they exist within the private sector.

The United States has the national health insurance it is willing to fund. Federal and state governments spend more than $560 billion a year on medical services, but coverage is not universal. Medicaid serves only a portion of the poor at an estimated $300 billion per year (in 2004 the federal share was $176 billion and the states spent $121 billion). Medicare is national health insurance for the aged at $265 billion per year, and employer-paid health insurance is national health insurance for middle- and high-income groups at more than $188 billion a year in lost federal, state, and Social Security taxes.[11]

The major redistributive policies in coming years will be those that attempt to lower the rate of increase in government health expenditures and rising health insurance premiums for the middle class. To achieve these twin objectives, there will be an ideological debate between those who favor relying on market competition in the private and Medicare markets (with continued consumer dissatisfaction over higher out-of-pocket payments and restricted provider access) and those who favor greater government regulation (limits on expenditure and/or premium increases), with its eventual (thus diffuse) decreased patient access to healthcare and to innovative medical technology.

To understand the debate underlying healthcare reform, it is necessary to appreciate the difference between its real versus its stated objectives. The public interest theory is *less* able to explain and predict the outcome of healthcare reform than is a theory based on how those who are politically powerful attempt to shift their costs onto those who are less politically powerful. The outcome will have little to do with improved equity or efficiency, as those were never the real objectives underlying national health insurance.

Study Questions

1. What are the objectives of national health insurance, according to the public interest and economic theories?
2. Do you agree with the following statement: The United States already has national health insurance for three different segments of the U.S. population, the really poor, middle- and high-income employees, and the aged.
3. Why do large employers, such as GM, have a concentrated interest in lowering rising healthcare costs?
4. What objectives would the middle class like to achieve through national health insurance?
5. Select a healthcare provider group and hypothesize what it would like to achieve through national health insurance.
6. Use the competing theories of government to describe the prospects for universal coverage based on an equitable financing mechanism.

Notes

1. U.S. Census Bureau, Current Population Reports, P60–226, *Income, Poverty, and Health Insurance Coverage in the United States: 2003*, http://www.census.gov/prod/2004pubs/p60-226.pdf.
2. U.S. Census Bureau, *Current Population Survey, 2004 Annual Social and Economic Supplement*, Table HI02. Health Insurance Coverage Status and Type of Coverage by Selected Characteristics

for People in the Poverty Universe, 2003,
http://pubdb3.census.gov/macro /032004/health/toc.htm.

3. The federal government establishes certain minimum eligibility lev-
    els and benefits under Medicaid. It is up to the individual states to
    determine whether those minimums are increased.

4. Lee Hawkins, Jr., and Karen Lundegaard, "GM Warns UAW on
    Health Benefits," *Wall Street Journal*, June 16, 2005, A3. See also,
    Lee Hawkins, Jr., "GM Plans to Cut Salaried Staff; Overhaul
    Looms," *Wall Street Journal*, March 21, 2005, A1, A6.

5. Hawkins and Lundegaard.

6. "The (Clinton) plan proposes that no firm pay more than 7.9 per-
    cent of its payroll toward the cost of workers' health premiums and
    that employees not be required to pay more than 3.9 percent of
    their wages." http://www.worldbank.org/html/extdr/
    hnp/hddflash/issues/00004.html .

7: Agency for Healthcare Research and Quality, 2002 Full Year
    Consolidated Data File (HC-070). Released December 2004.
    Medical Expenditure Panel Survey Household Component Data.
    Generated using MEPSnet/HC. http://www.meps.ahrq.gov/
    mepsnet/HC/MEPSnetHC.asp (August 23, 2005).

8. John Sheils and Randall Haught, "The Cost of Tax-Exempt Health
    Benefits in 2004," *Health Affairs-Web Exclusives*, February 25, 2004,
    content.healthaffairs.org/cgi/content/abstract/hlthaff.w4.106.

9. Robert Blendon, D. E. Altman, J. M. Benson, H. Taylor, M. James,
    and M. Smith, "The Implications of the 1992 Presidential Election
    for Health Care Reform," *Journal of the American Medical
    Association* 268 (1992): 3371–3375. (3374).

10. According to one study, "As a percentage of total spending (on
    maternity hospital costs) the legislation could increase charges by
    20.2 % if all women stayed longer . . ." Kristiana Raube and Katie
    Merrell, "Maternal Minimum-Stay Legislation: Cost and Policy
    Implications," *American Journal of Public Health* 89 (1999):
    922–923. See also, J. P. Kassirer, "Practicing Medicine without a
    License—The New Intrusions by Congress" (editorial), *The New
    England Journal of Medicine* 336 (1997): 1747.

11. Congressional Budget Office, *An Analysis of the President's
    Budgetary Proposals for Fiscal Year 2006*, Chapter 2, Table 2-2,
    http://www.cbo.gov/showdoc.cfm?index=6146&sequence=0.
    Centers for Medicare & Medicaid Services, Office of the Actuary:
    National Health Statistics Group, http://www.cms.hhs.gov/statis-
    tics/nhe/historical/.

THE SELF-INTEREST PARADIGM AND THE POLITICS OF HEALTH LEGISLATION

After completing this chapter, the reader should be able to

- describe how political markets are similar to economic markets,
- discuss how political markets differ from economic markets,
- explain whether competition or monopoly among demanders and suppliers of legislation are preferable in political markets,
- explain why regressive taxes are used to finance legislative benefits,
- discuss why the aged have been able to receive such large benefits from redistributive programs using the concept of "concentrated" and "diffuse" interests, and
- outline the ideological differences in designing the MMA.

The purpose of this book has been to use a self-interest paradigm (economic theory of regulation) to explain legislative outcomes in healthcare. The usefulness of this approach should be judged by its predictive ability. Although it is unlikely that any one theory will be able to explain all or even a very high percentage of all legislation, a theory is necessary for trying to understand why certain types of legislation were enacted and why others were not, unless one believes legislation is ad hoc. It is natural to try and organize what we observe in some meaningful manner. The criteria for selecting one theory over another should be based on pragmatic grounds: Which approach is better at explaining events under a broad range of circumstances? To reject a theory it is necessary to have a better theory.

The lack of coordination among the different types of health policies in this country has led many observers to decry the lack of rationality in the financing and provision of healthcare. Those with high incomes and those employed in large companies generally have adequate health coverage. The unemployed and those with low incomes do not. There is little or no coordination of policies and programs to care for the unemployed, the working poor, children, the low-income aged, and so on. The federal and state governments have failed to fill the gaps in insurance coverage to those least able to afford care. Many different agencies within the government provide medical services to the same people. For example, the elderly receive benefits from the Departments of Housing and Urban Development, the Department of Transportation, the Veterans Administration, the Social Security Administration, Medicare, Medicaid, and so on. This fragmentation and the gaps in coverage have led to inefficiencies in the provision of these services and inequities in how they are financed.

Yet the financing and delivery of health services in this country, in both the private and government sectors, are the result of a rational system. Although the outcome may not appear rational, the process was. To understand the resulting outcome it is necessary to have an approach by which the process can be understood. Health legislation was rational from the perspective of those who demand and supply legislation. Both the demanders and suppliers of legislative benefits knew what they wanted. The resulting outcome was determined by those able to provide the most political support. The outcome had little to do with what was an efficient use of scarce resources or what was best for the nation's health.

The self-interest paradigm assumes that human behavior is no different in political than in private markets. Individuals, groups, firms, and legislators seek to enhance their self-interests. They are assumed to be rational in assessing the benefits and costs to themselves of their actions. This behavioral assumption enables us to predict that firms in private markets will try to produce their products and services as efficiently as possible to keep their costs down and that they will set their prices so as to make as much profit as possible. They will be motivated to enter markets where the profit potential is greatest and, similarly, to leave markets where the profit potential is low.

It is merely an extension of the above discussion to include political markets. Individuals and firms use the power of the state to further their own interests. Firms try to gain competitive advantages in private markets by investing in technology and advertising. Why shouldn't firms also make political investments to be able to use the powers of government to increase or maintain profit?

The actions of organizations of individuals are no different from those of firms. Many people would like to use the power of the state to assist them in what they cannot otherwise achieve. For some, this may mean using the state to help them impose their religious or social preferences on others. Still other groups would like to use the state to provide them with monetary benefits that they could not earn in the market and that others would not voluntarily provide to them, such as low-cost medical schools for their children, pension payments in excess of their contributions, and subsidized medical benefits.

It is usually with regard to our public "servants" that the assumption of acting in one's self-interest becomes difficult to accept. After all, why would a person run for office if not to serve the public interest? However, to be successful in the electoral process requires legislators to behave in a manner that enhances their reelection prospects. Political support, votes, and contributions are the bases for reelection. Legislators must therefore be able to understand the sources of such support and the requirements for receiving it. A hungry person quickly realizes that if money buys food then one must have money to eat. Legislators act no differently than others.

Political markets have several characteristics that differentiate them from economic markets. These differences make it possible for organized interests to benefit at the expense of majorities. First, individuals are not as informed about political issues as they are about the goods and services on which they spend their own funds. In private markets individuals have an incentive to become informed when they make large purchases. In political markets many of the issues have such a minor impact on their economic well-being that it does not "pay" for them to do anything about it, let alone become informed on the issue.

Second, in private markets individuals make separate decisions about each item they purchase. They do not have to choose between sets of purchases, such as between one package that may include a particular brand of car, a certain size house in a particular neighborhood, several suits, and a certain quantity of food. Yet in political markets their choices are between two sets of votes by competing legislators on a wide variety of issues. Although individual voters may agree or disagree on parts of the package, they cannot register a vote on each issue, as they do in economic markets.

Third, voting-participation rates differ by age group. The young and future generations do not vote, and yet policies are enacted that impose costs on them. Future generations depend on current generations and voters to protect their interests. However, as has been the case many times, such as with respect to Social Security and Medicare, their interests have been sacrificed to current voters.

Fourth, legislators use different decision criteria from those used in the private sector. A firm or an individual making an investment considers both the benefits and the costs of that investment. Even though a project may offer very large benefits, profitability cannot be established unless its costs are also considered. Legislators, however, have a different time horizon, which not only affects the emphasis they place on costs and benefits but also when each is incurred. Because members of the House of Representatives run for reelection every two years, they are likely to favor programs that provide immediate benefits (presumably just before the election) while delaying the costs until after the election or years later.

Further, from the legislator's perspective, the program does not even have to meet the criterion that the benefits exceed its costs, only that the immediate benefits exceed any immediate costs. Future legislators can worry about future costs.

For these reasons organized groups are able to receive legislative benefits while imposing the costs of those benefits on the remainder of the population. For those bearing the costs of legislative benefits that others receive, it may be perfectly rational not to oppose such legislation. As long as the cost of changing political outcomes exceeds the lost wealth imposed by legislation, it is rational for voters to lose some wealth rather than to organize and bear the larger cost of changing the legislative outcome. (These costs are referred to as being "diffuse" and are even more so when the population paying them is unaware that they are bearing such costs.)

At times self-interest legislation may be in the "public interest." When this occurs, however, it is because it is a byproduct of the outcome rather than its intended effect.

Groups that are able to provide political support to legislators are those who have a *concentrated* interest in an issue and who are organized to represent their interests. These groups are often a minority of the population. A typical example of such a group would be the producers (and the union) of a particular product who perceive gains from legislation. In the health field the organized interests using the political process are likely to be members of a particular health profession, such as physicians and dentists. Although all health providers have an interest in legislation that provides them with economic benefits, only those who are able to organize themselves and overcome the free rider problem are likely to be successful in the legislative market.

The above discussion does not imply that all organized interest groups will receive legislative benefits. Organized groups will, however, represent their members' interests. Whether or not these groups are successful in that process is another matter.

Politics may be viewed as an exchange relationship, just like an economic market. And, as with any economic market, the resulting output depends on the relative market power of the various participants. When there is monopoly power on the demand side of a market, the monopolist is able to secure a better price than if there were more competitors, each with the same degree of market power. The same analogy occurs with respect to the demand for legislation; when there are no competitors for legislative benefits or when there is only limited opposition to its demands, an interest group demanding legislative benefits would not have to pay as high a price for those benefits (i.e., political support) and would be more likely to receive their benefits. Similarly, when there is competition among the suppliers of a good or service, the demanders are likely to be charged a lower price than if they were purchasing that service from a monopolist supplier. The same is likely to occur in political markets. Legislators who are assured of reelection are in less need of political support than those facing a strong challenge; monopolist legislators, therefore, can afford to exhibit greater independence and can "charge" demanders of legislative benefits a higher price for their services.

Just as in competitive economic markets, competition among demanders of legislative benefits and suppliers of those benefits is likely to result in a more efficient legislative outcome than when a monopoly exists on either the demand or supply side of the market. The greater the number of demanders, the less likely it is that any one will be able to receive large benefits (or all their demands) at the expense of others. Similarly, with respect to the supply side, the greater the competition among legislators for reelection, the less likely they will be to ignore some groups' demands, and their receptivity to those offering political support will be increased.

It has been generally assumed throughout that demanders of legislative benefits in healthcare have had some monopoly power. Similarly, it has been assumed that legislator suppliers have believed themselves to be competitors with regard to their reelection prospects. These assumptions lead to the legislative outcomes hypothesized.

The different types of health legislation may be distinguished according to the visibility of the legislation, the beneficiaries of the legislation, the groups bearing the cost of those legislative benefits, and the method of financing.

Producer Regulation

One form of health legislation relates to what will benefit providers. Legislative benefits to health providers are generally not obvious. Legislation has been enacted that provides some health professionals with a monopoly over the performance of certain tasks, thereby creating benefits for some practitioners at the expense of others. The legislative competition over tasks occurs at the state rather than at the more visible federal level. The stated justification set forth for restrictive provider legislation, whether it is on tasks, entry into the profession, or which providers should be reimbursed under public programs, is protection of the public. However, the only quality measures proposed by the health professions are those that enhance their members' incomes. The profession opposes quality measures that have an adverse effect on the profession's income, such as reexamination and relicensure.

The public bears the burden of producer regulation in two ways: the prices of medical services are higher than they would otherwise be, and second, the public is not as well protected from incompetent and unethical professionals as they are led to believe.

Thus, health provider regulation is financed by a hidden tax on the public. Those who use medical services pay higher prices. The government does not have to propose an explicit tax, which would make the cost of provider regulation more obvious. Instead, a regressive hidden tax is used. The higher prices are the same to all users, regardless of income level.

Although the movement toward market competition in healthcare was (and still is) opposed by physicians, hospitals, and dentists, its emergence was consistent with the self-interest paradigm. Business and government (including the administration), the two major payers of medical services, developed a concentrated interest in holding down the rise in medical expenditures and began to seek changes in the medical marketplace. As the cost of medical services to these large payers increased, their incentive to do something about it became stronger. The concern by business with their employee's insurance premiums and increased capacity among physicians and hospitals set the stage for market competition. The applicability of the antitrust laws was a necessary condition for competition to survive. It was no longer permissible for health professionals to engage in anticompetitive behavior.

Each administration had to limit the rise in hospital and physician payments under Medicare. Continued rapid rises in hospital payments for the aged, which are funded by a separate Medicare trust fund, based on payroll taxes, necessitated increases in Medicare payroll taxes. Medicare physician and outpatient payments, 75 percent of which are funded from general tax revenues, contributed (and still do) to the federal budget deficit, which was (and is) a political problem. An administration that has to keep proposing increased Medicare payroll taxes or is unable to resolve an increasing budget deficit loses political support. Given the choices of increasing payroll taxes, paying providers less, or making the aged pay higher premiums, each administration and Congress realized less political support would be lost by paying providers less.

The medical profession has become politically fragmented. The RBRVS the government adopted in the early 1990s to pay physicians under Medicare rearranged physician fees by specialty. The overall amount of physician payment under Medicare was to be unchanged ("budget-neutral") but some specialties benefited at the expense of other specialties. To represent their members' interests in these payment negotiations, each physician specialty developed a strong lobbying organization that also provided legislators with campaign contributions. The AMA could not take sides in this conflict over redistribution of fees among competing specialties. As a result, physicians look toward their own specialty society for legislative representation in a budget-neutral political environment.

The rise of competing specialty organizations to represent their members' economic interests has diminished the AMA's role as the principal spokesperson for organized medicine. Nevertheless, the AMA has sought out issues it believes will benefit all physicians. The AMA has proposed increased funding for all physicians under Medicare, lobbied to allow physicians to bargain collectively against insurance companies and managed care organizations, strongly favored malpractice reform that caps malpractice awards, and has been an important supporter of patient rights legislation that would increase the role of the physician over the HMO.

The rise of competing interest groups, namely government and business, as well as previously less successful health provider groups, such as nurses and chiropractors, suggests that the AMA and hospital associations are unlikely to be able to dominate the policy process as they have in the past.

Legislation Providing for Medical Research, Protection Against Epidemics, and a Clean Environment

Political support for legislation on health issues comes from the public and producers. When a crisis occurs, as when a flu epidemic appears imminent, a drug causes the death or illness of a number of people, or a particular pollution event causes illness among the population, the public demands leadership from its elected representatives to resolve the problem. Crises are obviously very visible. Failure by the legislature or by the administration to respond to these public concerns would result in a loss of political support. Political opponents would take the initiative and receive the political credit.

Unfortunately, as the crisis passes, public support begins to wane. The media turn to other issues. And legislators lose their interest in the subject as its visibility declines and public support diminishes. In their haste to respond to the public, legislators are likely to pass symbolic legislation; such legislation is unlikely to antagonize organized interests that would be adversely affected.

If, over time, the public and the media demand more stringent legislation to deal with an issue, as in the case of pollution, then legislation will be passed affecting new firms in the industry. Existing firms and unions are unlikely to be affected, as they represent an organized constituency that is able to provide political support. Instead, new firms are likely to bear the burden of new, more stringent legislation. Existing firms are thereby able to use the new legislation to gain a competitive advantage. An example of this approach was seen in the mandate for the use of scrubbers by electric utilities to reduce air pollution.

The other approach the legislature uses to reduce pollution is to allocate federal funds to the states for local building projects. An example of this approach is federal funding for waste-treatment facilities. The advantage of this approach is that all legislators can point with pride to the projects they have brought to their areas. For example, the Hill-Burton program, which provided federal funds for hospital construction, was considered immensely successful. Hospitals received free capital, and the funds were allocated according to a formula, which ensured that all congressional districts were rewarded. Although such an approach is politically popular, it is also wasteful in that funds are allocated regardless of need.

In the above examples, which illustrate the legislature's response to geographic requests for subsidies, all legislators had received a benefit for their districts. Although some areas are most in need of funds, other areas must also be subsidized. This approach obviously raises the cost of a program. Further, it is not clear that federal funds are the answer. For some types of projects, for which benefits are local, taxpayers in those specific states or regions should bear the cost. Further, rather than imposing costs on those causing pollution—for example, municipalities and businesses—and thereby incurring opposition and losing political support, the polluter's costs are imposed on the general public through the provision of subsidies to the polluter.

The beneficiaries of legislation with spillover effects are possibly the public (when legislation is truly meaningful and not merely symbolic), producers receiving a competitive advantage, and local governments that are able to substitute federal funds for their own in solving their waste-treatment problems. Those bearing the burden are typically new firms that are less able to offer political support, and the general public, which has to pay for these programs and even if its health concerns are not alleviated. (In those cases where legislation may be effective in reducing pollution, it will be achieved at a particularly high cost.)

Legislators' responses to public concerns over the environment and health crises are based on being able to receive public support for their actions. Thus, unless there is sufficient public support for an important issue, legislators will not respond. Further, monitoring both the health hazards and violators' compliance with health standards is a continuous process. However, if the public's interest declines, along with the visibility of the issue, legislators will no longer attach as much attention to the issue as it deserves and will be reluctant to impose costs on those industries able to offer political support.

Redistributive Legislation

Although all types of legislation result in redistribution of wealth, redistributive legislation is meant to be most explicit in its effects. There are two types of redistributive legislation. The first is based on a charitable motivation, that is, the public's desire to help the less fortunate. The second is universal redistribution, where the motivation of the voting public is primarily to help themselves at the expense of other taxpayers. What differentiates these two types of redistributive programs is whether a means test is involved.

The beneficiaries of charitable redistribution, such as Medicaid, are those with low incomes. Health providers also benefit. Providers are relieved of their bad debts and receive an increase in demand by those least able to pay for their services. Welfare-type programs are financed from general tax revenues.

Universal programs, such as Medicare, do not have a means test; therefore, everyone is eligible. The proponents of these types of redistributive programs often justify them by saying that unless groups other than the poor are included as beneficiaries there would not be sufficient political support to enact the program. The methods used to finance universal programs, however, are less equitable than the methods used for charitable programs. Usually an excise tax, such as an increase in payroll taxes, is used. These taxes are regressive in that all people must pay the same amount, regardless of income (typically everyone would pay either the same amount or a certain percentage of income up to a maximum level of income).

The most important medical redistributive program has been Medicare.[1] All the aged, regardless of income, are eligible, as eligibility is based on previous contributions to the Social Security system. In this manner higher-income aged qualified. If general tax revenues were used as the financing mechanism, it is likely that not all aged would have been eligible; Medicare would have become a welfare program. The basis for eligibility was debated for many years before Medicare was enacted in 1965. Once Social Security eligibility was accepted and an additional payroll tax was used as the financing mechanism for Medicare Part A, then physician benefits (Part B) were financed out of general tax revenues. General tax revenues for Part B was not opposed by the proponents of Social Security financing for Part A. The reason for this apparent contradiction is that eligibility for physician benefits was based on the initial eligibility for hospital benefits. The unions were willing to accept a more equitable method of financing Part B as long as all of their members were made eligible through the Social Security system.

Health providers, in addition to the aged, were important benefici-aries of Medicare. Providers were paid according to their own preferences; their prices rose rapidly, as did their incomes.

For groups to benefit from the legislative process, the benefits they receive must exceed any costs they incur from financing the program, even though the total costs of the program may exceed its benefits. The method by which this is accomplished is to finance the program by imposing a small cost on each person. In the case of provider benefits, this cost is often hidden; for example, restrictions may be placed on entry into the profession or on the tasks that other professionals can perform. The price of that profession's services is increased, but it is not obvious that the restrictions caused the increase. When benefits are provided to specific population groups, then the costs are more obvious to those bearing them. However, to minimize opposition, the costs are kept small on a per person basis (by spreading them over a large population base), and they are made to appear to be smaller than they really are. Underestimating future program costs and stating that the employer must pay part of those costs (as in the case of Social Security and Medicare payroll taxes) are two approaches for less-ening the visibility of the program's cost.

Funding for Medicare was provided by the working population through an additional Medicare payroll tax added to Social Security taxes. As the demand for medical services by the aged increased, medical prices increased sharply. The general public also bore the burden of this program by paying higher prices for their medical services. The aged (and near-aged) received Medicare benefits that were, in aggregate, in excess of their Medicare payroll taxes for that program, with the result that the major cost of Medicare is being borne by young workers and future generations. Few people would claim that Medicare is as equitable as it could be. Instead, Medicare benefits and payments are closely related to the political support each age group is able to provide.

Political support, not equity considerations, is the basis of another large medical redistributive program. Health insurance employers purchase for their employees is a nontaxable fringe benefit. The major beneficiaries of this government policy are those in the middle- and upper-income groups, by virtue of their being in higher tax brackets. It is estimated that the exclusion of health insurance premiums from taxable income will reduce income tax revenues and payroll tax revenues by a total of about $190 billion in 2004.[2] Middle- and upper-income groups receive most of this tax benefit.

Providers of health services, such as dental, physician, vision, and mental services are also important beneficiaries of the tax subsidy for the purchase of health insurance. If employees had to pay for health insurance with after-tax income, they would purchase less comprehensive medical services with a consequent decreased demand for the services of such providers. Health insurance companies also benefit in that the demand for health insurance is greater than it would be otherwise. It is difficult to reconcile the continuation of the open-ended tax subsidy for the purchase of health insurance with other than the self-interest paradigm.

The Emergence of Ideology in Visible Redistributive Programs

Previously, health policy was driven by groups with a concentrated interest. These groups were health providers, health insurers, and even large employers with unfunded liabilities for their retirees' health benefits. The middle class and the aged both had a concentrated interest in health legislation. Each group sought legislative benefits to enhance its economic interests.

However, primarily since the 1994 congressional elections, when Republicans took control of the House of Representatives for the first time in four decades, ideology has become a more important factor determining health policy. Ideological differences between the two political parties have had their greatest impact on visible redistributive programs; federal programs to assist the uninsured have been affected as well as programs to reduce rising health insurance premiums for the middle class and to provide the aged with a new prescription drug benefit.

The use of ideology (and politics) enhances the explanatory power of the economic theory of regulation; they represent differing economic preferences among voters over tax, expenditure, and equality (or inequality) of incomes. Both ideology and politics represent conflict over economic redistribution.

Conservative Republicans have favored strengthening the role of private health plans and allowing those eligible for federal subsidies to choose between competing private health plans. The proponents of market competition believe efficiency will be increased, innovation and quality will be greater, and healthcare costs will increase more slowly when patients have financial incentives to choose among competing health plans and providers must compete among themselves. To move toward a more competitive healthcare market, conservative Republicans have favored allowing Medicaid beneficiaries to choose among private health plans, providing refundable tax credits for those with low incomes, making HSAs available for the middle class, and instituting Medicare reform, that is having traditional Medicare compete with private health plans for Medicare beneficiaries who would be provided with a fixed dollar contribution toward the health plan of their choice.

Democratic liberals, on the other hand, have opposed changing Medicaid, Medicare, and the employer-based health insurance system; programs that they believe have worked well. Contrary to the Republicans, liberals would like to expand eligibility for government programs by increasing the income limits for Medicaid eligibility, while lowering the age limits (to 55 years of age) to become eligible for traditional Medicare. They have opposed HSAs, believing it would destroy the employer-based health insurance system by breaking up large risk pools. To reduce rising health insurance premiums, liberals would prefer to rely on government regulation of provider prices and government negotiation of drug prices with drug manufacturers.

The belief among conservative Republicans is that Democratic liberals are intent on expanding government programs; increasing government regulation of private health plans; and eventually, with expanded eligibility for government programs, combine expenditures from Medicare and Medicaid, together with employer-paid health insurance premiums into a single-payer system. By allowing individuals to have their own health accounts and make their own choices, conservatives also believe it would make it difficult for government to combine (by taxation) these individual health accounts to finance a single-payer system.

The ideological conflict revolves around expanding and maintaining traditional Medicare, Medicaid, and the employer-based health insurance system versus allowing beneficiaries of the above programs to have greater control over their choices of competing health plans. Several years ago, when the federal government had a budget surplus, these ideological differences forestalled programs to assist the uninsured and those with low incomes.

The Medicare Modernization Act of 2003

The emerging ideological conflicts in health policy and the role played by both politics and concentrated interest groups are best illustrated by the most recent example of visible redistributive legislation, the MMA, which was enacted in December 2003.

The new Medicare (Part C) prescription drug bill is a perfect illustration of how politics, ideology, and concentrated interests affect health policy.

The politics of the MMA.

Political considerations were paramount in making a drug benefit for the aged an important legislative issue. The year 2004 was a presidential election year and the two political parties expected the election to be very close. The aged are an important demographic group in Florida, a state that determined the 2000 presidential election and that President Bush won by fewer than 600 votes. Opinion polls showed that on health issues the public trusted Democrats more than Republicans, and the Democrats had been proposing a new drug benefit for the aged.

President Bush wanted to enact a drug benefit for the aged to remove it as a campaign issue; he wanted to neutralize the Democrats' political advantage with the elderly. The Republicans and President Bush made a Medicare prescription drug bill their number one domestic priority and believed they had to enact such a bill before the 2004 elections. The president further raised the visibility of a Medicare drug benefit by including it in his 2003 State of the Union address. If he succeeded in enacting such a bill, the president would be able to take credit for an issue important to the aged and an issue where the Democrats have been viewed more favorably by voters than Republicans.

The Democrats were concerned that if they did not back a new drug benefit for the aged, particularly after AARP came out in favor of it, they would be called obstructionists and be penalized for it at the coming election.

Ideological differences.

The ideological battles over Medicare were mainly between conservative Republicans in the House of Representatives and liberal Democrats in the Senate.

Conservative Republicans considered the drug benefit as *secondary* to reforming Medicare. They were opposed to adding a new entitlement to an existing entitlement that they believed was already out of control. They viewed Medicare as being unsustainable because of its rapidly rising costs and the increased number of aged being guaranteed benefits under Medicare. Financing these increased expenditures will place a huge financial obligation on a declining working population (relative to the number of aged). In designing the drug bill, the more important objective of conservative Republicans was slowing the growth in Medicare spending.

The Republicans wanted to change ("reform") Medicare by providing the aged with a fixed dollar contribution and having them choose among competing health plans; traditional Medicare would have to compete with other health plans to survive.

Democrats (and Republican Senators with rural constituencies) wanted to add a "stand-alone" drug benefit to traditional Medicare. They wanted to maintain traditional Medicare and were opposed to using the drug benefit as an inducement for the aged to join private health plans. They believed the Republican proposal for changing Medicare from a defined benefit to a defined contribution plan would destroy a program that had served seniors very well. The Democrats further believed that Medicare's political support derived from its principle of equal benefits and equal subsidies for all aged. To hold down the costs of the new drug benefit, liberals favored having the government use its huge purchasing power to negotiate lower drug prices with the drug companies.

For a new Medicare prescription drug bill to be enacted, it had to receive the support of Republicans in the House while also receiving sufficient support from Democrats in the Senate for it to be accepted by the Senate. An ideological compromise was necessary if both sides were to vote for the bill. The compromise bill was almost defeated by conservative House Republicans. Republicans lost their major objective, which was to restructure Medicare by having traditional Medicare compete with private health plans (premium support). Instead, they received a demonstration project, years in the future, that few expect to occur.

However, to secure the political support of conservative Republicans, the bill added features unrelated to prescription drugs that upset Senate liberals, who tried to filibuster the bill but lost. Senate liberals were opposed to even a competition demonstration project, to allowing tax-deductible HSAs for those younger than 65 years, to prohibiting the government from directly negotiating with drug companies, to adding a new cost-containment mechanism to Medicare to force the president and Congress to take action if federal tax revenues exceeded 45 percent of Medicare spending, and violating the equal benefits and equal subsidy principle, requiring higher-income seniors to pay higher Medicare Part B premiums.

Concentrated interests.

Organizations that perceived significant economic benefits accruing to their members were important advocates for a new Medicare prescription drug bill. By providing huge subsidies to these organizations (hospital, physician, health insurance, and drug company associations, as well as large employers), legislative proponents were able to build support for the bill. Lobbyists for these organizations played a significant role in persuading wavering legislators to vote in favor of the bill.

Economic interests outweigh ideological interests for groups with a concentrated interest. Such groups typically oppose government regulation of their own services and products; however, when it is in their economic interest, they support government intervention to benefit themselves.

As a Republican, committed to lessening the role of the federal government, President Bush proposed an enormous increase in federal expenditures. Political considerations overrode ideology. Ideological differences, however, could not be neglected and, after almost derailing the bill, compromises were reached that enabled the bill to pass but disappointed both Senate liberals and House conservatives. Concentrated interest groups were important beneficiaries of the new drug benefit and provided important political support for the bill.

The Legislative Outlook

Medicare's Financial Solvency

The most controversial health legislation in coming years are likely to be laws that deal with the explicit redistribution of medical services. Medicare reform will be at the top of the list of redistributive issues legislators will have to deal with. The baby boomers start to retire in 2011, and this will place great pressure on the Medicare Trust Fund. Medicare will have to be reformed to ensure the Medicare Trust Fund's financial solvency. The number of workers per aged person has declined from 16.5 in 1950 to 3.4 by 2000, and it is projected to decline to 3.2 by 2010 and to 2.2 by 2030.[3]

To maintain the same Medicare benefits for all future retirees as medical costs continue to rise rapidly will require large increases in the Medicare payroll tax as well as continued large deficits to fund Medicare Part B and the new Medicare prescription drug benefit (Medicare Part C).

The impending bankruptcy of the Medicare Trust Fund has been delayed by the enactment of the 1997 BBA, which reduced Medicare payments to hospitals and shifted home health care from Medicare Part A to Part B. This approach to increasing the solvency of the Medicare Trust Fund was meant to forestall difficult political choices. The Bipartisan Commission on the Future of Medicare considered Medicare reforms that would have provided the aged with more choices of health plans, although they would pay higher premiums for certain types of health plans. The Commission, however, was unable to have a "super majority" of its members agree on Medicare reform; consequently its recommendation was not adopted.

The MMA of 2003 similarly frustrated the attempts by proponents of Medicare Reform to include a "premium-support" proposal and have traditional Medicare compete against private health plans. Instead, a new stand-alone drug benefit was added to traditional Medicare, which lessens the incentive for the aged to switch to managed care plans. Providing all the aged with a new drug benefit will hasten the financial pressures requiring legislators to address the problem.

Solving Medicare's financial problem by imposing a large payroll tax on a smaller base of workers per Medicare beneficiary will result in political opposition. It is likely that reforming Medicare will have to impose costs on all elements of society: workers, healthcare providers, and the aged themselves. Each group will oppose having some of the costs of reform shifted to themselves. For this reason, legislators will postpone reform as long as possible. The political burden of proposing Medicare reform will fall on the administration in office.

Unless a bipartisan compromise can be reached between the two political parties, no party will be willing to propose restructuring and refinancing of Medicare as they would be attacked by the other political party.

The public interest and the self-interest theories lead to differing predictions as to the outcome of Medicare reform. The public interest theory would suggest that legislators, anticipating Medicare's impending financial problems, would enact legislation before the burden on the working population and the federal deficit worsens. Further, as part of the legislative solution, greater economic efficiency would be achieved if the aged had a financial incentive to choose less costly health plans, rather than remaining in the current, higher cost, nonmanaged fee-for-service system. Lastly, the financing required to maintain the solvency of the system (reducing benefits, delaying eligibility, and raising funds) would rely on a more equitable approach than the current financing system, which relies on huge intergenerational subsidies and provides the same benefits and subsidy to all the aged, regardless of income.

Self-interest paradigm predictions are not based on achieving greater equity or economic efficiency. Instead, calculations of forthcoming political support would determine the legislative outcome. The aged, particularly the middle- and high-income aged, have a concentrated interest in retaining as much of the status quo as possible, while also asking for additional benefits. To achieve their goals, the aged and near-aged are able to provide more political support for their interests than the young and future generations. Thus, the burden of reforming Medicare will likely not be equally shared among all groups.

Any burden imposed on the aged and near-aged will be phased in over a long time, minimizing the impact on these politically important groups. The main financial burden will again fall on the working population and on future generations. The disadvantage of this approach is that eventually the younger working population will develop a concentrated interest for limiting their payroll taxes. The conflict between the young and old, however, is unlikely to occur for a number of years, thereby still making it politically attractive for politicians to minimize the financial burden on the aged and near-aged.

Controlling Rising Health Insurance Premiums

A second important redistributive issue likely to arise in the near future is controlling rising health insurance premiums. As medical prices have risen, so have insurance premiums. As premiums increase, wages are reduced and the number of uninsured increase. The sharp increases in health insurance premiums have been a greater financial burden on those with lower incomes. Middle- and higher-income groups, however, have also been affected.

Two approaches are being used in the private market to limit the rise in premiums. Greater reliance is being placed on patient incentives, such as higher copayments and deductibles (and high-deductible policies).

Second, for those who want to minimize their out-of-pocket payments, there is beginning to be a return to greater reliance on managed care insurers to limit rising costs, such as utilization management, evidence-based medicine, and limited provider networks with less choice of provider.

Again, the public interest and self-interest theories provide different predictions as to the likely role of government to limit rising premiums on the middle class. The public interest theory would likely encourage market competition as the best way to achieve economic efficiency and the "appropriate" rate of increase in premiums.[4] Among the measures likely to be adopted to improve performance of medical care markets would be making available more information on provider performance, which insurers are beginning to develop, such as "report cards" to enable patients to make more informed choices. Similarly, insurers are experimenting with pay for performance, to be able to reward providers that meet higher-quality standards. And legislators would be expected to repeal anticompetitive restrictions, such as barriers to entry (CON laws) and any willing provider laws.

However, a competitive market, by itself, would not address the financial hardship of rising premiums on those with low incomes. In a price-competitive market, providers cannot subsidize the care of the poor by raising prices to the nonpoor. Thus, if one believed in the public interest theory, then reliance on a competitive market would also require the government to provide income-related subsidies for the purchase of health insurance for those for whom rising premiums are a financial burden.

The self-interest theory leads to an entirely different set of predictions.

As health insurance premiums continue to increase, along with greater out-of-pocket payments, and those who select HMOs for their lower premiums have less provider choice, the middle class is likely to become increasingly dissatisfied and want the government to "do something about it." (Large employers, such as GM, and their unions will likely be in the forefront of having the government intervene.)

There is no shortage of politicians who will attempt to gain middle-class support by offering them what is unattainable: free choice of provider, lower out-of-pocket payments, and a slower rise in their premiums. It is likely that under such circumstances legislators will propose regulatory solutions, such as "Medicare for All," namely, expand the current Medicare system to include everyone. The effect would be to have a single-payer system, similar to Canada. (Similar in its effects would be government regulation that would limit the rise in health insurance premiums and/or total medical expenditures.)

The effects of a single-payer system and/or government limits on premiums would not likely be felt for several years. Proponents of regulation to control rising expenditures would claim that additional taxes are not required, given the waste in the current system. However, expenditure or premium limits will affect access to care and incentives for the development of new medical technology. Two important reasons for the rise in medical expenditures over time have been increasing demands for medical services and very expensive medical advances, which enable people to have a higher quality of life and to live longer. But the middle class' dissatisfaction with such a regulatory system, as would inevitably occur, and as has happened in other countries with such a system, would be left for other politicians to deal with.

It may not be that many years before this ideological conflict occurs over the role of market competition versus government regulation in the organization and delivery of medical services.

Expanding Medical Coverage for the Uninsured

After more than 40 years of Medicare and Medicaid, and the expenditure of more than a trillion dollars, there is still no adequate system to finance care to the medically indigent, both young and old. The numbers of uninsured and underinsured are increasing. Yet little legislative progress is expected to assist these groups.

The poor and working poor have inadequate health insurance coverage. The aged want to maintain their Medicare coverage and choice of provider, reduce their medical costs further by having increased government subsidies for their prescription drugs, as well as reduce their risk of impoverishment if they require care in a nursing home for an extended illness. The middle class do not want to lose their health insurance if they become ill or if they change jobs; they would like greater choice of provider, and they do not want to keep paying an increasing percentage of their income for their health insurance. These population groups, the poor, the aged, and the middle class, are able to offer different levels of political support, hence legislators' responses to their concerns are also likely to differ.

The middle class determines the amount of taxes they are willing to pay for care of the medically indigent. Because the middle class is unwilling, according to numerous polls, to raise their taxes further to cover the poor and working uninsured, it is unlikely that this country will have any form of universal coverage any time soon. It would only occur if the middle class see greater benefits for themselves in expanding Medicare to include everyone ("Medicare for All").

To disguise an uncomfortably low level of altruism among middle-class voters, opponents of a competitive system place the blame for inadequate care to the poor on market competition, because it eliminates cross-subsidies. The amount of care provided to the poor, however, is the responsibility of society and not health providers. Health providers are willing to provide the amount of care that society is willing to fund.

The public interest theory cannot adequately explain why there is no adequate system for financing medical services for those with low incomes. Instead, a more accurate explanation for why this country has not had national health insurance nor is likely to have such a system in the foreseeable future is provided by the self-interest theory.

Although the uninsured remain a significant concern, the types of explicit redistributive health legislation enacted have been directed toward concerns of the middle class and the aged, those with health insurance. For example, in 1996 HIPPA was enacted, which included "guaranteed renewal," "portability," and "limitations on preexisting exclusions." These health insurance reforms require health insurers to renew all health insurance policies, precluding them from dropping individuals or groups that incur high medical costs and permit employees to change jobs without losing their health insurance. In addition, once a person has met the preexisting exclusion limit for any illness (usually 12 months), an insurer cannot reimpose another 12-month waiting period before the insurance benefits can be used.

The aforementioned health insurance reforms (together with restrictions placed on managed care companies by the Congress and state legislatures) addressed middle-class concerns. Further, the government does not bear any financing costs. The costs of these regulations are imposed on the insurers.

The Self-Interest Paradigm and Economic Efficiency and Equity

Self-interest has the potential for making redistributive programs more equitable and markets more efficient. As the costs of providing benefits become too great to those bearing the cost, changes will occur in the method of financing those costs. The process of achieving increased equity, however, occurs very gradually. Large costs cannot be immediately imposed on a group, nor can their benefits be quickly reduced, otherwise it would make it worthwhile for these groups to offer political opposition. There is some indication that certain redistributive programs are gradually becoming more equitable, that is, the benefits are inversely related to income. For example, up to 85 percent of Social Security benefits are taxable for taxpayers whose income exceeds $34,000 (single) or $44,000 (married couples).[5] And the Medicare portion of the Social Security tax is now on all earned income, making it more of a proportional tax. Further, the new Medicare prescription drug benefit imposed a higher Part B premium on high-income aged (although the number of current aged subject to this increased premium is extremely small). These changes will eventually decrease the intergenerational inequity that occurs.

A second trend that has occurred in healthcare is greater economic efficiency in the delivery of health services. This trend is not the result of a conscious decision on the part of legislators but is again the result of self-interest. As the cost of healthcare became too large, business and government pressed for innovative changes in methods of paying for and delivering health services. Incentives were provided for increased efficiency.[6]

The self-interest paradigm does not imply that equity and efficiency will continually worsen. Instead, there is often a self-correcting mechanism. As the costs to others of inequity and inefficiency increase, those bearing the burden have an increased incentive to organize and reduce those costs. Although self-interest is the initial motivating force for redistributing wealth, it is also self-interest that prevents the resulting inequities and inefficiencies from becoming too great.

Study Questions

1. In what way are political markets similar to economic markets?
2. How do political markets differ from economic markets?
3. Would competition or monopoly among demanders and suppliers of legislation be preferable in political markets?
4. Why are regressive costs or taxes usually used to finance legislative benefits, according to the economic theory?
5. Broad redistributive programs, such as Social Security and Medicare, have provided all aged with large net benefits. Using the concepts of "concentrated" and "diffuse" interests, explain first why the aged have been able to receive such large net benefits and, second, why benefits to future aged will be much lower than those received by previous aged groups.
6. What were the ideological differences in designing the MMA?

Notes

1. Legislators do not provide redistributive benefits for which the beneficiaries, such as the aged, bear the full costs. Otherwise, why would the beneficiaries not buy those benefits on their own? Only in a situation of market failure would there be a net benefit to the aged from having the government provide them with a benefit for which they would pay the full costs. Although lack of information, adverse selection, moral hazard, and economies of scale in the administra-

tion of any health insurance program all serve to make the insurance market less than perfect, few would claim that Medicare or any other visible redistributive benefit is based on grounds of market failure.

2. John Sheils and Randall Haught, "The Cost of Tax-Exempt Health Benefits in 2004," *Health Affairs-Web Exclusives*, February 25, 2004, content.healthaffairs.org/ cgi/content/abstract/hlthaff .w4.106.

3. The numbers after year 2000 are estimates based on intermediate assumption. Social Security Administration, *2005 Annual Report of the Board of Trustees of the Federal Old-Age and Survivors Insurance and Disability Insurance Trust Funds*, http://www.ssa.gov/OACT/TR/TR05/trLOT.html

4. "Appropriate rate of increase in premiums" means the amount people are willing to pay (based on their perceived value) for medical services that are efficiently produced. Among the assumptions of a competitive market achieving economic efficiency are that purchasers are informed and that there are no entry barriers limiting the number of suppliers.

5. Under the current law, there is a two-tier system for taxing Social Security benefits: 50 percent of Social Security benefits are taxable for taxpayers whose income plus one-half of Social Security benefits exceed $25,000 for an individual or $32,000 for a married couple filing a joint tax return. Up to 85 percent of Social Security benefits are taxable for taxpayers whose income exceed $34,000 (single) or $44,000 (married couples). http://www.lawprofessorblogs.com /taxprof/linkdocs/CRS.pdf.

6. This trend, however, may be reversed if the middle class becomes increasingly dissatisfied with high out-of-pocket payments and restricted provider choices, as discussed earlier. The demand for patient rights' legislation and greater choice of provider by the middle class, while still preferring the relatively lower HMO premiums, has led legislators to propose increased managed care regulation. These regulations increase the cost, hence premiums, of managed care firms. However, the resulting premium increases are not an obvious consequence of the regulation. If the public were more aware of the trade-off between increased regulation and increased premiums, it is likely that fewer such regulations would be demanded.

INDEX

AARP. *See* American Association of Retired Persons

Acid rain, 220–21

ACT UP. *See* AIDS Coalition to Unleash Power

ADA. *See* American Dental Association

Administrative agencies. *See* Regulatory agencies

Advertising issues, 165, 167, 179

AFDC. *See* Aid to Families with Dependent Children

AFL-CIO. *See* American Federation of Labor and Congress of Industrial Organizations

Aged. *See* Elderly

Age Discrimination in Employment Act, 254–56

Agricultural cooperatives, 47–48

AHA. *See* American Hospital Association

Aid to Families with Dependent Children, 242–44, 259

AIDS Coalition to Unleash Power, 211–12

AIDS epidemic, 210–12, 223

Airline Deregulation Act, 143

Airline industry, 140–45

Air pollution, 215–16

AMA. *See* American Medical Association

Ambulatory surgicenters, 112

American Academy of Family Practitioners, 104

American Academy of Pediatrics, 71

American Airlines, 142

American Association of Retired Persons: drug benefit support, 332–33; endorsement, 344; lobbying

revenues, *350n*; Medicare Catastrophic Coverage Act and, 294–97

American Bar Association, 178

American College of Cardiology, 109

American College of Physicians, 361

American College of Radiology, 109–10

American College of Surgeons, 361

American Dental Association: advertising issues, 96, 99; any willing provider laws, 99–100; Council on Dental Education, 117; demand-increasing legislation and, 91–92; dental care issues, 91–92; dental insurance and, 100; education issues, 116–17; foreign-trained dentist and, 114, *130–31n*; free rider problem, 71; Gies report, 117; House of Delegates, 78, *131n*; insurance issues, 91–92; legislative success of, 78–79; licensure issues, 116–17; membership structure, 71, 77, *83n*; PPO and, 76; price competition, 99; reimbursement legislation, 99–100; services, 71; substitute provider and, 110–11; supply-control policies, 116–17

American Federation of Labor and Congress of Industrial Organizations, 272–74, *288n*

American Federation of State, County, and Municipal Employees, 244

American Hospital Association: budget neutrality effect on, 360–61; complement provider and, 104; on educational subsidies, 104; free rider problem, 73; healthcare reform, 360–61; legislative success of, 67, 79;

ABOUT THE AUTHOR

Paul J. Feldstein, Ph.D. has been professor and Robert Gumbiner Chair in Healthcare Management at the Paul Merage School of Business, University of California, Irvine, since 1987. His previous position was at the University of Michigan as professor in both the Department of Economics and the School of Public Health. Before that, he was Director of the Division of Research at the American Hospital Association. Professor Feldstein received his Ph.D. from the University of Chicago.

Professor Feldstein has written six books and numerous articles on health economics. His book, *Health Care Economics*, 6th edition, 2004, is one of the most widely used texts on health economics. The third edition of his book, *Health Policy Issues: An Economic Perspective on Health Reform*, was published by the Health Administration Press in 2002.

During several leaves from the University, Professor Feldstein worked at the Office of Management and Budget, Social Security Administration, and the World Health Organization. He has been a consultant to many government and private health agencies; an expert witness on health antitrust issues; as well as serving on the Board of Directors of Sutter Health, a not-for-profit health system in California; Province Healthcare, a for-profit hospital company; and Odyssey HealthCare, a for-profit hospice company.